630492

Transfusion and Transplantation Science

D1477212

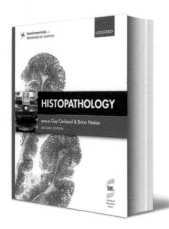

fundamentals of
biomedical science

OXFORD

HISTOPATHOLOGY

EDITED BY Guy Orchard & Brian Nation

SECOND EDITION

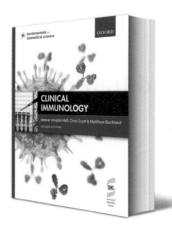

fundamentals of
biomedical science

OXFORD

CLINICAL
IMMUNOLOGY

EDITED BY Angela Hall, Chris Scott & Matthew Buckland

SECOND EDITION

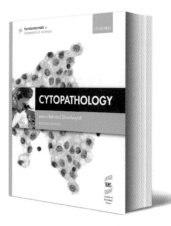

fundamentals of
biomedical science

OXFORD

CYTOPATHOLOGY

EDITED BY Behdad Shambayati

SECOND EDITION

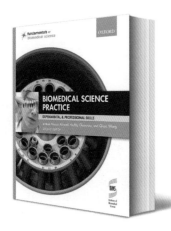

fundamentals of
biomedical science

OXFORD

BIOMEDICAL SCIENCE
PRACTICE

EXPERIMENTAL & PROFESSIONAL SKILLS

EDITED BY Nessar Ahmed, Hedley Glencross, and Qiuyu Wang

SECOND EDITION

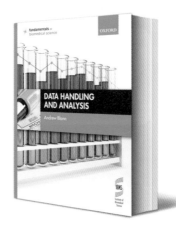

fundamentals of
biomedical science

OXFORD

DATA HANDLING
AND ANALYSIS

Andrew Blann

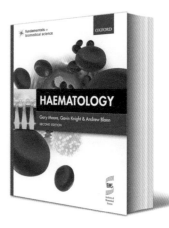

fundamentals of
biomedical science

OXFORD

HAEMATOLOGY

Gary Moore, Gavin Knight & Andrew Blann

SECOND EDITION

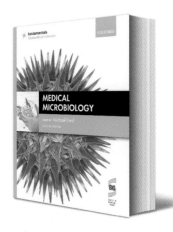

fundamentals
biomedical science

OXFORD

MEDICAL
MICROBIOLOGY

EDITED BY Michael Ford

SECOND EDITION

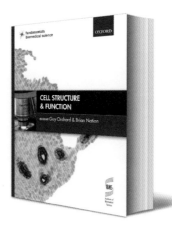

fundamentals
biomedical science

OXFORD

CELL STRUCTURE
& FUNCTION

EDITED BY Guy Orchard & Brian Nation

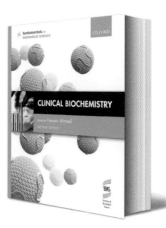

fundamentals of
biomedical science

OXFORD

CLINICAL BIOCHEMISTRY

EDITED BY Nessar Ahmed

SECOND EDITION

fundamentals OF
biomedical science

Fundamentals of Biomedical Science

Transfusion and Transplantation Science

Second edition

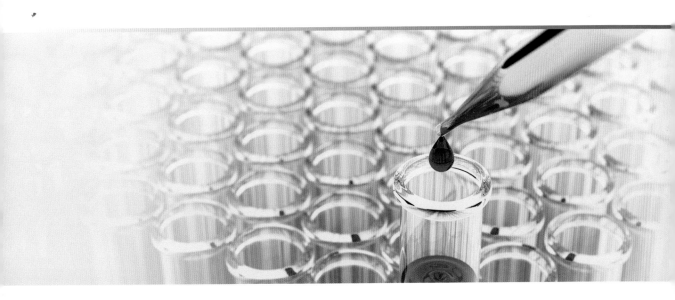

Edited by
Neil D. Avent

Professor of Molecular Diagnostics and
Transfusion Medicine, School of Biomedical &
Healthcare Sciences, Plymouth University
Peninsula Schools of Medicine and Dentistry

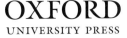

OXFORD
UNIVERSITY PRESS

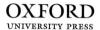

Great Clarendon Street, Oxford, OX2 6DP,
United Kingdom

Oxford University Press is a department of the University of Oxford.
It furthers the University's objective of excellence in research, scholarship,
and education by publishing worldwide. Oxford is a registered trade mark of
Oxford University Press in the UK and in certain other countries

First edition 2013

Impression: 1

Published in the United States of America by Oxford University Press
198 Madison Avenue, New York, NY 10016, United States of America

British Library Cataloguing in Publication Data
Data available

Library of Congress Control Number: 2017956303

ISBN 978-0-19-873573-1

Printed in Great Britain by
Bell & Bain Ltd., Glasgow

Acknowledgements

I am grateful to my previous and current colleagues and friends at the NHS Blood and Transplant, Welsh Blood Service, University of the West of England, Bristol and Plymouth University Peninsula Schools of Medicine and Dentistry for their input into the chapters that make up this book. Their expertise has been paramount to the success of this edition, and they are leaders and well renowned in their respective fields. I am also grateful for useful contributions of Malcolm Needs into Chapter 2, which in the first edition he authored. I also acknowledge the efforts of the previous editor, Robin Knight, who is now retired, and again a former colleague and friend at the NHSBT. It is with sadness that during the editing of this book, one of its authors, Dr Geoff Lucas, died. Geoff was a world expert in platelet immunohaematology and is sadly missed by the transfusion medicine community.

I am also, as always, grateful for the love and support of my family, my mother, my wife Sharon, my children Sophie, James, and Sian, and grandchildren Jack and Harry.

An introduction to the Fundamentals of Biomedical Science series

Biomedical scientists form the foundation of modern healthcare; from cancer screening to diagnosing HIV, from blood transfusion for surgery to food poisoning and infection control. Without biomedical scientists, the diagnosis of disease, the evaluation of the effectiveness of treatment, and research into the causes and cures of disease would not be possible.

However, the path to becoming a biomedical scientist is a challenging one; trainees must not only assimilate knowledge from a range of disciplines, but must understand—and demonstrate—how to apply this knowledge in a practical, hands-on environment.

The *Fundamentals of Biomedical Science* series is written to reflect the challenges of biomedical science education and training today. It blends essential basic science with insights into laboratory practice to show how an understanding of the biology of disease is coupled to the analytical approaches that lead to diagnosis.

The series provides coverage of the full range of disciplines to which a biomedical scientist may be exposed; from microbiology to cytopathology to transfusion science. Alongside volumes exploring specific biomedical themes and related laboratory diagnosis, an overarching *Biomedical Science Practice* volume provides a grounding in the general professional and experimental skills with which every biomedical scientist should be equipped.

Produced in collaboration with the Institute of Biomedical Science, the series:

- understands the complex roles of biomedical scientists in the modern practice of medicine,
- understands the development needs of employers and the profession,
- places the theoretical aspects of biomedical science in their practical context.

Learning from this series

The *Fundamentals of Biomedical Science* series draws on a range of learning features to help readers master both biomedical science theory and biomedical science practice.

Additional information to augment the main text appears in **boxes**.

Method boxes walk through the key protocols that the reader is likely to encounter in the laboratory on a regular basis.

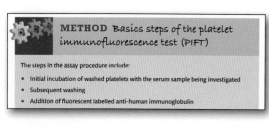

METHOD Basics steps of the platelet immunofluorescence test (PIFT)

The steps in the assay procedure include:

- Initial incubation of washed platelets with the serum sample being investigated
- Subsequent washing
- Addition of fluorescent labelled anti-human immunoglobulin

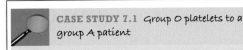

Case studies illustrate how the biomedical science theory and practice presented throughout the series relates to situations and experiences that are likely to be encountered routinely in the biomedical science laboratory.

> **CASE STUDY 7.1** Group O platelets to a group A patient
>
> • Three-year-old female with acute lymphoblastic leukaemia (ALL).
> • Given one adult therapeutic dose (ATD) of group O apheresis platelets, as no group A available.
> • Became unwell.

Clinical correlations bring relevance to the material by placing it in its clinical context.

> **Clinical correlation**
>
> **Hyperhaemolysis** is a rare complication of transfusion which has been mainly, but not exclusively, reported in patients with sickle cell disease (SCD). It has also been referred to as the sickle cell haemolytic transfusion reaction syndrome. It is characterized by the destruction of both the

Key points reinforce the key concepts that the reader should master from having read the material presented, while **Summary** points act as an end-of-chapter checklist for readers to verify that they have remembered correctly the principal themes and ideas presented within each chapter.

> **Key points**
>
> ■ Erythrocyte antigens arise as a result of evolutionary pressure, in most cases the drivers of which are unknown.
> ■ Any erythrocyte surface structure, both carbohydrate or protein may be expressed by polymorphic genes termed *alleles*.
> ■ Incompatible transfusion or pregnancy may lead to the production of blood group specific antibodies that may cause transfusion reactions or in pregnancy haemolytic disease of the newborn and fetus.

Key terms provide on-the-page explanations of terms that the reader may not be familiar with; in addition, each title in the series features a **glossary**, in which the key terms featured in that title are collated.

> **Immune response**
> The body's ability to recognize and defend itself against substances that appear foreign and harmful such as bacteria and viruses.
>
> **Window period**
> This is the period between the onset of the infection and the
>
> within the host and can reach a high viral load (i.e. re **immune response**. The speed of replication, or do varies with the different infectious agents. The forma results in a decline in the viral load, often to below the in the patients for varying times depending on the vir several TTIs the virus may not be eliminated by these
>
> The period between inoculation and detection of the i the **window period** (WP) (Figure 5.1 and Table 5.2) weeks and would depend on the test used and the te

Self-check questions throughout each chapter and extended questions at the end of each chapter provide the reader with a ready means of checking that they have understood the material they have just encountered. Answers to these questions are provided in the book's accompanying website; visit **www.oup.com/uk/avent2e**

> **SELF-CHECK 2.3**
>
> • Why is the D antigen so immunogenic?
> • What drives the huge variability in RH genetics?
> • What is the operational definition of partial and weak D and D-elute?

Online learning materials

The *Fundamentals of Biomedical Science* series doesn't end with the printed books. Each title in the series is supported by an accompanying website, which features additional materials for students, trainees, and lecturers.

www.oxfordtextbooks.co.uk/orc/fbs/

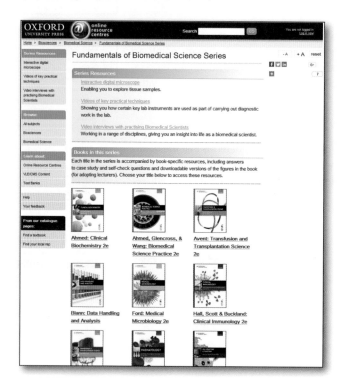

Guides to key experimental skills and methods

Multimedia walk-throughs of key experimental skills—including both animations and video—to help you master the essential skills that are the foundation of biomedical science practice.

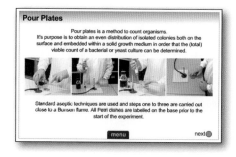

Biomedical science in practice

Interviews with practising biomedical scientists working in a range of disciplines, to give you valuable insights into the reality of work in a biomedical science laboratory.

Digital Microscope

A library of microscopic images for you to investigate using this powerful online microscope, to help you gain a deeper appreciation of cell and tissue morphology.

The Digital Microscope is used under licence from the Open University.

Answers to self-check, case study, and end-of-chapter questions

Answers to questions posed in the book are provided to aid self assessment.

> **Avent: Transfusion and Transplantation Science 2e**
>
> Answers to self-check questions
>
> Self-check 2.1
>
> How does the International Society of Blood Transfusion classify Blood Group systems? How does it classify a blood group antigen? Do the number of antigens per system indicate its clinical significance?
>
> **Answer:** The ISBT classifies a blood group system based on a gene that defines the system, and the molecular basis is known. In some instances (e.g. RH and MNS systems) there are more than one gene in the system – Rh=*RHD* and *RHCE*, MNS= *GYPA*, *GYPB* and *GYPE*.
>
> Self-check 2.2
>
> - How does the erythrocyte survive the extreme shear stresses imposed on it during its 120 day life cycle?
> - What are the major proteins of the erythrocyte membrane and its submembranous skeleton?
> - Apart from O2 and CO2 transport what other tasks do erythrocytes serve?

Lecturer support materials

The website for each title in the series also features figures from the book in electronic format, for registered adopters to download for use in lecture presentations, and other educational resources.

To register as an adopter visit **www.oup.com/uk/avent2e** and follow the on-screen instructions.

Any comments?

We welcome comments and feedback about any aspect of this series. Just visit www.oxfordtext-books.co.uk/orc/feedback/ and share your views.

Contributors

The second edition

Neil D. Avent, School of Biomedical and Healthcare Sciences, Plymouth University

John Barbara, formerly of NHS Blood and Transplant

Catherine Hyland, Australian Red Cross Blood Service

Joan Jones, Welsh Blood Service

Saeed Kabrah, Department of Biological, Biomedical and Analytical Sciences, University of the West of England

Richard Lomas, NHS Blood and Transplant

Geoff Lucas, NHS Blood and Transplant

Lionel Mohabir, Welsh Blood Service

Ruth Morse, Department of Biological, Biomedical and Analytical Sciences, University of the West of England

Malcolm Needs, NHS Blood and Transplant

Vehid Salih, Plymouth University Peninsula Schools of Medicine and Dentistry

The first edition

John Barker, Gateshead Health NHS Foundation Trust

Colin Brown, NHS Blood and Transplant

Carol Cantwell, St Mary's Hospital Imperial College Healthcare NHS Trust

Bill Chaffe, East Kent Hospitals University NHS Foundation Trust

Tony Davies, NHS Blood and Transplant

Joan Jones, Welsh Blood Service

Robin Knight, Former Head of NHS Blood and Transplant Red Cell Immunohaematology Division

Richard Lomas, NHS Blood and Transplant

Geoff Lucas, NHS Blood and Transplant

Karen Madgwick, North Middlesex Hospital NHS Trust

Lionel Mohabir, Welsh Blood Service

Malcolm Needs, NHS Blood and Transplant

Robert Walters, North West Wales NHS Trust

Contents

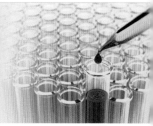

Introduction to Basic Immunology and Techniques

Neil D. Avent

Acknowledgements: the editor thanks Robin Knight who wrote an earlier version of this chapter in the book's first edition that forms the basis for this present update.

Learning objectives

After studying this chapter you should be able to:

- Outline the various components of the immune system.
- Outline the functioning of the humoral immune system.
- Describe antibody structure and function.
- Describe antigen–antibody reactions.
- Understand antibody-mediated red cell destruction.
- Understand the detection of red cell antigen–antibody reactions and agglutination.

Introduction

This book essentially covers the laboratory and scientific aspects of the transfusion of human blood and products or components made from blood, and the transplantation of tissues and stem cells, but not the clinical practice of transfusion and transplanting organs. This first chapter reviews the historical background to the science of transfusion and transplantation.

The history of both transfusion and transplantation can be traced back to ancient times, but the real advances have been made within the last 70 years. For many centuries, medicine was founded on the four body humours—blood, phlegm, yellow bile, and black bile—and it was thought that health could be restored by bloodletting, starving, vomiting, or purging. Such practices were still carried out in some places until the end of the nineteenth century.

The circulation of the blood and the function of valves in veins were described by the English physician William Harvey in a book published in 1628. A few years later (1669) another Englishman, Richard Lower, reported his experiments with the transfusion of blood from one dog to another and also between humans. About the same time in Paris, Jean Baptiste Denis also performed some transfusions of humans, but after a number of his subjects died the practice was banned in some European countries for the next 150 years.

In 1829, Dr James Blundell, a British obstetrician, first performed a successful human transfusion by taking four ounces of blood from the arm of a dying patient's husband with a syringe and transfusing it into the patient, who recovered. He had conducted a series of well-thought-out experiments using animals, where he showed that as long as the blood was transfused quickly after it had been taken then it would be successful even in resuscitating an animal dying of blood loss.

Many of Blundell's patients were women who were bleeding excessively after childbirth (post-partum haemorrhage) and he devised numerous instruments for the transfusion of blood, many of which we would recognize today. To honour the work of this pioneer the British Blood Transfusion Society still presents an annual James Blundell Award.

In 1849, Dr C Routh, physician to the St Pancras Royal Dispensary in London, reviewed the 44 examples of blood transfusion that had been reported at that time. He concluded that the procedure was one of the safest major operations which may be practised in surgery 'with the rate of mortality of one in three—rather less than that of hernia, or about the same as the average of amputations'.

In 1875, Landois reported that the red cells of one animal species clumped, or *agglutinated*, those of another if mixed together. Similar clumping had already been noticed when certain sera had been mixed with bacteria. It was suggested that this was due to antigens on the surface of the bacteria uniting with antibodies in the serum. Therefore, this knowledge of bacterial immunology was applied to the phenomenon of red cell agglutination.

One of the most important discoveries in the history of transfusion was made by the Austrian scientist Karl Landsteiner, who observed the agglutination of human red cells by serum of other humans—a difference within a species, rather than between species. He went on to describe the ABO blood group system in 1901. In 1930 he received the Nobel Prize for Physicians and Medicine and a decade later, together with Dr Wiener, described the *Rh-factor*, now known to be part of the Rh blood group system. In fact, the term Rh-factor arose when Landsteiner and Wiener raised an antibody against *Macacus rhesus* red cells in guinea pigs. The guinea pig antiserum was later shown to be not against Rh antigens at all, but the LW-glycoprotein (see Chapter 2).

Following the work of Landsteiner, and independently, Moss and Jansky, in describing the ABO groups, the reason why so many early transfusions were fatal was at last understood. The blood of one person can be *incompatible* with that of another, so before a transfusion can be given the donor's blood must be shown to be compatible with that of the potential recipient. Initially this was done by matching the ABO groups, but later more complex tests were devised, the so-called *crossmatch*.

A major contribution to the discovery of further blood groups was 'a new test' described in 1945 by Drs Robin Coombs, Arthur Mourant, and Rob Race: the antiglobulin test. This is still often referred to, erroneously, as the Coombs test. Using this technique IgG, or non-agglutinating antibodies, can be detected on the surface of red cells either as the result of being coated by antibody *in vivo*, or in an *in vitro* laboratory test.

Since then, more blood groups have been discovered, so that today there are some 36 human erythrocyte antigen (blood group) systems known. The whole arena of histocompatibility (tissue typing) and the human lymphocyte antigen (HLA), human platelet antigen (HPA), and human neutrophil antigen (HNA), systems have been described and their function understood. These, too, are described in greater detail in this book.

The two World Wars of the twentieth century were both times when advances were made in transfusion science and practice. During the First World War it was shown that if blood was collected into an *anticoagulant* to prevent clots from forming, the blood could be stored for a short time before being transfused. By adding dextrose to the sodium citrate anticoagulant, blood could be stored for several days in a refrigerator. Therefore, there was no need to have a donor available at the time blood was needed. The process of storing blood was improved during the Second World War when the first large-scale collection of blood from volunteers was started in the UK under the Emergency Medical Service. From this was born, in 1947, the National Blood Transfusion Service, which has grown to become, in England, by 2006, NHS Blood and Transplant. Scotland, Wales, and Northern Ireland have their own similar services.

There have been two other major developments that enabled advances to be made in transfusion practice. The first is the use of plastic bags for the collection of blood, instead of glass bottles. Dr Carl W Walter was instrumental in this development that has enabled whole blood, as collected from the donor, to be split into its component parts—red cells, plasma, platelets, and white cells. Each of these *blood components* can be stored separately and transfused to patients who require that specific component, for example red cells because they are anaemic.

In the 1940s Dr Edwin Cohn, a Harvard biochemist, developed a method for fractionating plasma into its different proteins, so that specific *blood products* could be produced. These include fibrinogen, gamma globulins, albumin, and various clotting factors. Some of the latter are now made using *recombinant technology*.

Another major advance has been the introduction of *monoclonal antibody technology*. Dr César Milstein and his co-workers showed that by fusing an antibody-producing cell with a myeloma cell, a clone of cells could be grown in culture that continued to produce antibody. The supernatant containing the specific antibody can be harvested and used as an antibody reagent. Prior to this, antibodies were obtained from humans or animals, often after deliberate immunization, but the required antibody had to be isolated or unwanted antibodies removed. Monoclonal antibodies, being obtained as a single specificity and in large volumes, do not need to undergo such lengthy treatment. Monoclonal antibodies are now used not just for *in vitro* tests, but also for *in vivo* treatment.

Transplantation has a shorter history, although in Roman times Saints Cosmas and Damian are attributed to have grafted the leg of a recently deceased black Ethiopian to replace the ulcerated leg of a white patient. The major problem of tissue transplantation is that of rejection—the transplanted cells are seen by the recipient's immune system as foreign and mount an 'immune attack' to reject them.

It was the realization that graft rejection was due to incompatibility of antigens on human white cells that lead to the discovery of the HLA system and the *major histocompatibility locus* that has enabled the great advances to be made with transplantation.

Kidney (renal) transplants were first carried out successfully in 1954 and the world's first heart transplant was done in 1967, since which time most organs have been transplanted. Not only can solid organs (e.g. kidneys, heart, lungs) be transplanted, but also bone marrow and stem cells. Stem cell transplantation is a fast growing science, but not without ethical controversy. Some tissues, such as corneas, skin, and bone, can be collected and stored and then transplanted without the problems of rejection associated with more cellular organs. These, too, are covered in this book.

Over the past few years there has been an increase in legislation from the European Union affecting many aspects of our lives, including transfusion and transplantation. Reference will be made to some of these directives in the text and you will learn that this clinical/scientific discipline is now highly regulated by a number of statutory agencies. Details of where you can find the more important directives and guidelines are given at the end of the final chapter, which deals with quality (Chapter 12).

1.1 Basic immunology and techniques

The human immune response will not be considered in detail in this book as it is covered adequately elsewhere. However, the main features that are directly relevant to topics in this book, such as immune cell destruction, are reviewed below. The immune response can be considered as two broadly defined arms, the **innate immune response** and the **adaptive immune response**. The innate immune response is regarded as non-specific and includes the epithelial linings of the skin, digestive tract, and blood vessels. These provide a physical barrier to potential pathogens, and tight junctions between these epithelial cells form an effective 'wall' of cells. The colonization of the surface of epithelial cells is also inhibited by mucus production, and its removal by beating cilia. Within mucus are mucins (large complex glycoproteins) and defensins, which are short peptides, and naturally occurring antibiotics. Some external secretions (e.g. tears, sweat) contain antibacterial substances such as the enzyme lysozyme. In peripheral blood, the complement cascade (see Section 1.5) destroys invading pathogens, but one pathway requires that IgG or IgM (adaptive immune response, see below) are bound to the bacteria. The origin of the term 'complement' is just that—the cascade is able to complement the binding of immunoglobulins. However, the **lectin** and **alternative** pathways are activated directly by bacterial components, not requiring bound immunoglobulin.

Certain pathogen specific sequences (e.g. lipopolysaccharide, teichoic acids, bacterial flagella, and DNA sequences found more frequently in bacteria) are recognized by receptors on immune cells that are part of the innate response. These include **Toll-like receptors** on **macrophages** and neutrophils, which phagocytose invading bacteria rapidly, even without prior exposure to them. **Natural killer (NK) cells** are part of the innate immune system, and are stimulated by interferons. These innate immune cells scan other cell types to monitor their expression of major histocompatibility complex (MHC) class 1 molecules (for MHC see Chapter 9). When they detect low levels of MHC-1 (a hallmark of virally infected and some cancer cells) it induces them to undergo **apoptosis** (cell death). Cytotoxic T cells behave in a similar way to infected and cancer cells, but they are part of the adaptive immune response.

The adaptive immune response is usually divided into **humoral immunity** and **cellular immunity**. Both are initiated by the recognition of a foreign protein or cell and lead to its removal or destruction, either through the interaction of a specific antibody, in the case of humoral immunity, or by the interaction of complement or cytokines produced by cytotoxic or killer T cells, in cellular immunity.

When considering transfusion of blood and blood components, we are concerned mainly with the humoral response to **antigens** on erythrocytes, platelets, and leucocytes that enter the circulation either by transfusion, with a transplanted organ or during pregnancy, where some of the fetal cells pass into the maternal circulation. In the transplant situation, although antibodies do play a role in graft rejection, the cellular immune response is more important.

The immune system

For an individual to survive in an immunologically hostile world, the cells of its own immune system have to be able to distinguish 'self' from 'non-self' as any foreign cell, virus particle, or protein might cause that individual harm. Once recognized as foreign then it has to be eliminated from the body if possible before it can cause harm. See Figure 1.1.

During fetal and early development B and T lymphocytes learn what is 'self' so that they can then spot what is non-self and potentially harmful. Essentially, B and T cells have HLA receptor

Macrophage

A major immune phagocytic cell that is associated with red cell turnover or destruction. Found in huge numbers in the spleen.

Apoptosis

Programmed cell death—the process in which cells control their own demise.

Humoral immunity

That part of the immune system that is initiated by the recognition of a foreign protein or cell and leads to its removal or destruction through the interaction of a specific antibody.

Cellular immunity

The part of the immune system that is initiated by the recognition of a foreign protein or cell and leads to its removal or destruction by the interaction of complement, or cytokines produced by cytotoxic or killer T cells.

Antigen

Any foreign structure capable of eliciting an immune response to both T and B cells.

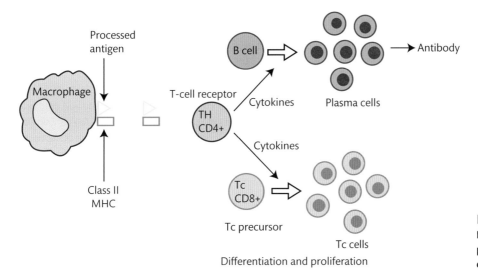

FIGURE 1.1
Immune response: antigen processing and activation of T cells and B cells.

molecules that enable each of the millions of lymphocytes to recognize a specific antigen. If something foreign enters the body, then antigen presenting cells (APC) isolate the antigen molecules and present them on their cell surface to be recognized by the unique receptors on T or B cells. If seen as non-self then the APC initiates cellular events that lead to the activation of clones of lymphocytes that will in turn deal with the foreign antigen.

Activated T cells, cytotoxic CD8+ Tc cells, secrete an array of cytokines that can lead to the death of the foreign cells. This is the main immune reaction that causes graft rejection and **graft versus host disease**. B cells, with the help of CD4+ T helper cells, transform into antibody-secreting plasma cells. More than one plasma cell line is activated, each producing an antibody with a slightly different reactivity against the initiating antigen, although the general specificity is the same. The resulting antibodies are said to be **polyclonal antibodies**—the product of more than one clone of cells. In some disease states and *in vitro*, antibodies can be produced from a single clone—a **monoclonal antibody**.

The clonal expansion that follows initiation takes time and it might be several days, or even weeks, before there is any detectable antibody. At first IgM antibodies are secreted, then the plasma cells 'switch class' and produce IgG molecules. If there is no further exposure to the new antigen then the IgM production peaks and then declines so that IgM antibodies are no longer detectable. However, the IgG antibody production continues and antibodies can be detected many years after the initial exposure, which can, as we shall see, be important when looking for compatible blood for a patient.

Once initiated to a new antigen, some T and B cells become non-secreting memory cells that retain that 'knowledge' and, because of the clonal expansion there will be a large number of primed **memory cells**, so that if there is another contact with that foreign antigen they will be able to respond much quicker than when that antigen was first encountered. Also, the dose of the antigen can be much smaller than that needed for an initial or primary response. Whereas it might take several weeks or months for an antibody to become detectable initially, in a secondary response there is no lag phase as IgG antibody molecules are produced immediately.

It was stated above that for B lymphocytes to be transformed into antibody-producing plasma cells the interaction of T helper cells is required. However, some antibodies are produced without T-cell involvement. B cells have some antigen receptors that are able to interact directly with sugar-based antigens. A number of polysaccharides, but not polypeptides, especially if

Graft versus host disease (GVHD)
The most common cause of graft failure that is caused by donor immune cells, especially T lymphocytes, reacting against recipient tissue. The characteristic symptoms are the presence of a rash, diarrhoea, and abnormal liver function tests.

Polyclonal antibodies
These are produced by more than one clone of B cells.

Monoclonal antibody
Produced from a single clone of B cells.

they have multiple identical repeats in their molecular structure, can initiate B cells and the proliferation of plasma cells. The antibodies produced are IgM and because of the absence of T helper cell involvement class-switching does not occur and IgM antibodies continue to be produced. Because there are no memory cells produced, antibody production continues only as long as there is continuing exposure to the antigen.

The ABO antibodies are an example of this T-independent immune response. The IgM antibodies are really directed to antigens on bacteria in the gut but they cross-react with the very similar A and B antigens on the red cells. Because these antibodies are produced as a result of exposure to antigens in nature and not as a result of stimulation by foreign red cells entering the circulation, those with blood group activity are often referred to as **naturally acquired** antibodies.

> ### Key points
>
> The immune system recognizes and responds to foreign, or non-self, proteins (antigens) by producing antibodies or cells that interact directly with that protein.

SELF-CHECK 1.1

What are the differences between a primary and secondary immune antibody response?

1.2 Antibody structure

The **humoral immune response** results in the production of specific antibodies that interact with the corresponding, initiating antigen on the target cell, but what is an antibody and how does it bring about cell destruction or removal?

Antibodies are proteins, gamma-globulins, with specific characteristics collectively known as immunoglobulins. An immunoglobulin molecule is composed of two 'heavy-' and two 'light-' type chains, held together by non-covalent interactions and disulphide bonds. There are five classes of immunoglobulins (Ig) each with their own specific heavy chain:

- IgG-gamma (G or γ)
- IgM mu (M or μ)
- IgA alpha (A or α)
- IgD delta (D or δ)
- IgE epsilon (E or ε).

These heavy chain types differ in the number of amino acid residues and carbohydrate content, giving each class different characteristics and biological activity. The gamma chain has four variations, producing four subtypes of IgG—IgG1, IgG2, IgG3, and IgG4—which results in variations in their biological activity. Most immune IgG blood group antibodies are a mixture of IgG1 and IgG3, and only rarely are they IgG2 or IgG4. There are two classes of IgA: IgA1 and IgA2.

There are two types of light chain, kappa (K or κ) and lambda (L or λ). The light chains of antibody molecules produced by each clone of antibody-producing plasma cells will be the same type. Each IgG immunoglobulin molecule has the two light chains and two γ heavy chains, held together by disulphide bonds between cysteine amino acids and by non-covalent hydrophobic interactions. See Figure 1.2.

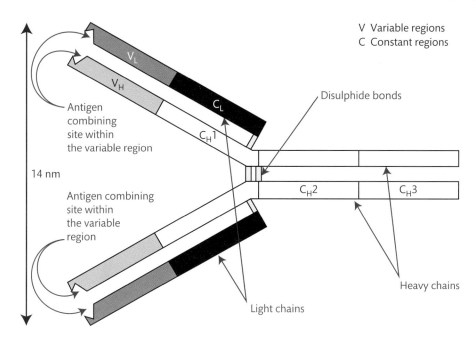

V Variable regions
C Constant regions

FIGURE 1.2
Basic structure of an IgG antibody molecule.

An IgG molecule can be broken down by the use of proteolytic enzymes into two Fab fragments, and one Fc fragment. The Fab (fragment antigen binding) is composed of an intact light chain and the amino-terminal end of the γ heavy chain, linked together by interchain disulphide bonding, and acts as the specific antigen binding site.

The Fc (fragment crystalline) is composed of a dimer of the carboxy terminal portions of the two γ heavy chains linked by disulphide bonding. It is associated with some of the IgG molecule's biological functions (e.g. complement activation and macrophage binding). The Fc fragment of the IgG molecule contains most of the carbohydrate content.

The IgM molecule is a pentamer, with the five sections, each comprising two light chains and two μ heavy chains, being held together by a J-chain, as shown in Figure 1.3. See Tables 1.1 and 1.2.

TABLE 1.1 Properties of IgG and IgM antibody molecules.

Property	IgG*	IgM
Placental transfer	Yes	No
Complement activation	Yes	Yes
Treatment with dithiothreitol (DTT)	Unaffected	Reduced
Optimal reaction temperature	37°C	4–20°C
Primary immune response involvement	(+)	+++
Secondary immune response involvement	+++	(+)

*See Table 1.2.

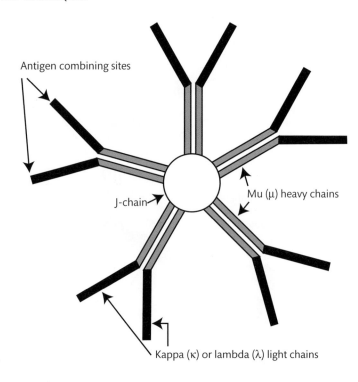

FIGURE 1.3
Basic structure of an IgM antibody molecule.

TABLE 1.2 **Properties of blood group antibody IgG subclasses.**

Property	IgG1	IgG2	IgG3	IgG4
Mean percentage of total IgG	~70%	~18%	~8%	~4%
Complement activation (via the classic pathway)	+++	+	+++	–
Placental transfer	++	±	++	+
Macrophage binding	+++	–	+++	–

1.3 **Antibody function**

The polypeptide chains of immunoglobulin molecules are not straight, linear molecules but are folded and held in place by intrachain disulphide bonds. The specificity of the antibody is determined by the variable regions of the heavy and light chains in the Fab part of the molecule; composed of 110 variable amino acid sequences, and containing the 'hyper-variable' regions where the antigen binding sites are located, sometimes termed the **paratope**. With some 500–1,000 heavy chain and over 200 light chain variable region genes, there are more than 10 million potential antibody specificities that can be produced by any individual.

The other biological functions of the antibody—complement activation, placental transfer, and the ability to bind to macrophages—are located on the constant regions of the Fc part on the immunoglobulin molecule.

The hinge region (two closely associated triplets of proline amino acids) provides the heavy chain with a degree of flexibility, enabling it to bend. An IgG molecule has a 'T' shape with the

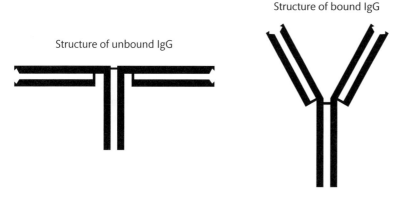

Structure of unbound IgG

Structure of bound IgG

FIGURE 1.4
Possible structure of unbound and bound IgG molecule.

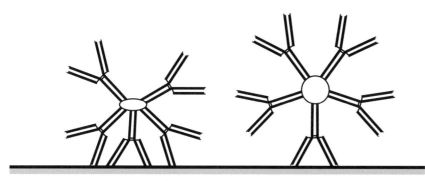

Red cell membrane—antigens

FIGURE 1.5
Possible structures of bound IgM molecules.

antigen binding sites about 14 nm apart but becomes a 'Y' shape on binding with its antigen. This change in shape also allows the effector functions, associated with the Fc portion, to become activated.

Immunoglobulin M molecules have a diameter of about 30 nm, and as well as being flexible at the hinge regions they can change shape on binding with an antigen by movement of the J-chain. Photomicrographs show them as various 'crab-like' shapes when bound to antigens on a cell surface. IgM antibodies can agglutinate red cells when they are suspended in plasma or saline, by binding to antigens on cells next to one another.

SELF-CHECK 1.2

What are the functions of antibody molecules? See Figures 1.4 and 1.5.

1.4 **Antigen–antibody reactions**

The reaction of an antibody and antigen occurs very quickly. It is a reversible reaction governed by the **law of mass action** and will eventually come to equilibrium, when the formation of Ag:Ab complexes is at the same rate as the dissociation.

$$Ag + Ab = AgAb$$

The antigen and antibody are held together by relatively weak attracting forces, involving hydrogen, ionic, and hydrophobic bonding, as well as van der Waal's forces. As antibodies are produced to a specific antigen by a number of clones of plasma cells the affinity, or association constant, for the antigen will vary within those polyclonal antibodies. Greater differences will be found between antibodies of different specificities. The greater the affinity of an antibody the more likely it is to bind with an antigen. Likewise the greater the amount of antibody that is present for a given amount of antigen, then more antibody will become bound to that cell and the more likely that the antibody-coated or sensitized cells will be recognized and removed *in vivo* or detected in *in vitro* tests.

Key points

Of the five immunoglobulin classes, IgM and IgG antibodies are the most important in transfusion. Antigen binding is a function of the Fab portion, and other effector mechanisms—complement activation, placental transfer, and macrophage binding—are functions of the Fc portion of the molecule.

1.5 Antibody-mediated red cell destruction

Antibodies do not destroy red cells directly *in vivo*, but initiate their destruction in two ways by:

- The activation of complement
- Macrophage recognition of red cell-bound antibody.

Complement

The role of complement is essentially to destroy invading cells, such as bacteria, but antibodies to blood cells can also initiate this pathway. The complement system has nine main components, C1–C9, working in a sequential manner; each one, once activated, is capable of activating the next in the cascade. The complement cascade is actually three different pathways (classical, lectin, and alternate) that utilize identical end-stage components but are activated differently. The alternate and **lectin pathways** are activated by bacterial proteins/lectins, whereas the 'classic' complement cascade is activated by the Fc portions of immunoglobulin molecules when bound to a cell surface antigen. Two Fc molecules are required to activate C1. This can be by one IgM antibody molecule or two IgG molecules, very close together on the cell membrane.

The order of the reaction sequence is:

$$C1-C4-C2-C3-C5-C6-C7-C8-C9$$

The final steps of the cascade cause 'channels' to be formed through the cell membrane, allowing water to move into the red cell, resulting in cell lysis or haemolysis of red cells.

The classical complement pathway has three distinct phases:

Lectin pathway

An arm of the complement pathway where mannose binding lectin and proteins binds to bacterial or viral mannose containing oligosaccharides and initiates the binding of further complement components and activation of the cascade.

1. *Activation phase*

   C1 is activated by a red cell antigen–antibody reaction, followed by the activation of C4 and C2 molecules to form the C4b2b complex (C3 convertase); in the alternate and lectin pathways C3bBb is the substrate for C3 convertase).

2. *Amplification phase*

   The activation of C3 by C3 convertase, which leads to the binding of C3b to the C4b2b complex and C3b binding to other sites on the cell membrane.

3. *Membrane attack phase*

   The activation of C5 by the C4b2b3b complex and the subsequent activation of C6, C7, C8, and C9 leading to cell lysis.

Once activated, complement needs to be carefully regulated so that it does not cause damage to the body itself. There are several regulators that interact with C3b and C4b to inhibit their activity by further splitting the molecules into C3d and C4d, which do not have any effector capabilities. Because of the limited number of complement molecules bound initially to the cell or the action of regulatory mechanisms, the cascade often stops at the C3 (effectively C3b) stage and does not proceed to cell lysis. However, cells coated with C3b can be removed from the circulation by macrophages in the liver, but cells with C3d are not recognized and are therefore not removed.

Complement fragments C3a and C5a have properties that are important parts of the overall inflammatory response mechanism. They are chemotactic for neutrophils, attracting them to the site where complement is activated so they can phagocytose cells coated with C3b. The two complement fragments are also anaphylatoxins that bind to basophils in the blood and tissue mast cells, causing them to degranulate and release histamine. This in turn causes the blood vessels to dilate, allowing more blood containing complement and antibodies to get to the site of inflammation. C5a can also bind to macrophages, inducing them to release cytokines such as IL-1 (interleukin) and IL-6, which increase the expression of cell adhesion molecules (CAM) lining the endothelial cells of the blood vessels. Neutrophils attracted to the site then bind to the vessel walls and can be migrated to the inflamed site.

However, when considering antigen–antibody reactions of blood cells these are not localized as, for example, a cut to the skin, so therefore the effects of complement and cytokine activity are not localized, as will be considered later.

Figure 1.6 also indicates the actions of the various complement control proteins (CCPs), including CD55 (decay accelerating factor), which interacts with C4b and C3b of both the alternate and **classical pathways**, and inhibits the formation of their respective convertases. CD46 (membrane cofactor protein, MCP), which inhibits the cleavage by serum factor 1 of C3b and C4b; and CD59 (membrane inhibitor of reactive lysis, MIRL) prevents C9 from polymerizing and thus prevents formation of the membrane attack complex. Further details on CD55 and CD59 are found in Chapter 2, and the inappropriate interactions of xenotransplanted organ CCPs in Chapter 9.

Classical pathway

The primary arm of the complement cascade that leads to red cell destruction when complement components bind to immunoglobulin bound to red cells and other cell types (e.g. bacteria).

Macrophages

As blood cells are not localized but circulating, the effector cells, macrophages, for removing old or damaged blood cells are found mainly in the spleen. As the blood circulates through the spleen IgG antibody-coated cells will adhere to IgG receptors (FcR; for more details see Chapter 3)

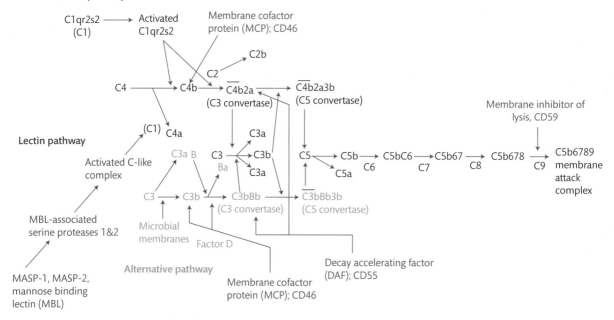

FIGURE 1.6

The 'classical, alternative, and lectin' complement pathways. The lectin pathway (brown) and alternative pathway (green) 'feed' into a common pathway (black). The membrane components that inhibit the complement cascade are shown in blue, and their site of action.

on the surface of the macrophages that will then engulf the cell, effectively removing it from the circulation. With red cells, the cell is not always engulfed, but a part of the membrane is removed allowing the rest of the red cell to break away as a **spherocyte**.

Of the four sub-classes of IgG immunoglobulin, IgG2 and IgG4 seem not to be recognized by these macrophages, whereas IgG1 and IgG3 are. It has been shown that 1,000 IgG1 molecules are required per red cell for it to be sequestered, but only 100 molecules of IgG3 are required.

Cells with C3b on their surface are recognized by macrophages in the liver and they, too, are removed from the circulation. However, C3b is quickly broken down *in vivo* to C3d that is not recognized by macrophages, so cells thus coated have a nearly normal life span. The presence of both IgG and complement C3b on the red cell increases the likelihood of the red cells being removed from the circulation, by the 'additive' effect of the removal of complement-coated cells in the liver and IgG-coated cells in the spleen.

This mechanism is called **extravascular haemolysis** as the immune-mediated cell removal takes place outside the circulation in the liver or spleen.

Some antibodies, especially anti-A and anti-B, can activate the complement pathway, or 'fix complement' as it is sometimes called, which leads directly to the cells being lysed within the circulation; this is called **intravascular haemolysis**.

Therefore, antibodies are produced in response to an external antigenic stimulus. The primary response is slow and IgM antibodies are formed first with the plasma cells then switching production to IgG. In a secondary response, IgG antibodies are produced from the outset with little or no lag phase.

Extravascular haemolysis

Immune-mediated cell removal that takes place outside the circulation in the liver or spleen.

Intravascular haemolysis

Cells being lysed within the circulation by antibodies that activate the complement pathway, especially anti-A and anti-B.

Antibodies by themselves do not cause cell destruction, but they activate the complement cascade that might result in either cell lysis within the circulation or removal by macrophages in the liver of cells coated with C3b. If complement is not activated then cells coated with IgG antibody will be recognized by macrophages in the spleen and removed from the circulation. There are then two types of lysis: intra-and extravascular lysis.

SELF-CHECK 1.3

How does complement bring about red cell destruction?

1.6 *In vitro* detection of antigen-antibody reactions

To detect red cell antigen-antibody reactions the cells themselves can be used as markers, as most routine blood bank techniques produce agglutination (antibody-induced clumping). The same technique cannot be used for platelets or granulocyte work and here antibodies are detected by indirect methods such as using flow cytometry. Whatever technique is used it is important to get as much antibody onto the cells as possible as there is a minimum threshold of antibody molecules per cell that will be detectable in routine tests. For the antiglobulin test, for example, this minimum figure is about 100 antibodies per red cell.

Factors affecting antigen-antibody reactions *in vitro*:

- Antigen-antibody ratio
- Time
- Temperature
- pH
- Ionic strength.
  - Increasing the ratio of plasma used in a test to the number of cells will maximize the chances of there being sufficient antibody molecules per cell to be detectable. There are, of course, practicable limits to the volume of plasma that can be used, and other factors such as ionic strength to be taken into account.
  - All reactions need time to come to equilibrium, but in most routine techniques it is unlikely that true equilibrium is reached in the incubation times used. Experience has shown what minimum times can be used. In any test the set parameters should not be changed without proper re-evaluation of the technique.
  - Most immune antibodies react better at 37°C than at lower temperatures. But naturally acquired, IgM, T-independent antibodies tend to react better at lower temperatures. As these latter antibodies, with the exception of anti-A/B are not generally clinically significant then most tests are incubated at 37°C.
  - Immune antibodies have a pH optimum around 7.2; therefore, tests are performed using buffers to maintain this pH.
  - Lowering the ionic strength of the reactants in a red cell antigen-antibody test from that of physiologically normal saline, 0.45 M, to an equivalent of 0.15 M, increases the rate of antigen uptake of most antibodies. Incubation times in 'normal' ionic conditions are typically 60 minutes but when using low ionic strength conditions 15 minutes is sufficient.

Red cell agglutination

When the red cells are joined together by cross-linking of antibody molecules they become agglutinated. Red cell agglutination occurs in two distinct, but inter-related stages, the primary antibody sensitization stage and the secondary agglutination stage.

The factors affecting antibody sensitization of red cells have already been considered. In the second stage, the rate of red cell agglutination is determined by the frequency with which the antibody-sensitized red cells collide. Red cells come closer by the action of gravity, which can be increased by centrifugation and by surface tension, or interfacial energy. However, these aggregating forces are balanced by a repelling force associated with an 'ion cloud' around each red cell.

Red cells have an overall net negative charge due to the negative charges on a major constituent of the membrane, the glycoproteins. The negatively charged red cells attract a 'cloud' of positively charged ions from the suspending saline (NaCl) medium. The intensity of the ionic cloud that moves with the red cell decreases with increasing distance from the cell surface. The resulting charge is known as the zeta-potential, and this determines the minimum distance that the red cells are able to approach each other. A number of other forces acting on the red cell membrane, including the movement of water molecules at the membrane surface, are also believed to affect red cell attraction and repulsion.

The repulsive force of the positively charged ion cloud around each cell means that red cells cannot approach close enough to allow an IgG molecule to span the gap between them. An IgM antibody molecule is, however, large enough to span this gap and is therefore capable of causing agglutination of red cells in plasma without any further manipulations. For IgG antibody molecules to agglutinate red cells an alteration in the environment of the red cells is required to enable them to cross-link. Methods employed include the addition of macromolecules (such as albumin), enzyme treatment of the red cells, or the use of an anti-human globulin (AHG) reagent. See Figure 1.7.

Red cell agglutination by IgM antibodies

As IgM antibodies can 'span' the gap between red cells they are capable of agglutinating red cells suspended in saline. The first antibodies described in the ABO blood group system were

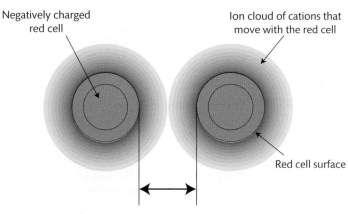

Negatively charged red cell

Ion cloud of cations that move with the red cell

Red cell surface

FIGURE 1.7
Ion cloud affecting the minimum distance between red cells (not to scale).

Minimum distance between red cell surfaces (>14 nm)

IgM antibodies and until the development of techniques to detect the so-called 'incomplete antibodies' we now know to be IgG, all blood-banking techniques used red cells either in their own plasma or suspended in saline. Tests were carried out on glass slides or tiles, or in later years in tubes, and more recently in microplates (microtitre plates) that are effectively 96 small tubes in one easy-to-use plastic tray. Because the interaction of IgM antibodies, especially anti-A and anti-B, with their antigens is very quick, incubation times can be short or, indeed, 'immediate'. The **immediate spin technique**, in which the tube containing the reactants is centrifuged without incubation, is widely used when working with ABO antibodies.

In 1990 details of a new test system were published, and this method has subsequently come into widespread use. It uses small microtubes, or columns, containing a gel or bead matrix, to which can be added blood grouping or antiglobulin reagents. There are several commercial systems on the market, for example Bio-Rad ID-System, Grifols DG Gel, and Ortho BioVue, each with six or eight columns being presented in a single card. For routine grouping, cards with antisera (e.g. anti-A, anti-B, anti-D) incorporated into the matrix are available. A small volume of a red cell suspension is added to the appropriate column, the card is then centrifuged, and red cells that are agglutinated by the antiserum are trapped in the matrix as visible agglutinates.

For reverse ABO grouping, or detecting alloantibodies, a small volume of plasma and the appropriate cells are incubated in the chamber above the microtube that contains a neutral matrix. The card containing the columns is centrifuged after incubation, and any agglutinated cells are trapped within the matrix.

Monoclonal antibodies produced by *in vitro* cell culture for use as grouping or phenotyping reagents are, wherever possible, IgM molecules so that they can be easily used in the laboratory by saline or direct agglutinating techniques, without having to resort to more complex methods that are needed when using IgG reagents.

Red cell agglutination by IgG antibodies

Addition of macromolecules

Macromolecules such as 20% bovine albumin effectively reduce the 'charge density' (the dielectric constant) around the red cells, thereby reducing the net repulsive force between cells. This allows the red cells to approach closer together than is possible in a saline environment, so that IgG antibody molecules can span the gap between red cells, producing cross-linkage and therefore agglutination. It is thought that some macromolecules may also act by binding to the outer surface of the red cell membrane, affecting membrane water and therefore altering interfacial tension. Methods using different macromolecules have variable sensitivity and do not enable all IgG red antibodies to produce agglutination. Although once widely used, especially in the days before monoclonal IgM RhD typing reagents, these techniques are rarely used today.

One exception is the use of Polybrene, (hexadimethrine bromide), which causes red cells to aggregate. In the low ionic Polybrene (LIP) technique, red cells and plasma are incubated for only 1 minute at room temperature in a very low ionic strength medium so that antibody uptake is very quick. Polybrene is added to 'aggregate' the red cells, then the non-specific aggregation is dispersed leaving antibody mediate agglutination. This rapid technique is not, however, suitable with some antibody specificities (e.g. anti-K) and has a limited, but valuable, use.

Use of enzymes

As the negative charge of a red cell is carried on the glycophorin A molecules of the red cell membrane, proteolytic enzymes, such as papain, can be used to remove some of these molecules. This effectively reduces the net negative charge on the red cell membrane, enabling red cells to come closer together, allowing some IgG antibody molecules to agglutinate red cells. The enzyme treatment also increases the exposure of some antigens by reducing steric hindrance caused by surrounding molecules, thereby improving antibody uptake. Enzyme techniques are particularly good for the detection of Rh antibodies. However, antigens which are present on glycophorins A, such as M and N, and on the Duffy glycoprotein, Fy^a and Fy^b are destroyed by the enzyme treatment, so antibodies to these antigens cannot be detected by using enzyme techniques.

Use of anti-human globulin (AHG) reagents

By using an antibody, anti-human IgG, red cells that are coated with IgG protein can be agglutinated. The Fab portion of the anti-human globulin antibody reacts with the Fc portion of the IgG antibody present on the sensitized red cells. This effectively overcomes the problem of the minimum distance between red cells, which individual IgG antibodies are incapable of spanning. See Figure 1.8.

The early AHG reagents were made by injecting a rabbit with a crude human globulin preparation so that they produced anti-human globulin antibodies. The rabbit was then bled and the serum containing the antibodies, after some manipulation, used in the **antiglobulin (Coombs) test**. These AHG reagents contained a mixture of antibodies to IgG, IgM, IgA, and to complement C3 and C4. Later work showed that C4 can be adsorbed onto red cells *in vitro* in a non-specific manner and could lead to a false-positive reaction if anti-C4 were present in the AHG reagent. Modern reagents are usually made from anti-IgG raised in rabbits by using a purer IgG preparation, and a monoclonal anti-C3d; these are called **polyspecific AHG reagents**. Monospecific anti-IgG, anti-IgM, anti-IgA, C3d, and anti-C4 are also available and are widely used when investigating cases of immune red cell destruction.

In the direct antiglobulin test (DAT) red cells are taken from a patient, then washed in saline to remove all traces of plasma and immunoglobulins, except those already bound *in vivo* to the cells. The AHG reagent is then added and if bound IgG antibodies or C3 are present then the test is positive.

> **Polyspecific AHG (anti-human globulin) reagents**
> A blend of antibodies that recognize immunoglobulins and anti-C3d of complement used in the Coomb's (antiglobulin) test.

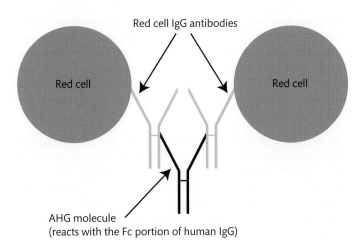

Red cell IgG antibodies

Red cell

Red cell

AHG molecule
(reacts with the Fc portion of human IgG)

FIGURE 1.8

Action of antiglobulin molecules agglutinating red cells coated with IgG antibody.

The indirect antiglobulin test (IAT) is the most widely used test in immunohaematology for the detection of antibodies in an antibody screening test and to identify the specificity of any antibodies thus found. It is also used in the serological phase of compatibility testing or crossmatching.

Plasma, or a known antibody (antiserum), is incubated with red cells, usually in a low ionic strength solution (LISS) so that any antibodies present can bind to their corresponding antigens. If a tube technique is used the cells are then washed in saline, AHG reagent added, and a positive reaction indicates the presence of antibodies. For many years antiglobulin tests were carried out in test tubes, but now column (microtube) systems are widely used. The major advantage of these systems is that there is no need to wash the red cells after the incubation phase. The cells and plasma under test are incubated in a chamber above the matrix containing the antiglobulin reagent. After incubation, the cards are centrifuged and only the red cells not the plasma are forced through the matrix, and if coated with IgG they are trapped in the matrix as visible agglutinates.

These systems can be used in conjunction with columns for grouping (ABO, RhD) using IgM, directly agglutinating antibodies in the matrix either manually or in automated, computer controlled systems. Most laboratories in the UK now use some form of automation for routine ABO and D grouping, and antibody screening of patient samples for both pre-transfusion and antenatal cases.

Key points

IgM antibodies can agglutinate red cells directly in a saline medium but IgG antibodies do not and are usually detected by using the antiglobulin test or enzyme-treated red cells.

1.7 Techniques

Molecular techniques are widely used for testing for human leucocyte and platelet antigens, but most blood transfusion laboratories still employ serological techniques as outlined above. Although not yet widely used, DNA microarrays are available to determine the presence or absence of a wide range of blood group genes, especially single nucleotide **polymorphisms** (SNPs). Also, next generation sequencing for blood group antigens has begun to emerge as a technique that can genotype both donors and patients. For antibody detection the corresponding antigen, or the appropriate **epitope**, is required. Some recombinant blood group proteins and synthetic peptide **mimotopes** (short synthetic peptides that mimic natural epitopes of the individual blood group antigens) are being developed to be used in microarray antibody detection systems without the need for intact red cells.

Details of techniques have not been given in this chapter as most blood banks or transfusion departments now employ commercial test systems. Therefore the manufacturer's instructions must be followed. Each laboratory will have its own set of standard operating procedures (SOPs) that detail the techniques that have been **validated** for use by that laboratory. But all serological techniques follow the general principles outlined in this chapter and will be referred to in other chapters.

The basic purpose of laboratory testing pre transfusion or transplantation is to ensure compatibility between the donor cells and the recipient. Where this cannot be achieved then any

Polymorphism
The occurrence of more than one form of the antigen.

Mimotopes
Short synthetic peptides that mimic natural epitopes of the individual blood group antigens that are being developed to be used in microarray antibody detection systems without the need for intact red cells.

Validated
Having documentary evidence to show that a system/ equipment or process meets pre-defined requirements for its intended use.

incompatibility should be as little as possible so that the advantages of the donor cells transfused or transplanted outweigh the adverse effects. Transfusion/transplantation laboratories also have to be able to investigate untoward reactions and other cases of immune cell destruction such as that found in haemolytic disease of the newborn; these are considered in the following chapters.

SELF-CHECK 1.4

What methods can be used to detect IgG antibodies?

 ## Chapter summary

- Although there has been a long history of attempts at transfusing blood and transplanting tissues the real advances were made in the second half of the twentieth century.

- In both transfusion and transplantation 'foreign' antigens are introduced into the body; therefore, an immune response can be expected.

- The immune response can be either 'innate' or 'adaptive'. The adaptive immune response can be further divided into two divisions 'humoral' and 'cellular'.

- In the humoral response antibodies are produced in response to an external antigenic stimulus.

- The primary response is slow; IgM antibodies are produced first with the plasma cells then switching production to IgG.

- In a secondary response IgG antibodies are produced from the outset with little or no lag phase.

- Antibodies by themselves do not cause cell destruction; some can activate the complement cascade that might result in cell lysis within the circulation—intravascular lysis, or removal of cells coated with C3b by macrophages in the liver.

- Red cells coated with IgG antibody will be recognized by macrophages in the spleen and removed from the circulation—extravascular lysis.

- The main techniques used for blood grouping involve the formation and visualization of agglutination either by direct agglutination (IgM antibodies) or by using the antiglobulin test (IgG antibodies).

Answers to the questions in this chapter are provided on the book's accompanying website:

 Go to www.oup.com/uk/avent2e

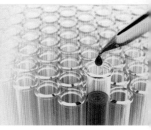

2

Human Blood Group Antigens

Neil D. Avent

Learning objectives

After studying this chapter you should be able to:

- Understand the ultrastructure of the erythrocyte membrane and its skeleton.
- Differentiate between the molecular basis of carbohydrate and protein-based blood group antigens.
- Gain an understanding of the genetics and resultant proteins that govern antigen expression.
- Understand what genetic mutations contribute to weakening and silencing of blood group antigens.
- Understand how blood group active molecules contribute to the structure and function of the normal erythrocyte, and abnormalities when they are deficient.
- Form an appreciation of DNA-based methods for defining blood group genotype and prediction of phenotype.

Introduction

Blood groups perhaps represent some of the best examples of the clinical implications of human polymorphism. The 1930 Nobel prize winner Karl Landsteiner first identified the existence of blood-group antigens and antisera in 1901. Throughout the remainder of the twentieth century serology revealed all clinically significant blood groups. In the 1980s new molecular techniques emerged that permitted the identification of protein species involved in blood group antigen expression by the small-scale purification (immunoprecipitation) of those involved. Prior to this, the first membrane protein to be sequenced, glycophorin A (GPA), was completed in 1975. GPA, a major erythrocyte protein is responsible for expression of M and N blood group antigen expression. Conventional protein sequence analysis then revealed that two amino acid changes in the N terminus of GPA (Ser1Leu and Gly5Glu) confer the difference between the M and N blood group antigens.

Throughout the 1990s gene cloning technology successfully investigated the major clinically significant blood group active genes, and established the molecular basis of most blood group polymorphisms. This knowledge is discussed in some depth here, but it is first important to consider what constitutes a polymorphic trait.

2.1 **Human polymorphism and evolution**

For most human genetic traits, an incidence of 1% or greater within the population is regarded as true polymorphism, but as we shall see this is hardly appropriate in blood transfusion. Most blood group antigens are considered low frequency or high frequency, with comparatively few antigens balanced in the population. Examples of balanced polymorphisms include the Rh C/c; E/e of the RH system; Fy^a/Fy^b of the Duffy system; and Jk^a/Jk^b of the Kidd system.

Polymorphism is driven by evolution—a mutation will only increase in frequency if beneficial to the individual, for the most part it is not, and gradually disappears over a number of generations. The evolution of blood groups is indeed an interesting question for which we only have some clues, and for many we have no idea why these polymorphic traits emerged. In the ABO system, the blood group active A, B, and H antigens are not just expressed on erythroid cells, but throughout the body, including the gut lumen. It is possible therefore that the simple switching of structures to which gut flora bind was an innate immune response to pathogenic gut flora. In the Rh system, as we shall see later, the D-negative phenotype appears to have arisen by genomic mutation independently in several regions worldwide, most widespread in Western Europe, reaching some 15–20% of the population (indeed, in the Basque region it is almost 40%). In Africa, a different genetic mutation caused the D-negative phenotype, and in most African populations the D-negative frequency is around 7–10%. Why was this the case? When these D-negative mutations first arose in the population, they would be positively selected for, because non-existent obstetric care in ancient times meant that D-negative babies carried by D-negative mothers would have a selective advantage. As we shall see in the FY system the Fy(a-b-) phenotype is dominant in West Africa, most probably because Duffy-negative erythrocytes are resistant to invasion by malarial parasites. These three examples are hypotheses, with in some cases strong circumstantial evidence. What is unclear, however, is why a number of other polymorphisms (e.g. Rh C/c, E/e, and the VS/V polymorphisms found in high prevalence in Africans) impart any selective advantage.

The International Society of Blood Transfusion (ISBT) nomenclature committee governs the classification of blood group systems and the antigens classified within each system, and at the time of writing there are currently 36 (Figure 2.1). To become a blood group, the genetic basis of blood group antigen expression must have been defined. These are two broad groups: (1) carbohydrate antigens—exclusively defined by the Golgi-localized glycosyltransferases that catalyse the transfer of a monosaccharide moiety from a nucleoside-sugar precursor to a growing carbohydrate chain; (2) protein antigens, where the differences in the sequence or configuration of the protein causes recognition as an antigenic determinant. In several instances the complete absence of a protein causes the negative phenotype within a blood group system. For example D-negative erythrocytes (RH system) lack the D polypeptide; and Fy(a-b-) erythrocytes lack the Fy (Duffy) glycoprotein. The current (2017) ISBT nomenclature, commonly used names, genes, numbers of assigned antigens, and chromosomal location are presented in Table 2.1.

The ISBT also classifies blood group alleles using both a numeric and letter notation. This is written as thus *RHD*01W.20* where italics representing an allelic gene, *RHD* indicates the affected

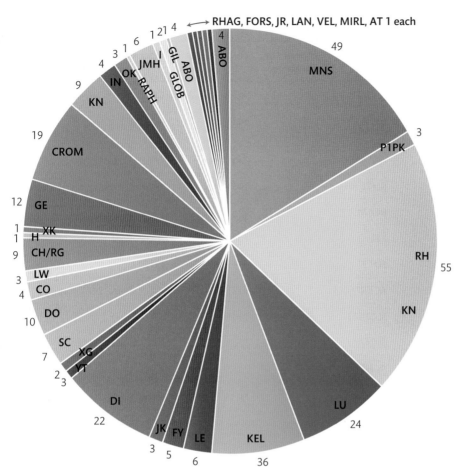

FIGURE 2.1
The blood group systems 2017.
The pie chart illustrates the numbers of blood group antigens assigned to each of the 36 blood group systems. In a clockwise direction the segments of the pie chart are ordered from ABO (ISBT001) to the most recently defined blood group system, AUG (ISBT036).

gene, *01 the original wild-type allele, and W.20 indicates a weakening allele of RHD. In null alleles (otherwise known as silencing mutations) the W (weak) suffix is replaced with N for null.

Blood group antigens—an overview

In theory, any structure that presents itself to the immune system and is not recognized as self has the potential to be antigenic. In general, this variation can include either carbohydrate structures attached to either lipids or proteins (hence glycolipid or glycoprotein). From here on the chapter is organized by the functional significance of the antigen carriers (protein antigens) or the specific structures (carbohydrate). All carbohydrate antigens are synthesized by a family of Golgi-localized enzymes called glycosyltransferases; the specific substrates and antigens they generate are the resultant antigens. A description of the molecular background of all of the current 36 blood group systems is provided, and arranged with respect to the functional significance of the antigen carriers themselves. As protein-based antigens are the key players in regulating red cell contents and interactions with other cell types, several broad categories (e.g. membrane transporters, receptors, enzymes, complement control proteins) have been identified. It is highly useful to remember the functional significance of the antigen carrier as this often relates to the clinical significance of the antigens carried by polymorphic variation in them.

TABLE 2.1   The 36 blood group systems as defined by the International Society of Blood Transfusion (ISBT).

ISBT number	ISBT symbol	Common name	Gene symbol	No. of Antigens	Chromosome	Biochemistry
001	ABO	ABO	*ABO*	4	9q34.1-q34.2	CHO
002	MNS	MNS	*GYPA GYPB GYPE*	48	4q28-q31	AA changes/hybrids
003	P1PK	P	*A4GALT*	3	22q11-ter	A4GALT transferase
004	RH	Rh	*RHCE RHD*	56	1p34-36.2	AA changes/hybrids/deletions
005	LU	Lutheran	*BCAM*	21	19q12-q13	AA changes
006	KEL	Kell	*KEL*	21	7q33	AA changes
007	LE	Lewis	*FUT3*	6	19p13.3	CHO
008	FY	Duffy	*ACKR1*	5	1q21-q22	AA changes, GATA mutation
009	JK	Kidd	*SLC14A1*	3	18q11-q12	AA changes
010	DI	Diego	*SLC4AE1*	22	17q21-q22	AA changes
011	YT	Cartwright	*ACHE*	2	7q22	AA change
012	XG	XG	*XG, CD99*	2	Xp22; Y	Quantitative
013	SC	Scianna	*ERMAP*	7	1p22.1	AA changes
014	DO	Dombrock	*ART4*	8	12q13.2-q13.3	AA changes
015	CO	Colton	*AQP1*	4	7p14	AA changes
016	LW	Landsteiner–Weiner	*ICAM4 (LW)*	3	19p13.2-cen	AA changes
017	CH/RG	Chido/Rodgers	*C4A,C4B*	7	6p21.3	Quantitative
018	H	H	*FUT1*	1	19q13.3	Mutations causing null phenotypes
019	XK	Kx	*XK*	1	Xp21.1	Mutations/deletions causing null phenotypes
020	GE	Gerbich	*GYPC*	11	2q14-21	Mutations, hybrids
021	CROM	Cromer	*CD55*	18	1q32.2	AA changes
022	KN	Knops	*CD35*	9	1q32.2	AA changes, quantitative
023	IN	Indian	*CD44*	4	11p13	AA change
024	OK	OK	*BSG (CD147)*	3	19p13.3	Ok(a-) lack CD147
025	RAPH	Raph	*CD151*	1	11p15.5	
026	JMH	John Milton Hagen	*SEMA7A*	6	15q22.2-23	AA changes

ISBT number	ISBT symbol	Common name	Gene symbol	No. of Antigens	Chromosome	Biochemistry
027	I	I	GCNT2	1	6p24.2	
028	GLOB	Globoside	B3GALT3	2	3q26.1	B3GALT3 transferase
029	GIL	Gill	AQP3	1	9p13.3	
030	RHAG	RhAG	RHAG	4	6p12.3	AA changes
031	FORS	Forssman	GBGT1	1	9q32.2	GBGT1 transferase
032	JR	Junior	ABCG2	1	4q22.1	
033	LAN	Lan	ABCB6	1	2q36	
034	VEL	Vel	SMIM1	1	1p36.32	Small 17 nt deletion in exon 3
035	CD59	MIRL	CD59	1	11p13	
036	AUG	Augustine	SLC29A1	1	6p21.1	

Key points

■ Erythrocyte antigens arise as a result of evolutionary pressure, in most cases the drivers of which are unknown.

■ Any erythrocyte surface structure, both carbohydrate or protein may be expressed by polymorphic genes termed *alleles*.

■ Incompatible transfusion or pregnancy may lead to the production of blood group specific antibodies that may cause transfusion reactions or in pregnancy haemolytic disease of the newborn and fetus.

SELF-CHECK 2.1

• How does the International Society of Blood Transfusion classify blood group systems?

• How does it classify a blood group antigen?

• Do the number of antigens per system indicate its clinical significance?

2.2 The erythrocyte membrane

All blood group active structures arise from the erythrocyte membrane, with one exception. The Chido/Rogers blood group arises from variation in C4A/C4B complement components that are absorbed onto erythrocytes from plasma. All others arise mainly from both variations in protein and carbohydrate sequences (apart from D-negative and Fy(a-b-) mentioned previously). On average, individuals have approximately five litres of blood, and the concentration (haemocrit) differs between males and females (males $4.7–6.1\times10^9$/ml and females $4.2–5.4\times10^9$/ml).

Erythrocyte membranes are highly specialized structurally; the cells travel approximately 300 miles in their average 120 day lifespan (a range of 100–140 days), and must be extremely flexible to do so. This equates to approximately 700,000 circuits of the vasculature. Erythrocytes are approximately 6.5–8 μm in diameter *in vivo* yet they actively transit through microcapillaries 3–4 μm in diameter. Therefore, they must be extremely flexible (termed **deformability**), and when aged become less so, losing their biconcave disc shape. Aged (effete or senescent) erythrocytes are rapidly removed from the circulation by splenic macrophages, there is huge turnover of erythrocytes—our bodies have approximately $2–3 \times 10^{13}$ erythrocytes, the most numerous cell type by far. Erythrocyte concentration in the circulation is controlled by the kidney hormone erythropoietin (EPO). EPO production is regulated by a sophisticated oxygen-sensing system that is regulated by a transcription factor called hypoxia-inducible transcription factor (HIF). The EPO gene has a hypoxia responsive element (HRE) to which HIF binds, triggering its transcription. EPO then induces erythropoiesis in the bone marrow, a process that takes approximately 7 days to produce mature red blood cells. Erythropoiesis is considered in more depth in Chapter 10. Approximately 2.2 million new erythrocytes are produced *per second*, giving some indication of both the scale and importance of them in maintaining a highly active metabolism. Erythrocytes are critical for function in most animals, and life on Earth would not have evolved without the development of the erythrocyte.

Deformability

The elastic ability of the erythrocyte imparted by its membrane. Erythrocytes can negotiate microcapillaries half their diameter due to their deformability.

Deformability of erythrocytes is entirely due to a highly evolved **membrane skeleton**, which lies beneath the plasma membrane, which has a conventional assembly of integral membrane proteins, peripheral proteins, phospholipids, and cholesterol. The membrane skeleton gains a high degree of elasticity by a spectrin-actin meshwork. Spectrin is a large filamentous molecule made up of 106 amino acid repeats and has both α and β sub-units. Spectrin forms a junctional complex with actin and several other protein components (Figure 2.2), and forms cross links to other spectrin dimers.

Membrane skeleton

The mesh-like network of proteins that give erythrocytes their extreme flexibility. Comprising predominantly of α-and β-spectrins, protein 4.1R, ankyrin, actin, and p55.

The erythroid membrane skeleton maintains many linkage or anchorage points to the plasma membrane. Two major linkages exist. The first is through the major erythrocyte membrane protein band 3 (1.1 million copies per erythrocyte), otherwise known as the anion exchange protein. Band 3 is a transport molecule that exchanges one anion for another (in–out mechanism) to maintain electroneutrality. These anions are Cl^- and HCO_3^-, and thus the protein is of prime importance in the transport of CO_2 in its hydrated form, bicarbonate. The protein is able to switch the direction of transport of these anions; in the lungs HCO_3^- moves out of the erythrocyte and is expelled as gaseous CO_2 in lung alveoli, whereas in metabolizing tissue, HCO_3^- is transported inside erythrocytes for binding to haemoglobin. This switch is governed by the local pH in the lungs and tissue. It is called the *Bohr shift*, which also governs O_2 and CO_2 binding to haemoglobin. Band 3 has an anion transport domain of 14 membrane-spanning segments and a large N-terminal tail that is cytoplasmically located. This cytoplasmic domain binds the skeletal protein ankyrin-R. The second attachment point is through the interaction with another major membrane protein called glycophorin C (200,000 copies per erythrocyte). This protein is a single-pass integral membrane protein with its N-terminus outside and cytoplasmic C-terminus. The C-terminal domain forms a tight interaction with the skeletal proteins protein 4.1R and p55, and is termed a **ternary complex**. Both the band 3 and glycophorin C interactions are termed *vertical interactions* with the membrane skeleton. *Horizontal interactions* of the spectrin dimers and protein 4.1R with phosphatidylserine, a cytoplasmically localized phospholipid, also occur.

Ternary complex

The key protein–protein interactions that govern the assembly of the erythrocyte membrane, comprising the major players: spectrin, actin, protein 4.1R, p55 and ankyrin.

Erythrocyte phospholipids are essentially identical to those found in other plasma membranes, namely phosphatidycholine (PC), phosphotidylethanolamine (PE), phosphatidylserine (PS) and sphingomyelin (SM). These phospholipids are asymmetrically distributed, the choline phospholipids (PC and SM) located toward the extracellular leaflet, and the serine phospholipids (PS

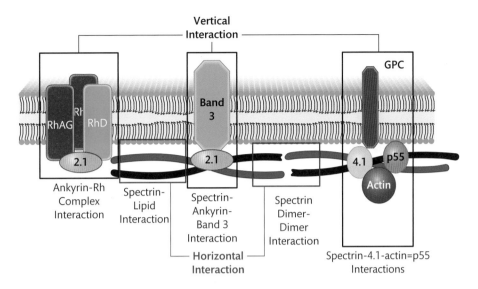

FIGURE 2.2

The key components of erythrocyte membranes and membrane skeleton

The major players in the erythrocyte membrane membrane skeleton are shown in this cartoon. The membrane bilayer is studded with a number of transmembrane proteins which have some form of attachment with the submembranous membrane skeleton. Only three are shown here for clarity, the N-terminus of band 3 (SLC14A1) forms an association with Ankyrin (synonym band 2.1), whilst glycophorin C (GPC) associates with the protein 4.1 (p4.1R) – p55-actin junctional (ternary) complex. Band 3 and GPC are major components quantitatively in the erythrocyte membrane with 1,100,000 and 200,000 copies per erythrocyte respectively. The Rh core complex (a trimer of RhAG2- RhD or RhCE) has approximately 100,000 copies per erythrocyte. These interactions are termed *vertical interactions* and are the primary reason for the extreme elasticity of the erythrocyte membrane. Both band 3 and the Rh core complex have interactions with Ankyrin (protein 2.1), but with different domains of it. Rh complex binds to the D2 domain and band 3 to the D3 and D4 domains. This may reflect a functional role, perhaps related to CO_2/HCO_3- transport.

and PE) **intracellular**. Phospholipid flippases generate this asymmetry and expend ATP in the process, confirming that the phenomenon must be of importance to the structural integrity of the cell. Plasma membranes contain considerable amounts of cholesterol, up to 25% by mass. This acts as a **membrane plasticizer** without which the plasma membrane would be too rigid at cold temperatures and erythrocytes would be unable to circulate to extremities where blood temperature is lower than 37°C.

> **Intracellular**
> Within the cellular milieu.
>
> **Membrane plasticizer**
> The presence of cholesterol in membranes, inducing the physical characteristic that they maintain their fluidity in the microcirculation by prevention of gelling in the extremities.

Functional significance of erythrocyte membrane proteins

Almost all erythrocyte membrane proteins are polymorphic and thus express blood group antigens, but there are exceptions that will be mentioned later. Here we describe the broad functional groups of proteins in the erythrocyte and, where known, any associated blood group system, and, where known, their function in erythrocytes.

Membrane transporters

- Anion exchanger (one for exchange Cl⁻/HCO₃) SLC4A1, CD233 *Diego (DI) blood group system* ISBT 010

- Ammonium transporter RhAG CD241– *Rh associated glycoprotein (RHAG) Blood group system* ISBT 034
- Possible CO_2 channel – RhD CD240D and RhCcEe CD240CE proteins – *RH blood group system* ISBT 004
- Water channel –Aquaporin 1 – *Colton (CO) blood group system* ISBT 015
- Urea transporter – UT-B, SLC14A1– *Kidd (JK) blood group system* ISBT 009
- Peptide transporter? – Kx protein – *XK Blood group system* ISBT 019
- Water and urea transporter, Aquaporin-3 – *Gill (GIL) blood group system* ISBT 029
- ATP binding cassette containing transporter ABCG2, CD338 – *Junior (JR) blood group system* ISBT 032
- ATP-binding cassette containing transporter ABCB6, - *Lan (LAN) Blood group system* ISBT 033
- Equalibrative nucleoside transporter, ENT1/SLC29A1 – *Augustine (AT) blood group system,* ISBT 036.

Erythrocyte enzymes

Huge numbers of circulating erythrocytes represent a suitable platform on which to locate an enzyme which may process biomolecules released into the peripheral circulation.

- Zinc metalloproteinase, Kell glycoprotein (processes big endothelin-3) CD238 – *Kell (KEL) blood group system* ISBT 007
- Erythrocyte acetylcholinesterase- *Cartwright (YT) blood group system* ISBT 011
- ADP ribosyltransferase (ART4) CD297–*Dombrock (DO) blood group system* ISBT 014.

Complement control proteins

Erythrocytes are highly susceptible to lysis following binding complement components; however, they have evolved sophisticated mechanisms to avoid 'bystander' events where activated complement is produced, for example sites of infection. Twenty-five per cent of our cells are erythrocytes, and they represent a huge reservoir to attenuate potentially harmful biomolecules from destruction of other cell types and tissues.

- Decay accelerating factor (DAF; CD55) – *Cromer (CROM) blood group system* ISBT 021
- Complement receptor 1 (CR1; CD35) – *Knops (KN) blood group system* ISBT 022
- Membrane inhibitor of reactive lysis (MIRL; CD59) – *CD59 blood group system* ISBT 035
- C4A and C4B of complement – *Chido/Rodgers (CH/RG) blood group system* (adsorbed onto the surface of erythrocytes from plasma) ISBT 017.

Erythrocyte adhesion molecules

Throughout their 120-day lifespan erythrocytes interact with a variety of other cell types. Mature erythrocytes lack integrins, which are widespread amongst leucocytes and platelets, but instead have a collection of cell adhesion molecules that are associated with erythropoiesis and erythrocyte turnover (**eryptosis**).

Eryptosis
The process by which senescent red cells are removed by splenic macrophages.

- Intercellular adhesion molecule 4 (ICAM-4) CD242 – *Landsteiner-Weiner (LW) blood group system* 016
- Basal cell adhesion molecule (B-CAM) CD239 – *Lutheran (LU) blood group system* ISBT 005
- Erythroid membrane associated protein (ERMAP) (CD number not assigned) – *Scianna (SC) Blood group system* ISBT 013

- CD44 – *Indian (IN) Blood group system* ISBT 023
- Extracellular matrix metalloproteinase inhibitor EMMPRIN CD147 – *OK Blood group system* ISBT 024
- Semaphorin Sema7A CD108 – *John Milton Hagen blood group system* ISBT 026
- MER2 (RAPH) CD151 – *RAPH blood group system* ISBT 025
- MIC2 and CD99 – *XG blood group system* ISBT 012
- VEL and *SMIM1* – *VEL blood group system* ISBT 034.

Receptors/signalling/structural molecules

- Glycophorin A (GPA) CD235A and glycophorin B CD235B: *MNS blood group system* ISBT 002
- Glycophorin C (GPC) CD236 and glycophorin D: *Gerbich (GE) blood group system* ISBT 020
- Duffy antigen receptor for chemokines (DARC) CD234: *Duffy (FY) blood group system* ISBT 008.

SELF-CHECK 2.2

- How does the erythrocyte survive the extreme shear stresses imposed on it during its 120-day life cycle?
- What are the major proteins of the erythrocyte membrane and its submembranous skeleton?
- Apart from O_2 and CO_2 transport what other tasks do erythrocytes serve?

Null phenotypes and non-polymorphic erythrocyte proteins

A major contribution that the study of erythrocyte antigens made to understanding the functional significance of their carrier molecules was the existence of null phenotypes. These are erythrocytes that lack all antigens of a particular system (or systems). For example, Rh_{null} erythrocytes lacks all RH, RHAG, and LW system antigens, indicating a phenotypic relationship between these genes and their protein products. Other null phenotype cells include the very common blood group O phenotype. Aside from blood group O, most null phenotypes are rare (Rh_{null}, e.g., is reported to be one in six million individuals). Many other blood group systems have null phenotypes (e.g. Kell, Gerbich) that are caused by the homozygous inheritance of mutated genes caused by a variety of genetic mutations—called *silencing mutations*. These include gene deletions, frameshift, missense, and nonsense mutations.

2.3 Blood group systems dependent on carbohydrate structures

ABO

Although there are only four antigens (A; B; A,B; and A1) in the ABO system, it is by far the most clinically significant blood group and the major cause of death due to mismatched transfusions. The main reason is because antigen-negative individuals all have *pre-formed* antibodies to A and B antigens. This is not due to pre-exposure of individuals to ABO incompatible erythrocytes, but to naturally occurring antibodies to bacterial antigens. These antigens are similar in structure to human A and B antigens so that antibodies to them (mainly of IgM subclass) cross-react,

TABLE 2.2 ABO phenotype frequencies from selected countries.

ABO phenotype	Possible genotypes	UK (2014)	USA (2011)	Japan (2012)	China (1999)	India (2014)	Australia (2016)	South Africa (2010)	Brazil (2010)	Saudi Arabia (2010)	Sweden (2007)
A	AA, AO	42%	42%	40%	28%	22.9%	38%	36%	42%	26%	44%
B	BB, BO	10%	10%	20%	19%	32.2%	10%	14%	10%	18%	12%
AB	AB	4%	4%	9.95%	5%	7.7%	3%	4%	3%	4%	6%
O	OO	44%	44%	30.05%	48%	37.2%	49%	46%	45%	52%	38%

producing severe transfusion reactions in incompatible hosts. Pre-formed antibodies are the main reason why ABO incompatibility is of prime clinical significance; all transfused blood is cross matched with a sample of recipient serum, as a final check of compatibility. Most transfusion-related deaths due to ABO incompatibility are caused by clerical errors (e.g. blood destined for transfusion into Mr Jones being transfused into the wrong Mr Jones), and cross-matching ensures the final preventative test to avoid tragedy.

The A and B antigen structures were described in the 1950s. Table 2.2 shows ABO phenotypes for certain selected countries. Biochemical studies performed by the late Sir Walter Morgan and Winifred Watkins in the UK and Elvin Kabat in the USA identified the terminal trisaccharide carbohydrate structures of the antigenic determinants of the A, B, and H structures.

ABO glycosyltransferases and synthesis of the A, B, and H structures

It was established shortly following the cloning of the A transferase gene in 1990 that polymorphisms in it were responsible for amino acid changes and frameshift mutations that cause the change in enzyme specificity to a B-transferase (galactosyltransferase) and an inactive transferase (in blood group O individuals). The A and B transferases are localized in the Golgi apparatus and they are enzymes that catalyse the transfer of monosaccharide from its nucleoside–sugar precursor to a nascent carbohydrate chain (moiety) (see Figure 2.3). The carbohydrate moieties are synthesised in a step-wise manner in the Golgi to newly synthesized lipids (glycolipids) and proteins (glycoproteins). The precursor substance that gives rise to A and B antigens is the H-substance that is synthesised by fucosyltransferase I (FUT-1). Blood group O individuals lack the A or B substance at the termini of their glycolipids and glycoproteins, only having the H substance. The H structure structure is not (normally) **immunogenic** as A, B, and AB phenotype individuals still retain a small amount of unconverted H-substance. The ends of the carbohydrate structures are immunogenic and form the blood group antigens. ABO, Hh, and Lewis system antigens are formed by such syntheses, and as such their biochemical origins share common precursors.

Molecular genetics

The ABO gene is located on chromosome 9 (position 133.25-133.28Mb), comprising seven exons (see Figure 2.4). It encodes a glycosyltransferase of 353 amino acids in length. The difference between A and B transferases is seven nucleotide changes, three silent mutations and the remainder cause four amino acid differences in the protein (Arg176Gly; Gly235Ser; Leu266Met; and Gly268Ala). Of these four, it was found by chimeric glycosyltransferases expression that only the 266 and 268 exchanges were critical for enzyme activity and substrate specificity. In blood group O phenotype individuals a mutation in the ABO gene that ablates the expression of the A,B glycosyltransferase is causative. In the first described O allele O[1], a single base deletion (G261) causes a frameshift mutation at **codon** 88 resulting in a truncated (118 amino acid

Glycosyltransferase

Golgi membrane bound enzyme that catalyses the transfer of a monosaccharide from its nucleoside derivative to a growing carbohydrate chain

Immunogenic

The likelihood that an antigen will stimulate an immunological response.

Codons

Three base pairs that code for a particular amino acid.

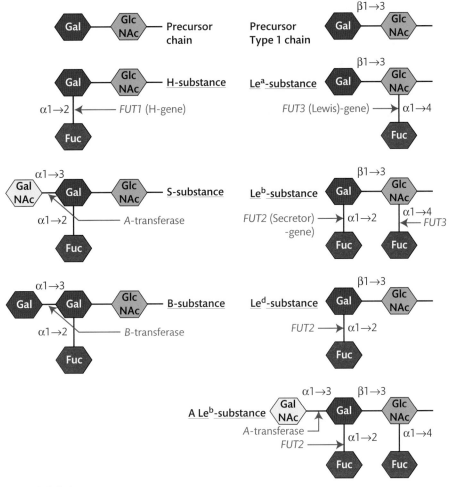

FIGURE 2.3

Structures of the ABH and Lewis blood group active glycoconjugates

Depicted are the biosynthetic precursors and ultimate products of the various glycosyltransferases involved in the synthesis of the A,B, H and Lewis antigens within the Golgi lumen. The left hand panel illustrates both the structures and key glycosyltransferases involved in the biosynthesis of A, B and H structures (involving FUT-1 and A or B transferases). The right hand panel illustrates the enzymes involved in the synthesis of the secreted ABH active glycoproteins (via the action of FUT-2) and biosynthesis of the Lewis antigens (action of FUT-3). GlcNAc=N-acetyl glucosamine; Gal=Galactose; Fuc=Fucose; GalNAc=N-acetyl galactosamine. The sugar linkages to the backbone are shown relating to the carbon atoms involved (e.g. α1-2; α1-3).

predicted), inactive transferase. Another common O allele is O^{1v}, which has the identical G261 deletion with nine further nucleotide differences between it and the derivative *A1* allele. Another common family of O alleles, previously termed O^2, has a number of mutations that differ from each other (dubbed O^2-1 to O^2-4), but all have a G802A mutation affecting codon 268 (glycine to arginine). This missense mutation, while encoding a full-length transferase, is inactive as the amino acid exchange occurs at the active site of the enzyme.

ABO variants

Variation in A, B, and O alleles of the ABO system produce (in the case of A,B) quantitative rather than qualitative variance in the numbers of A and B antigens on the surface of the erythrocyte.

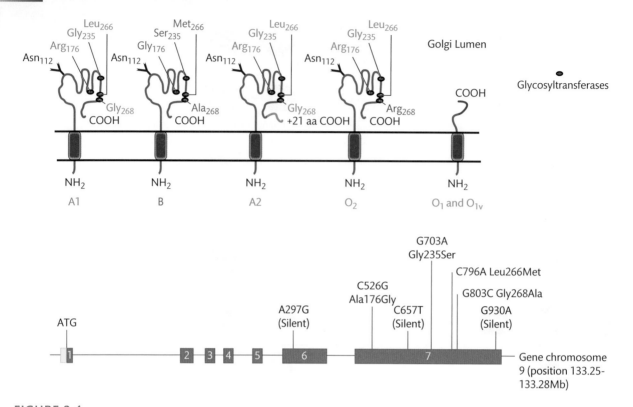

FIGURE 2.4
Cartoon structures of the various Golgi-localized glycosyltransferases.
The A and B transferases (top left) differ by four amino acid exchanges of which only Leu266Met and Gly268Ala are critical for substrate specificity. The A2 transferase differs from A1 in having a larger 21 amino acid C-terminal tail, caused by a frameshift mutation. Three representative inactive O-transferases are shown, O2, O1, and O1v. O2 has a missense mutation Gly268Arg at the active site of the enzyme abolishing its activity, whereas O1 and O1v have a frameshift mutation predicting a truncated 118 amino acid transferase, with no catalytic site. The lower panel depicts the gene structure, located on chromosome 9q34.2, which comprises seven exons, and the positions of the blood group-specific mutations are highlighted within exons 6 and 7.

The most common (approximately 10% of A+ individuals) is A2, which is caused by a deletion at nucleotide position C1061 resulting in a A2 glycosyltransferase that has a C-terminal tail 21 amino acids longer. This change is thought to alter the processing capacity of the enzyme leading to less A antigen production in erythroid cells. Other A2 alleles have been described, which include missense mutations (e.g. Arg352Trp), which will have a similar impact on A transferase activity producing quantitatively fewer erythrocyte A antigens. Over 200 different ABO alleles also cause weakening of expression either A or B antigens (A_{weak} and B_{weak}) and the interested reader is referred to the Blood Group Antigens Factsbook (Reid, Lomas-Francis & Olsson, 2012) or the BGMut database (see Further Reading).

Other carbohydrate-dependent blood group systems interacting with ABO

A complex interplay between multiple glycosyltransferases in cells of different lineages generate a variety of blood group active substances, including those with ABH activity. It is important to appreciate that there are a number of different precursor saccharide structures that can be processed, and found in different tissues. As can be seen from the following list, these precursors differ in the sequences of sugar monosaccharide connected to the carrier molecule and also different carbon atoms of the glycosidic bond.

Terminal disaccharide structures of the various precursor substances:

Type 1: Galβ1→3GlcNAcβ1→R (present in secretions, plasma, and endodermal tissue)

Type 2: Galβ1→4GlcNAcβ1→R (present on ectodermal and mesodermal tissues, major erythrocyte ABH active structures)

Type 3: Galβ1→3GalNAcα1→R (mucins, both erythrocytic and secreted)

Type 4: Galβ1→3GalNAcβ1→R (globo-A and globo-H glycolipids in small quantities on erythrocytes)

Type 5: Galβ1→3Galβ1→R (not found in humans, only chemically synthesized)

Type 6: Galβ1→4Glcβ1→R (secretions in milk and urine)

The addition of either *N*-acetylgalactosamine or galactose to the terminal disaccharide of a nascent carbohydrate chain forms the A or B antigens, respectively. Monosaccharides are added in a stepwise manner to this nascent chain by the sequential action of other glycosyl-transferases in the Golgi apparatus. The ABH antigens derived from ceramide derivatives can be tracked by analysis of Figure 2.5 later in this chapter.

H (FUT-1, ISBT 018) The H antigen is formed by the addition of L-fucose linked α1,2 to the penultimate sugar; in ABH active substances this is galactose (linked β1-3). The gene responsible for the synthesis of the H antigen is the erythroid *FUT-1* gene. In non-erythroid cells (ecto-dermal lineage) another fucosyltransferase, FUT-2, has identical activity and is responsible for the presence of ABH-active substances in secretions, and is also known as the secretor gene or Se. The H antigen remains present on the surface of all erythrocytes, regardless of ABO phenotype, as previously mentioned. Thus, anti-H is rare and is only found where *FUT1* genes are mutated and are unable to produce H antigen, producing the *Bombay phenotype*. The production of anti-H therefore warrants its own blood group system, H (ISBT 018). Secretor-negative individuals have mutations in Se (*FUT2*).

Lewis antigens (ISBT 007) are synthesized by the sequential actions of fucosyltransferases. FUT-3 is the Lewis gene, and catalyses the transfer of fucose α1-4 to *N*-acetylglucosamine (see Figure 2.3). The Le^a antigen is formed by this synthesis, and if the FUT2 (secretor) gene is active then an addition fucose is linked α1,2 to the terminal galactose residue. A or B active Lewis antigens (A-Le^b; B-Le^b) are then formed by the activity of the A or B transferases, respectively.

Other carbohydrate-dependent blood group systems

I blood group system ISBT 0027

The I blood group antigen is generated by the action of a β1-6 *N*-acetylglucosaminyltransferase (IGnT), which produces branches in glycan chains. Small i-active glycans lack branched oli-gosaccharide moieties. During fetal development, the i-active carbohydrate chains predominate, and the I antigen is produced during adult life and full expression is reached after 18 months. The defined molecular basis of the rare I$_{null}$ phenotype, where i expression continues throughout adult life and results in the resolution of the genetic origins of I/i. Missense mutations and a genomic deletion in the IGNT (*GCNT2*) gene is causative of the adult i-phenotype. IGNT became the twenty-seventh blood group system in 2002.

P1PK (ISBT 003); Globoside (GLOB, ISBT 028); Forssman (FORS, ISBT 031)

These three blood groups can be considered together as the antigens within these systems derive from common precursors. Ceramide (made up of sphingosine and a fatty acid) forms the ultimate precursor, and actions of various glycosyltransferases lead to the formation of glycolipids in the erythrocyte membrane that carry antigens, including ABH. Figure 2.5 depicts a simplified diagram of the biosynthesis and active glycosyltransferases that give rise to the antigens of these three systems and are analogous to the actions of FUT1, FUT2, FUT3, and the A & B glycosyltransferases shown in Figure 2.3.

The actions of A4GALT, a 4-α-galactosyltransferase, add galactose to the glycosylated ceramide precursors lactosylceramide and paragloboside, respectively, to form the P^k and P1 antigens. Defects leading to the inactivation of A4GALT are classed as null phenotypes (p phenotype) of which 29 mutant alleles have been described. A mutation Gln211Glu alters the

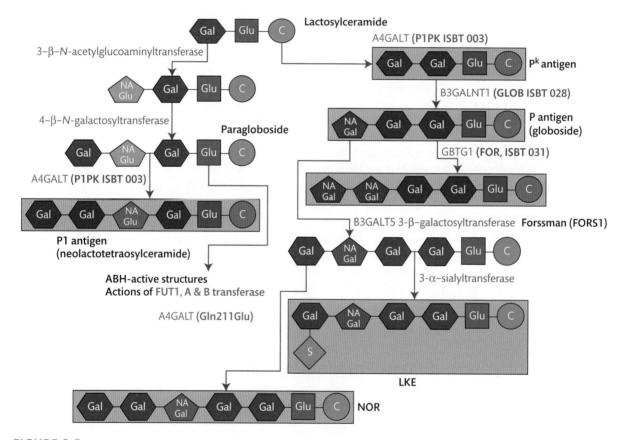

FIGURE 2.5
Simplified diagram illustrating the biosynthesis of the glycolipid antigens, P1, P^K, P, and Forssman (FORS1), and key involved glycosyltransferases.
All antigenic glycolipids are derived from the common precursor ceramide (labelled C). The sequential action of numerous glycosyltransferases then give rise to the various blood group active substances, the structures of which are shown (in shaded boxes). Each carbohydrate is shown by a different shape (Glu = Glucose; Gal = Galactose; NAGlu = N-acetylglucosamine; NAGal = N-acetylgalactosamine; S = sialic acid). The key transferases for each of the three blood group systems are shown in red. Paragloboside can serve as a substrate for FUT1 and the A and B transferases to give rise to blood group active glycolipids. Adapted from Reid, Lomas-Francis and Olsson, 2012.

substrate specificity of A4GALT converting the P substance by adding a galactose and forming the NOR antigen. The Pk antigen serves as a substrate for the B3GALNT1 transferase (a 3-β-N-acetylgalactosaminyltransferase), which adds a N-acetylgalactosamine to the terminus giving rise to the P antigen (the sole antigen of the GLOB, ISBT 028 system). Silencing mutations of B3GALNT1 abolish expression of P. The P antigen in turns serves as substrate for the A3GALN1 transferase (a 3-α-N-acetylgalactosaminyltransferase), which transfers N-acetylgalactosamine (linked α1-3) to the terminus and creates the Forssman (FORS1) antigen. Inactivating mutations of A3GALN1 causes FORS1 phenotypes.

Key points

- ABO is the most clinically significant blood group system due to the existence of preformed antibodies.
- Carbohydrate antigens depend on the sequences of oligosaccharides synthesized in the Golgi.
- Alleles of carbohydrate antigens are caused by mutations in glycosyltransferases that synthesize them in the Golgi.

2.4 Blood group systems dependent on protein structures

Rh blood group system (ISBT 004)

Rh was first described in 1939 by Levine and Stetson when they found an antiserum from a pregnant mother who had delivered a stillborn infant that had died from haemolytic disease of the fetus and newborn (HDFN). It agglutinated 80% of random samples from the New York blood bank. It was later surmised (incorrectly) that the human serum reacted identically to a guinea pig serum that had been raised to *Macacus rhesus* erythrocytes. The term anti-Rh (for Rhesus) was then coined throughout the 1940s based on this observation. It later transpired that Levine's guinea pig serum reacted against LW blood group antigens, which has a phenotypic relationship with RhD in that the LW glycoprotein (ICAM-4) is expressed less on RhD negative erythrocytes. Therefore, Rh is a classic misnomer, and when this was realized it was decided that renaming would be too challenging with the growing number of publications on this critical blood group system.

Rh antigen classification

The Rh system is generally classified using the CDE (Fisher-Race) nomenclature or a shorthand version where R denotes the presence of the D antigen or its absence. In the USA the CDE nomenclature is replaced by DCE to reflect gene order, strictly more correct as the Fisher-Race system predicted (incorrectly) that there were three *RH* genes, C, D, and E. The common Rh haplotypes are shown in Table 2.3

The proteins involved: Rh molecular era

The Rh molecular era arrived in the late 1980s/early 1990s with the identification, purification, and cloning of the Rh polypeptides and the Rh-associated glycoprotein (RhAG), with key

TABLE 2.3 The classification of the common Rh antigens Rh, CcEe, and D.

D-positive haplotypes		Phenotype	Notes
Fisher-Race	Wiener notation		
Cde	R_1	C+c-D+E-e+	Most common D+ haplotype in Europeans
cDE	R_2	C-c+D+E+e-	Greatest D antigen site density in common D+ haplotypes
cDe	R_0	C-c+D+E-e+	Most common D+ haplotype in Africans
CDE	R_Z	C+c-D+E+e-	Rare
-D-	-	C-c-D+E-e-	Very rare, elevated D antigen sites
D-negative haplotypes			
cde	r	C-c+D-E-e+	Most common D-negative haplotype in Europeans and Africans
Cde	r'	C+c-D-E-e+	Most common in South East Asians
cdE	r''	C-c+D-E+e-	
CdE	r^Y	C+c-D-E+e-	Rare

research papers describing this work appearing between 1990 and 1992. The author of this chapter was fortunate to be personally involved in this work during his PhD studies at the University of Bristol. This and subsequent work revealed that Rh proteins are an ancient transport protein species found both in erythrocytes and other tissues in higher vertebrates and all species on the planet. All Rh proteins and related plant Mep/Amt ammonium transporters have a conserved 'ammonium transporter fold'. They span the membrane bilayer multiple times, but vary in number—the human Rh proteins span the membrane 12 times and *Escherichia coli* ammonium transporter AmtB 11 times. Humans have five different Rh proteins, the blood group active proteins Rh, CcEe, and D, and three, Rh-associated proteins, named RhAG, RhBG, and RhCG. The latter two protein species are beyond the scope of this chapter; however, they are widely expressed in other tissues, namely the sex organs, kidney, brain, liver, and others. The erythrocyte protein RhAG is critical for assembly of what is termed the erythroid *Rh core complex*. This complex comprises a trimer of proteins—two RhAG molecules associated with one Rh protein, either RhCcEe or D (Figure 2.6). RhAG is known to be critical as Rh-deficient individuals (known as **Rh$_{null}$ phenotype**) have missense and nonsense mutations in the *RHAG* gene and express no Rh antigens whatsoever. Rh$_{null}$ cells indicate that the Rh core complex has a structural and transport role in the mature erythrocyte as these cells are stomatocytic, and have defective cation co-transport activity. In fact, there are other mutations in *RHAG* that are less catastrophic and result in blood group antigen expression on the molecule—gaining the recognition of its own blood group system RHAG (ISBT 030).

Rh$_{null}$ (regulator type)

The null phenotype of the RH system, with red cells expressing no Rh or LW antigens, and have a defect in the Rh-associated glycoprotein gene *RHAG*.

The D antigen

D is the most immunogenic antigen of the Rh system. It is the major cause of Rh HDFN, and of transfusion reactions in D-incompatible blood transfusions. The culprit is the absence of the RhD protein

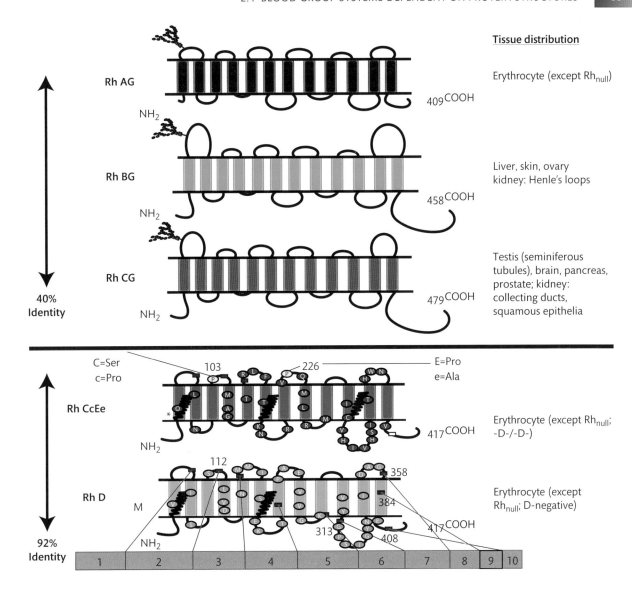

FIGURE 2.6

The two-dimensional structures of the human erythroid and non-erythroid Rh proteins.

In the top panel the erythroid, blood group active RhAG (Rh-associated glycoprotein) and non-erythroid RhBG and RhCG proteins are shown. All have 12 membrane-spanning segments and cytoplasmically localized N-and C-termini. The sequences of all three of these proteins is highly conserved (~40%), and they possess the *ammonium transport fold*, which is a conserved membrane domain. The bottom panel illustrates the blood group active Rh proteins, RhD and RhCcEe, and shows the amino acid (35 or 36 depending on RhCE status) changes between RhD and RhCcEe. The critical amino acids for Rh C/c (Ser103Pro) and Rh E/e (Pro226Ala) are highlighted in yellow. The figure also shows the segments of the proteins encoded by each respective exon—all RH genes have a similar structure comprising 10 exons. **Palmitoylation** sites (3 in RhCcEe; 2 in RhD) are shown as black zig-zag lines and are located at the boundary of the inner phospholipid leaflet.

from the surface of erythrocytes on D-negative individuals, and exposure of D-positive erythrocytes from feto-maternal transfer or transfusion induces the immune response to the D antigen. As the molecular basis is the absence of the RhD protein, almost any structural difference between it and the closely related RhCcEe protein can elicit such an immune response. As the humoral immune response results in the generation of antibodies, the polyclonal anti-D response includes many anti-bodies that react with different externalized regions of the RhD protein, which are referred to as **D epitopes (epD)**. There are only nine amino acid differences between the RhD and RhCcEe proteins and lie in regions of the RhD protein that are accessible to anti-D, yet there are known to be over 50 different specificity monoclonal anti-D, which recognize distinct (but in most cases overlapping) epitopes. In partial D and some weak D phenotypes some of these epitopes are missing due to mutations affecting the configuration of these external regions of the molecule—these are discussed in more detail shortly.

One of the almost unique features of erythrocyte Rh proteins is that their external regions are not glycosylated, giving less steric hindrance to D epitopes being more accessible to antibodies and B-cell-bound antibody receptors. Three-dimensional modeling of the RhD protein suggests that regions located deep within the membrane bilayer are accessible to antibodies and B cells (Figure 2.7). This structure has been termed the *RhD* **antigenic vestibule** which is a rather open structure analogous to the cone of a volcano (on a molecular scale!). Although immunoglobulins are large molecules (in comparison to erythrocyte membrane antigens), they only make contact at the very tip of their Fab region (the hypervariable regions), termed the **paratope**. The structures to which the paratope binds is known as its corresponding epitope.

RH genetics

At the turn of the millennium the structure of the RH locus was finally resolved, and settled a near 40-year controversy as to the numbers of RH genes and their arrangement on chromosome 1. A fierce controversy raged throughout the 1960s as to whether there were three RH genes (C, D, and E) or two (D and CE). The two-gene theory was correct, but interestingly the *RHD* gene is arranged in a tail-to-tail configuration to the closely related (96% sequence homology) *RHCE* gene (see Figure 2.8). Both genes comprise 10 exons and this strange tail-to-tail configuration may explain the relatively common occurrence of hybrid *RHD–RHCE* genes that have been known to cause Rh-variant and RHD-negative phenotypes.

Simultaneously with the determination of the structure of the RH complex, the molecular basis of the common 'deletion-type' RHD-negative genotype was defined. It had been known since 1991 that the prevalent D-negative phenotype in Europeans was caused by a complete

---

Epitope

The specific region on an antigen that the immunoglobulin binds via its paratope. Also known as an *antigenic determinant.*

Antigenic vestibule (RhD)

The open domain of the RhD protein responsible for expression of all D epitopes.

Paratope

The epitope binding region of the immunoglobulin molecule.

FIGURE 2.7

The predicted structure of the trimeric Rh core complex.
Based on predictive models based on the related *E. coli* AmtB and human RhCG crystal structures, the membrane configuration of RhAG, RhD, and RhCcEe have been predicted. The molecules are shown in plan view, viewing perpendicular to the plane of the erythrocyte membrane. The dimension of each monomer is approximately 46 Ångström in diameter, and the trimer is arranged in a cloverleaf structure and comprises two molecules of RhAG and one either RhD or RhCcEe. Locations of epitope critical amino acids located on external loop 4 (shown as red residues) or loop 6 (shown in purple) illustrate the accessibility of each loop, and the fact that the centre of both RhD and RhCcEe proteins have externalized loops that penetrate the membrane at some depth—known as the *antigenic vestibule*. Adapted from Conroy MJ, Bullough PA, Merrick M, Avent ND (2005) Modelling the human rhesus proteins: Implications for structure and function. British Journal of Haematology 131: 543-551. Reproduced with permission from John Wiley & Sons.

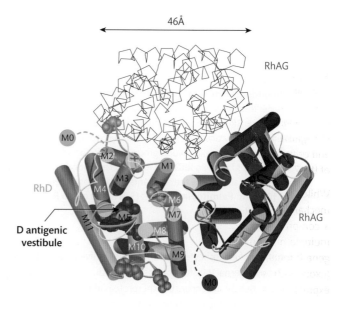

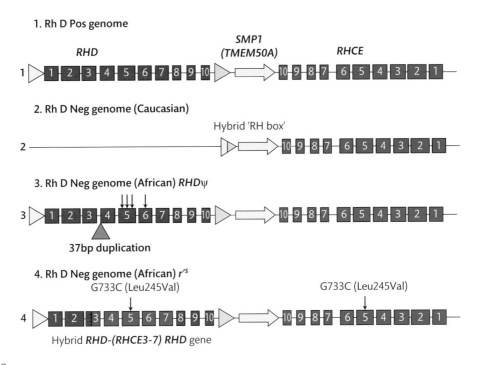

FIGURE 2.8

The genomic structure of the blood group active *RH* genes in D-positive and D-negative individuals.
1. The RH gene complex is located on chromosome 1p36.11; both *RHD* and *RHCE* genes are comprise 10 exons. *RHCE* is positioned in reverse orientation to *RHD*, and the pair of genes has an additional gene of unknown function (*SMP*1 or *TMEM50A*) but predicts a transmembrane protein. The *RHD* gene is flanked by two homologous repeat sequences of 20 kb in size, dubbed upstream and downstream Rhesus boxes. 2. It is likely that a gene deletion event, caused by unequal crossover between the Rhesus boxes, generated the 'deletion type' D-negative haplotype prevalent in European and African populations. The crossover event is evidenced by the fact that a hybrid Rhesus box is present in D-negative haplotypes of this type. 3. In African populations, at least two further mutated RHD genes cause D-negative phenotypes. RHDψ is a pseudogene of high prevalence, and found within a normal cde haplotype. RHDψ has a 37 bp duplication, three missense mutations in exon 5, and a nonsense mutation in exon 6. Consequently, It does not express any valid product. 4. A further high-prevalence haplotype is Cde^s (r's) found in individuals with African ancestry. The haplotype expresses a weakened C antigen and partial c and e antigens, although it is D negative. It is associated with expression of the V and VS antigens. A hybrid *RHD-RHCE-RHD* gene is responsible for expression of the weakened C antigens, and both the hybrid and ce gene encode Val245, the residue critical for V and VS antigen expression.

RHD gene deletion. This is, indeed, the case, but two highly homologous 7 kb segments of DNA that flank the *RHD* gene, termed **Rhesus boxes**, appear are evidence that the *RHD* gene was deleted owing to an unequal crossover event in D-negative (deletion) genotypes. The flanking Rhesus boxes (dubbed upstream and downstream boxes) are replaced in deletion type D-negative genomes with a hybrid Rhesus box, comprising the 5′ end of the upstream and 3′ end of the downstream box. It would appear that an unequal crossover event involving both of the 7 kb Rhesus boxes resulted in the deletion of the *RHD* gene from D-negative genomes.

While the 'RHD deletion type' D-negative genotype is the most prevalent, different genetic mechanisms have emerged. Two of the most common in Africans are a pseudogene, *RHD*ψ, a compromised *RHD* gene (containing a 37 bp insertion inducing a frameshift mutation, multiple missense and a nonsense mutation). Furthermore a common hybrid *RHD–RHCE* gene is found, named Ce^s (r's), where part of the *RHD* gene is replaced by *RHCE* equivalents (exons 3–7) (see Figure 2.7). Serologically D-negative individuals that inherit *RHD*ψ or Ce^s express no D epitopes whatsoever.

> **Rhesus box**
>
> Repeated 9 kb DNA sequences that flank the *RHD* gene in D-positive individuals. The *RHD* deletion type D-negative genotype results in a hybrid Rhesus box where crossover that generated the deletion produces a hybrid *Rhesus box*.

Rh CcEe antigens

The Rh C/c and E/e blood group polymorphisms are simple amino acid changes on the surface of the Rh CcEe protein, this directly inferring that these residues are active components of the C/c and E/e antigens. Rh C/c involves a Ser103Pro change and Rh E/e a Pro226Ala change. Three other amino acids were originally implicated in C/c antigenicity (Cys16Trp; Ile60Leu; and Ser68Asn); however, these exchanges are not completely conserved. The three dimensional configuration of the Rh CcEe protein is such that residues 103 and 226 (located on the second and fourth **exoloops**, respectively—(the cytoplasmic localized loops and termed **endoloops**) are located physically close, and readily explain 'compound' Rh antigens (e.g. those that bind anti-Rh Ce, cE, ce (also known as anti-f)).

Other Rh system antigens are located exclusively on the Rh CcEe polypeptide. Two low-frequency antigens, C^X (RH9, ISBT 004009) and C^W (RH8, ISBT 004008), which have frequencies within the Caucasian population of 0.01% and 2%, respectively, are caused by *RHCE* mutations causing amino acid exchanges in the RhCE protein (C^X = Ala36Thr, C^W = Gln41Arg). In Africans, the common cde^s phenotype i carries the Rh antigens VS and V and partial c and e phenotypes. VS and V are caused by a C733G mutation of exon 5 altering amino acid Leu245Val. Often the cde^s haplotype is inherited with a hybrid *RHD–RHCE–RHD* gene comprising exons 1-(5'portion)3 *RHD*, (3' portion) 3–7 *RHCE*, and *RHD* 8–10 (Figure 2.8), where exon 5 of this hybrid gene also encodes the V/VS mutation G733. Because exon 2 of this hybrid gene is *RHD* derived, and identical in sequence to *RHC* exon 2, the hybrid gene expresses a partial C phenotype. Where this hybrid exists the entire gene complex is termed Cde^s (or r's). In another complex turn of events, an exon 7 mutation in both the hybrid gene and the cde^s gene, G1006T (Gly336Cys) either abolishes the V antigen or results in it being expressed in weakened form, but has no effect on the VS antigen. Such complexities of the Rh system are common in individuals of African descent, and make matching of blood for patients with sickle cell disease a significant challenge.

Other Rh antigens—Rh variants

Partial and weak D phenotypes (see Daniels, 2013) Partial D phenotypes are operationally defined in that the erythrocytes react positively with some monoclonal anti-D, but fail to react with others. Strictly, partial D phenotype individuals were classified on their ability to make anti-D. Weak D individuals by definition have only a weakening of some (or all) D epitopes but lack none and do not make anti-D. There has been debate in the literature as to whether the terms weak D and partial D should be simply renamed as variants rather than two different subclasses. However, the terms weak and partial D have some meaning. Weak D has traditionally been regarded as a simple reduction in the levels of D antigen site density on erythrocytes leading to problems in the serological typing of these individuals as blood donors, but these individuals do not normally make anti-D when exposed to normal D-positive erythrocytes. Partial D could have severe consequences if these individuals are typed as D-positive and they receive normal D-positive erythrocytes during transfusion or carry a normal D-positive child during pregnancy (see Chapter 3). These definitions have proved problematic, as some individuals classified as weak D have, in fact, made anti-D. These have included weak D types 1, 2, 4.2.2, and 15, whereas there is controversy that some of these anti-D maybe autoantibodies, or perhaps these individuals lack some D epitopes, the classic definition of a partial D.

Very weak D (D-elute) To complicate issues yet further, there is another D variant class. Known initially as 'D-elute', based on the ability to be only able to detect anti-D binding by complex adsorption/elution serological testing, these erythrocytes have barely detectable D antigen. D elute is caused by various mutations in the *RHD* gene and are common in Asians, especially of Chinese ancestry.

Endoloop

A cytoplasmic localized loop structure of a **polytopic** membrane protein.

Exoloop

An externally localized loop domain of a membrane protein.

Genetic basis of Rh variants There are over 300 catalogued D variants, and for a comprehensive list the reader is referred to the Rhesus base resource (see Further Reading) maintained by Dr Franz Wagner (Springe Blood Centre, Germany). A comprehensive review of the variants could fill this entire chapter, suffice to say that hybrid *RHD–RHCE–RHD* genes (analogous to the situation that creates the r^s **haplotype** seen in Figure 2.8), point mutations causing missense, mutations and premature termination codons form D variants. These mutations may have a profound effect on D antigenicity, ablating a large number of D epitopes, or may have little or no discernable difference to the wild-type RhD protein having almost normal D epitope expression. This massive variation in D antigenicity (site density) has been termed the RhD continuum (Figure 2.9), and reflects the fact that homozygous expression of *RHD* results in greater site densities (R_2R_2 approximately 30,000 sites, R_1R_1 approximately 16,000 sites).

In some instances, and in common with the MNS blood group system, the same Rh antigen can be detected on erythrocytes of partial D phenotypes with different genetic backgrounds. Examples are illustrated in Figure 2.10. In all of these unusual Rh variants, the hybrid RHD–RHCE proteins generate structures that are novel to the immune system in incompatible individuals. These antigenic structures involve the close approach of one exofacial domain derived from the *RHD* gene with one derived from *RHCE*. Molecular modelling suggests that exofacial loops 3 and 4 of the Rh proteins are of sufficient distances from one another to be able to form **discontinuous epitopes**. The FPTT antigen (Rh50) is expressed on all subtypes of the partial D phenotype DFR, which possesses a hybrid *RHD–RHCE–RHD* gene whereby all or part of exon 4

> **Haplotypes**
> Linked genes, the alleles contributed from one or the other parent, in a blood group system that are passed on together.

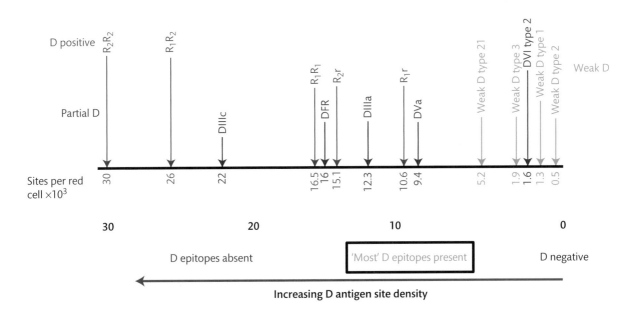

FIGURE 2.9

The RhD continuum of D antigen density.

This depicts the huge range in D antigen site densities of various D-positive (red), partial D (blue), and weak D (green) phenotype erythrocytes. The homozygous expression of D, as would be expected, shows increased expression; however, one partial D (DIIIc) shows expression levels even higher than homozygous R_1R_1 cells. Partial D shows a huge range in D antigen density, and selected examples are shown; the y-axis depicts site numbers in thousands. Weak D site densities are normally less than 1000 per erythrocyte, but the exception is weak D type 21. D-elute erythrocytes, with barely detectable D antigens (>100 sites per cell), are omitted for clarity. 'Super D' phenotype erythrocytes (-D-) are essentially where the *RHCE* gene is replaced by another *RHD* gene. Homozygous expression (-D-/-D-) results in highly elevated D antigen sites, 200,000 per erythrocyte.

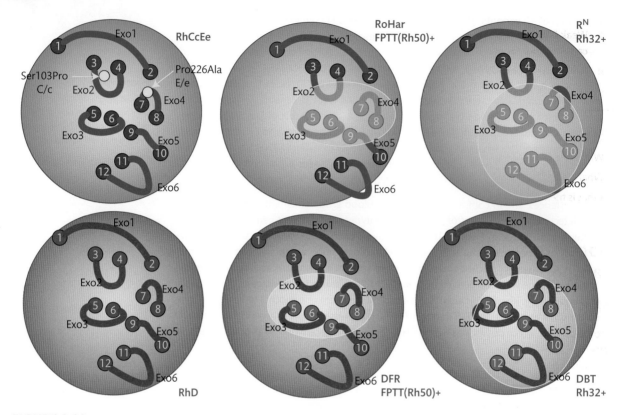

FIGURE 2.10

Low-frequency RH antigens expressed on D variants—discontinuous epitope structural basis.

Certain Rh system antigens can be detected on erythrocytes that have been obtained from individuals with different Rh genetic backgrounds. Examples of these antigens include RH50 (FPTT) found on DFR and R_oHar phenotype erythrocytes; RH32 found on R^N and DBT variant erythrocytes and also (not shown) the Evans (RH37) antigen found on both D (a –D– like gene rearrangement with essentially two copies of *RHD* per haplotype) and DIVb variant erythrocytes. Analysis of the predicted structure of the result hybrid molecules reveals close approaches of both RHD-derived (depicted in red) and *RHCE*-derived (in blue) exofacial loops (numbered exo1–exo6), close enough to form a discontinuous epitope. The figure shows the close approach of these hybrid loop structures as a yellow-shaded circle. The positions of the exofacial loops are derived from the published predicted structures of both RhD and RhCcEe proteins. A **continuous epitope** is dependent on just one region of a protein and may be independent of tertiary structure.

is replaced by *RHCE* equivalents. Exon 4 of both Rh proteins encodes epitope critical amino acids required for expression of loop 3 of Rh proteins, whilst exon 5 encodes those required for exofacial loop 4. In the *RHCE* variant Ro_{Har} there is a very different genetic background; here a *RHCE.ce* gene has exon 5 replaced by a *RHD* equivalent, and as a result expresses only limited numbers of D epitopes at low site density.

Key points

- D-positive individuals express all D epitopes, and have varying levels of RhD protein based on Rh genotype $-D-<R_2<R_1/R_O$.

- Partial D lack D epitopes and consequently such individuals, when exposed to normal D-positive blood through transfusion or pregnancy, can become alloimmunized.

- Weak D individuals have difficult-to-detect D antigen, although most routine anti-D can—they do not normally produce anti-D.
- D-elute have ultra depressed levels of D antigens.
- D-negative individuals lack the RhD protein and thus all D epitopes.

SELF-CHECK 2.3

- Why is the D antigen so immunogenic?
- What drives the huge variability in RH genetics?
- What is the operational definition of partial and weak D and D-elute?

Blood group antigens on other erythrocyte transporter molecules

Kidd (JK) blood group system (ISBT 009)

Incompatibility for the Jk^a antigen is a leading cause of delayed haemolytic transfusion reactions. The JK blood group antigens (Jk^a, Jk^b, and Jk3) are expressed on the erythrocyte urea transporter UT-B (synonym SLC14A1) and its gene, *SLC14A1*, is located on chromosome 18.

The molecular basis of the JK (Kidd) antigens was resolved in 1997, but the involvement of the JK protein in urea transport was known for three decades, when Jk_{null} (Jk(a-b-)) erythrocytes were shown to resist haemolysis in 2M urea. Jk^a, Jk^b, and Jk3 antigens are carried by the erythrocyte urea transporter SLC14A1 with the *JK*A* and *JK*B* alleles being caused by a **single nucleotide polymorphism (SNP)** at codon 280 (Asp→Asn).

SLC14A1 on erythrocytes permits them to lose urea rapidly as they negotiate the ascending vasa recta, which has a very high local concentration of urea. This minimizes the loss of urea from the renal medulla, and allows the concentration of urea in urine. The initial correlation of the Kidd blood group antigen carrier as a possible urea transporter resulted in experiments that examined urine concentrating ability in Jk_{null} (Jk(a-b-)) individuals who showed reduction in this process. SLC14A1 is expressed on endothelial cells lining the descending vasa recta and erythrocytes (defined by immunocytochemistry), and within kidney, bladder, prostate, testis, brain, and thymus. The urea transporter within kidney is found within the inner medullary collecting ducts, and is a different molecular species to SLC14A1. Studies using UT-B (the murine equivalent of SLC14A1) knockout mice has confirmed that the erythrocyte urea transporter contributes to the urea concentrating mechanism, as urine urea concentration in UT-B knockout mice was 35% lower. Evidence gleaned from studies of double-knockout (UT-B and AQP1) mice has suggested that UT-B is capable of water transport. These mice had defective urine concentrating ability, and decreased survival rates and growth, but had normal erythrocyte morphology. It is possible therefore that the erythroid urea transporter maintains an aqueous pore through which urea passes.

Jk_{null} (Jk(a-b-)) individuals are extremely rare, but found in Finnish, Polynesian, and South American populations. Several genetic mechanisms have been described that generate Jk(a-b-) phenotypes. In Polynesians, splice site mutations that causes exon 6 and exon 7 skipping has been found, whereas in Finnish people a T871C SNP disrupts an N-glycosylation motif Ser291Pro (NSS→NSP). Further, Jk(a-b-) alleles have been subsequently described and are listed in the BGMut database.

Single nucleotide polymorphism (SNP)
A single nucleotide substitution in the DNA reading frame that encodes a particular inherited characteristic.

Diego and band 3 SLC4A1 (ISBT 010)

Diego system antigens are carried by the aforementioned band 3 glycoprotein SLC4A1. Almost all of the 22 Di system antigens are low frequency, with the exception of Di^b, Wr^b, and DISK. Di(a+) individuals are rare amongst most ethnic groups, but among South American indigenous peoples up to 36% are Di (a+), and in Asians up to 10% are. As a consequence of Di^a incompatibility, HDFN can occur due to anti-Di^a. Almost all Di(a+) individuals have the *Memphis variant* of band 3. This is caused by a Lys56Glu amino acid change due to a mutated *SLC4A1* gene altering its apparent molecular weight during gel electrophoresis. The role of band 3 in maintaining erythrocyte shape and anion exchange has been discussed earlier in this chapter; however, here we consider one important variant of it that occurs in South East Asia: South Asian **ovalocytosis** (SAO). SAO is a hereditary condition, relatively frequent in the Southern Pacific, and confers resistance to cerebral malaria. SAO is caused by a 27-bp deletion in the *SLC4A1* gene, resulting in a deletion of nine amino acids at the junction of the proteins N-terminal and membrane domains. This results in a less flexible 'hinge', causing the ovalocytosis. This mutation has no effect on Di antigens, but nevertheless illustrates the power of Malaria in driving evolution. SAO erythrocytes have a shortened circulation half-life, but the selective advantage of conferring resistance to severe malaria has driven its stability in the South Asian population.

Colton (ISBT 015)

Colton system antigens are carried by the erythrocyte water transporter aquaporin 1 (AQP-1). AQP-1 was the first human membrane protein to be crystallized, and has given incredible insight into how a transporter selectively transports water across cell membranes. This is a crucial function for erythrocytes as they are exposed to variations in osmotic pressure (e.g. the kidney). AQP-1 has a classic 'hourglass' constrictional pore within its membrane domain of 3 Ångströms in diameter, slightly larger than the diameter of the water molecule (2.8 öngströms). This high degree of selectivity allows the single-file transit of H_2O, and nothing else, for example the hydroxonium ion H_3O- is excluded. AQP-1 is arranged in a tetrameric configuration in erythrocyte membranes. For many years it had been known that a null phenotype of the Colton system existed, Co(a-b-) or Co_{null}, and initially when Colton antigens were assigned to AQP-1, the complete absence of AQP-1 from their membranes was a puzzle, especially as AQP-1 is also expressed in the kidney (proximal tubule and thin descending loop of Henle) and pulmonary vascular endothelium, indicating an important role in the lungs. As it turned out, another water transporter, AQP-3 (carrier of the GIL blood group antigens), is present in erythrocyte membranes and can compensate for the absence of AQP-1. Co_{null} individuals have no change in airway wall thickness when infused with 3 litres of saline (in contrast controls had a 40% increase in thickness, indicating the onset of peribronchial oedema). In the kidney, AQP-1 deficiency contributes to the inability to concentrate urine.

The four Colton system antigens, Co^a, Co^b, Co3, and Co4, are high frequency with the exception of Co^b, which is present in about 10% of populations worldwide. The Co^a/Co^b polymorphism is associated with a C134T mutation in the *AQP1* gene, resulting in Ala45Val, which is localized to the first external loop of the protein. Co_{null} individuals all lack the Co3 antigen, and all CO system antigens, which are caused by the homozygous or compound heterozygote inheritance of a mutated *AQP1* gene. Examples include a deletion of part of exon 1; 307insT (Gly104 frameshift and premature stop codon mutation); C576A Asn192Lys; 232delG Ala78 frameshift and premature stop; C113T Pro38Ser and 601delG Val201Stop. Interestingly, one mutation, A140G (Gln47Arg), abolishes expression of the Co^a antigen (conferred on a *CO*A* (*CO*01*) allele but not the Co3 antigen). Homozygote individuals for this mutant allele make a novel CO alloantibody, termed Co4.

GIL Gill Blood group system (ISBT 029)

A single antigen of this system GIL is expressed almost universally, and a GIL–individual has a mutated *AQP3* gene resulting in exon 5 skipping and a subsequent stop codon. The aquaglycerporin aquaporin-3 is absent from the erythrocyte membrane. AQP-3 is a member of the aquaporin family, but unlike AQP-1 is able to transport small biomolecules such as glycerol and urea in addition to water. Of five patients with anti-GIL, there may have been possible haemolytic transfusion reactions and mild HDFN. GIL was classified as a blood group system in 2002.

Junior (JR) and Lan (LAN) (ISBT 032 and ISBT 033)

Both Junior and Lan (short for Langereis) are carried by ABC-(ATP-binding cassette) containing transporters ABCG2 and ABCB6. Both proteins have a wide tissue distribution; ABCG2 may be of particular importance in the placenta. All Jr(a–) and Lan–individuals are homozygous for *ABCG2* and *ABCB6* genes that have silencing mutations.

Augustine (AUG) ISBT 036

Since the 1960s At(a–) individuals have been known, but it is only recently (2015) that the molecular background of the At^a antigen and a null phenotype have been described. Anti-At^a has caused severe haemolytic transfusion reactions and mild HDFN. At(a–) individuals have a mutation in the *ENT1* gene (*SLC29A1*), which encodes the equalibrative nucleoside transporter ENT1. The mutation Glu391Lys is located on the fifth external loop of the protein, which has 11 transmembrane domains, a cytoplasmic N-terminus, and an extracellular C-terminus. All known individuals that have produced allo anti-At^a have African ancestry. The three described null phenotype individuals are of European descent and are all homozygous for a splice site mutation (589+1 G>C) silencing the *SLC29A1* gene. These individuals have periarticular and ectopic bone mineralization (psuedogout), indicating an important role of SLC29A1 in bone mineralization.

Key points

- Erythrocytes transport a variety of solutes, and help maintain concentration gradients throughout key organs, for example the kidney.
- Water transport is rigorously controlled by the erythrocyte and avoids osmotic lysis.
- Membrane transporters are often grouped together (termed a metabolon) to coordinate their actions (e.g. the anion exchange protein and the Rh complex).

SELF-CHECK 2.4

- What are the key 'back up' systems erythrocytes have in place to maintain water and urea balance?
- How are membrane transporters attached to the erythrocyte membrane skeleton?
- Why are some null phenotypes extremely rare (e.g. Co (a-b-); Jk(a-b-))?

Blood group antigens expressed on membrane receptors

MNS blood group system (ISBT 004)

MNS is one of the most complex of the blood group systems. Currently there are 56 different alleles described in the literature that give rise to 48 different MNS antigens, a few of which are described here. In this chapter the MNS-critical amino acid residues are described with respect to the mature polypeptide for clarity; however, it should be noted that the nascent polypeptides of both GPA and GPB contain a 19-amino acid leader peptide.

As mentioned earlier in the chapter, the M and N antigens were the first blood groups to be defined at the molecular level by conventional protein sequence analysis of the carrier molecule glycophorin A. It was established that two amino acid changes at positions 1 and 5 of the mature protein are responsible for the M and N antigens (Ser1Leu and Gly5Glu). The gene that harbours these mutations is *GYPA* and thus gives rise to M and N alleles (ISBT nomenclature *GYPA*M* and *GYPA*N*). The relative frequencies of the different alleles are as follows: in Europeans MM 28%, MN 50%, and NN 22%, and in Africans MM 25%; MN 48%, and NN 27%. The Ss antigens are carried by the related protein glycophorin B (GPB), which actually shares a common sequence at the N-terminus with the N form of GPA. Consequently, some 'anti-N' will react with M+N−erythrocytes because they cross react with the GPB form of N (as well as the N form of GPA)—this antigen is thereby noted as 'N' (ISBT MNS30). The S to s blood group polymorphism is a change (Met to Thr) affecting amino acid 29 of the mature protein.

Three null phenotypes are associated with the MNS system. En(a−) erythrocytes normally have no GPA but normal GPB expression, thus they react with anti-'N'. The rarest null phenotype in the system is named M^kM^k, lacking both GPA and GPB. Finally, there is a normal GPA but deficient GPB phenotype, S−s−.

Variant MNS alleles

In common with the Rh blood group system a variety of genetic mechanisms generate the MNS system antigens. Mutations in both the *GYPA* and *GYPB* genes cause enough structural changes in the external configuration of both GPA and GPB proteins to illicit immune responses when exposed to incompatible antigens. In *GYPA* point mutations cause the expression of low frequency antigens—for example Mt(a+) is caused by a codon change to Thr56Ile in GPA, and Hut+ individuals have a mutation affecting codon 26 (Thr26Lys). In the *GYPB* gene the Henshaw (He+) antigen, relatively common in Africans and found on both S+ or s+ genetic backgrounds, involves point mutations affecting codons 1, 4, and 5. The amino acid changes involved are Leu1Trp, Thr4Ser, and Glu21Gly (see Figure 2.11).

Hybrid glycophorin A and B proteins

Analogous to the RH system, genetic rearrangements between the *GYPA*, *GYPB*, and closely related *GYPE* genes (which does not apparently produce a viable protein product found on erythrocytes) produce hybrid GPA–GPB molecules, which generate novel junctional structures that can illicit immune responses during incompatible transfusion or pregnancy. One such example is the Hil antigen, an interesting case study for the molecular background of antigens. At least five genetically different hybrid molecules (GPA–GPB, GPB–GPA–GPB (three types), GPA-GPB–GPA) express the Hil antigen. Interestingly, the Dantu antigen is formed by a hybrid 99 amino acid GPB–GPA, (39GPB–60GPA), and where individuals are homozygous for this variant, the incidence of severe malaria is decreased by 40% (see Leffler et al., 2017).

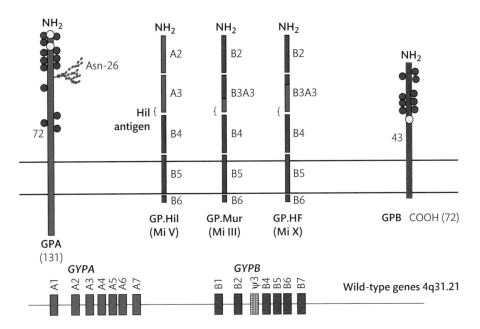

FIGURE 2.11

Erythrocyte glycophorins A and B, membrane topology, variant antigens, and gene structures.
Both GPA (blue) and GPB (red) are homologous single-pass membrane proteins with extensively O-sialylated serine and threonine residues in their externalized N-terminal domains. GPA has a single N-glycan (Asn-26) attached. The genes are arranged in tandem on 4q31.21, each having seven exons, but GPB has a pseudoexon 3 not incorporated into the mature transcript. Recombination or gene conversion between the *GYPA* and *GYPB* genes producing hybrids are common causes of variants of which three are shown in the figure. Hybrid *GYPA–GYPB* genes producing the GP.Mur, GP.HIL, and GP.HF glycophorins are shown; all three variants express the Hil antigen, which most probably is a novel structure created by joining the amino acid sequences derived from *GYPA* exon 3 to *GYPB* exon 4, whose hybrid gene structures are omitted for clarity.

Gerbich blood group system (ISBT 020)

Gerbich is a relatively 'old' blood group system named first in 1960. Gerbich system antigens are carried by the highly related glycophorins C and D (GPC and GPD) of which GPC has been mentioned previously as an important attachment site to the erythrocyte membrane. Both GPC and GPD are the products of the same gene, *GYPC*, located on chromosome 2q14.3, GPD being derived from a second ATG start codon, resulting in a protein 21 amino acids shorter than GPC. Like GPA and GPB (to which they *are not* related at the genetic level), they have extensively O-sialylated serine and threonine residues at their externalized N-terminal domain 13 and 8 residues, respectively (GPC and GPD). Both proteins span the bilayer once, and have short but identical C-terminal tails.

The Gerbich antigens are of high prevalence (Ge2, Ge3, Ge4 GEPL, GEAT, GET1) or low prevalence (Wb (Webb) Ls^a, An^a, Dh^a, and GEIS). The molecular basis of some of these antigens is described in Figure 2.12. Anti-Ge2 is the most commonly occurring antibody largely in Melanesian populations, generated by incompatible transfusion or pregnancy. The Gerbich and Yus variants of Melanesians are associated with partial deletions of the *GYPC* gene (see Figure 2.12), and interestingly are unable to stimulate phosphatidylserine exposure with anti-GPC monoclonal antibodies (an attribute of normal erythrocytes with wild-type GPC). This may possibly signal that these variants, rare in the rest of the world, may impart resistance to malaria, endemic in Melanesia. The Leach phenotype is the null phenotype of the Gerbich system (referred to as Ge-2, -3, -4) and erythrocytes have ovalocytosis, indicating the structural role GPC (and GPD) has in maintaining the structure of the erythrocyte, described earlier in this chapter.

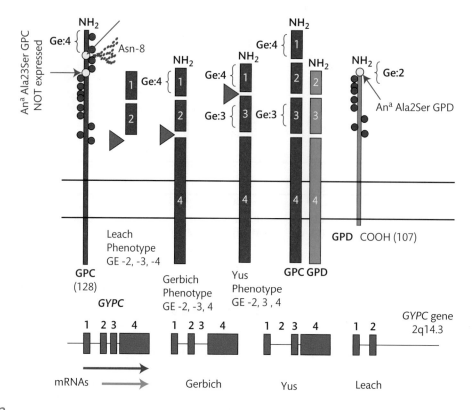

FIGURE 2.12

Gerbich blood group antigens molecular basis and variant phenotypes.
This figure depicts a cartoon of the GPC (red) and GPD (green) erythrocyte proteins (top panel far left and right) and the *GYPC* wild-type gene structure (bottom panel far left). The green and red arrows illustrate the transcription start sites for *GYPC* and *GYPD*, respectively—being products the same gene, the AUG start signal for GPD is at codon 22 corresponding to GYPC. Top panel centre illustrates the truncated protein species that are derived from the Gerbich and Yus mutated *GYPC* genes, indicating regions encoded by each exon, exon 2 deleted from Gerbich and exon 3 deleted from Yus. The corresponding gene structures are shown on the lower panel. Gerbich and Yus mutated genes produce a single truncated product, and no GPC and GPD; thus, both phenotypes lack the Ge2 antigen located on GPD. The An^a antigen is also unique to GPD, despite having a corresponding amino acid change on GPC it is only expressed at the N-terminus of GPD. The Webb (Ge5) (Wb+) antigen is an amino acid change (Asn8Ser) only found on GPC. The exon 3 deleted Gerbich gene, despite having the AUG start codon for GPD, does not express it, probably due to stability issues of the truncated GPD protein. The Leach phenotype has been shown to be due to a deleted *GYPC* gene, and is shown on the left of the variant glycophorins. Again, no stable product is inserted into the membrane as it lacks the membrane domain encoded by exon 4.

Blood group systems expressed by erythrocyte membrane-bound enzymes

Kell (KEL) blood group system (ISBT 007) and Kx (ISBT 019)

Kell blood group incompatibility can not only cause transfusion reactions, but is also a prevalent cause of HDFN (see Chapter 3). The major clinically significant polymorphism is K/k (K1/K2; KEL*01/KEL*02; Kell/Cellano). K+ individuals represent approximately 9% of the European/North American population. Twenty-one antigens are currently classified in the Kell system (see Figure 2.13). The Kell glycoprotein is a membrane-bound enzyme, a zinc metalloproteinase with an apparent molecular weight of 93 KDa by SDS-PAGE. The protein has a small cytoplasmic N-terminal domain, single membrane-spanning segment, and a large C-terminal catalytic domain, which carries four or five N-glycans (Figure 2.13). Interestingly, the K/k polymorphism is due to a single amino acid exchange Met193Thr. Thr193 (k) forms part of an Asn-Arg-Thr$_{193}$ sequence motif that serves as an N-glycan addition signal in the Golgi apparatus during synthesis, resulting in Asn191 becoming glycosylated. In K+ individuals this motif is disrupted (Asn-Arg-Met$_{193}$) resulting in no N-glycan addition. Table 2.4 denotes the major KEL system antigens, their molecular basis, and frequencies in different populations.

Clinically, K is the most important erythrocyte antigen outside the ABO and Rh system; anti-K can cause haemolytic transfusion reactions and a severe form of HDFN (see Chapter 3). Anti-Kp^a and anti-Js^a has been reported as a cause of HDFN. Anti-Js^b has only been reported in individuals of African ancestry, and has caused severe HDFN.

The function of the Kell glycoprotein is that it processes peptide hormones that have vasoconstrictive activity. The Kell glycoprotein has significant homology to neprilysin family endopeptidases, including endothelium converting enzymes ECE-1 and ECE-2, and neutral

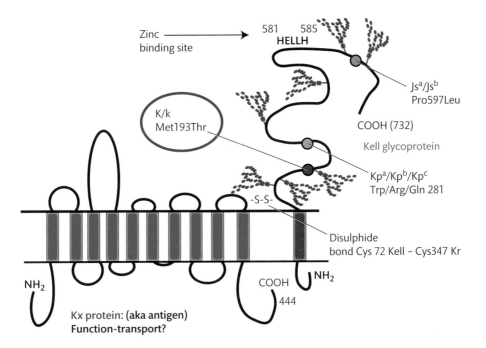

FIGURE 2.13
Membrane assembly of the Kell and Kx protein complex.
Depicted is the membrane organization of the Kell glycoprotein, directly attached by a disulphide bridge to the Kx protein via a Cys72 (Kell) – Cys 372 (Kx) bond. The location and identities of the various clinically significant KEL antigens are shown, and the position of the zinc binding site 581 HELLH 585 critical for the metalloproteinase activity of the glycoprotein. Kell has seven (or six for K+) predicted N-glycans shown as red-branched structures. The Kx protein has 10 membrane-spanning segments and is responsible for expression of the Kx antigen.

TABLE 2.4 The major clinically significant KEL antigens.

Kell system antigen	ISBT notation	Molecular basis (nucleotide/amino acid change)	Frequency
K/k	007.001/002	C578T; Thr193Met	K+ 9% Caucasians; 2% Blacks; Iranian Jews 12%
Kp^a/Kp^b/Kp^c	007.003/004/021	C841T (Kp^a); G842A(Kp^c); Arg281Trp (Kp^a); Arg281Gln (Kp^c)	Kp^a 2% Caucasians
Js^a/Js^b	007.006/007	T1790C; Leu597Pro	Js^a 20% Africans

endopeptidase 24.11 (CD10) and PHEX, which is an enzyme deficient in X-linked hypophos-phatemia (XLH) (known as X-linked vitamin D-resistant rickets). All these enzymes possess a zinc binding motif, HEXXH, in Kell this sequence is $H_{581}ELLH_{585}$. Expression studies using Kell glycoprotein have shown that it is able to cleave the substrates of ECE-1 and ECE-2 (namely big endothelins (ET)-1, big ET-2, and big-ET3), which are inactive peptides of around 40 amino acids, to their potent vasoconstrictive forms of endothelins, which are 21 amino acid peptides. However, Kell has a much stronger affinity for big-ET3 than other big endothelins, and it has been shown that there is no difference in the Km of its enzyme activity in K+ or Js^{b+} (KEL6) in *in vitro* expression and intact erythrocyte assays.

Kell$_{null}$ (or K$_o$) individuals are extremely rare. All are caused by homozygosity or compound heterozygosity for mutations that prevent the expression of the *KEL* gene. Examples include missense mutations (e.g. Pro560Ala in *KEL*01N.01*), splice site mutations at consensus splice site boundaries (e.g. intron 8 IVS8 +1g>a in *KEL*01N.12*; intron 8 IVS8 +1g>t in *KEL*01N.13*), and premature stop codons (e.g. Gln348Stop in *KEL*01N.04*). Here in the ISBT nomenclature the inclusion of *N* denotes a null phenotype.

KX, McLeod syndrome, and phenotypic relationship with Kell The XK protein (that encodes the Kx antigen) is a 37 KDa (444 amino acid) product emanating from the XK gene initially defined by positional cloning. Defects in the XK gene (deletions, splice site mutations) generate the McLeod phenotype, which is typified by neurological disorders, late-onset muscle wasting, elevated levels of the enzyme creatine phosphokinase and **acanthocytic** erythrocyte mor-phology, and depression of Kell antigen expression. McLeod phenotype individuals sometimes also have chronic granulomatous disease (CGD), but this is not always the case. Normally, per-sons with **McLeod syndrome** but without CGD may make anti-Km instead of anti-Kx when exposed to non-McLeod phenotype blood, but there has been an exception. *XK* transcripts/XK protein are expressed not only in erythroid tissues, but also in brain, skeletal muscle, heart, and pancreas, but the function of the XK protein is unknown. *XK* has some homology with a rab-bit glutamate transporter, and maintains an N-in C-in topology with 10 membrane-spanning domains (Figure 2.13). This may indicate that the XK protein is involved in processing/trans-porting the neurotransmitter glutamate, perhaps via the glutamate/glutamine cycle.

> **McLeod syndrome**
>
> Caused by a gene defect in the *XK* gene (and others) leading to acanthocytic red cells and depression of Kell system antigens. Individuals have neural defects leading to peripheral neuropathy, cardiomyopathy, and anaemia.

Kell$_{null}$ (Ko) phenotype erythrocytes have substantially elevated Kx antigen, and it has long been proposed that the absence of Kell glycoprotein in Ko individuals makes the Kx antigen more accessible. This hypothesis appears attractive when one considers that XK protein expression in Ko erythrocyte membranes is reduced (as defined using immunoblot analysis with anti-XK antipeptide sera). Also, the XK protein contains 14 potential phosphorylation sites of which 10 are localized at the cytoplasmic face of the membrane bilayer and is also palmitoylated; thus XK may be involved in multiple regulatory protein–protein interactions and membrane signal-ling events in a manner analogous to that of the anion exchange protein.

Cartwright YT (ISBT 011)

The Cartwright (YT) antigens are expressed on erythrocyte acetylcholinesterase (AChE). A single SNP in the *ACHE* gene C1057A causing a His322Asn change is the cause of the Yt^a/Yt^b polymorphism. Yt^a is of high prevalence, almost 92% of people are Yt(a+b–), although in the Israeli population the figure is around 75%. Acetylcholinesterase is one of a number of proteins linked to the membrane via a glycophosphoinositol (GPI) tail. As a consequence it is deficient from erythrocytes of individuals with type III paroxysmal nocturnal haemoglobinuria (PNH III). PNH III results in defects in the *PIGA* gene, which is critical for attachment of the GPI tail.

Erythrocyte AChE may serve to inactivate stray acetylcholine that enters the bloodstream, which maybe analogous to the function of the Duffy chemokine receptor. No known functional difference between Yt(a+b-) and Yt(a-b+) erythrocytes are known. The clinical significance of anti-Yt^a is unclear, with at least one report of it causing a fatal delayed haemolytic transfusion reaction. Anti-Yt^b is very uncommon and has unknown clinical consequences.

Dombrock DO (ISBT 014)

DO system antigens are expressed on this 314-amino acid GPI-linked membrane protein. It carries Do^a/Do^b antigens and the high-incidence antigens Gy^a (Gregory), Holley (Hy), and Joseph (Jo^a). The molecular origins of DO expression was described with the identification of the *DOK* gene as erythrocyte membrane-bound adenosine triphosphate ribosyltransferase 4 (*ART-4*). The protein has no known function, but ADP-ribosylation is known to be a post-translational modification and, interestingly, ART-4 enzymes have been implicated in modification of α4 integrin in skeletal muscle. The DO glycoprotein does indeed possess an RGD (Arg-Gly-Asp) motif that is involved in integrin binding. Most ART enzymes have specificity for arginine modification, but the bovine erythrocyte ART appears to have specificity for cysteine residues, which may actually confirm an earlier study identifying such a protein (possibly DO) in humans. However, on turkey erythrocytes, the enzyme appears to modify arginine residues. Thus the activity and substrate(s) of the human DO protein remain to be studied in detail.

Do^a/Do^b antigenicity is induced by a SNP altering codon 265 (Asn→Asp), which disrupts the RGD motif in Do(a+) individuals, which may have function consequences. Do$_{null}$ individuals exist, and are caused by a variety of genetic mechanisms, including small genomic deletions, splice site mutations, and a nonsense mutation. The Gy^a, Hy, and Jo^a antigens are caused by the SNPs in the *DO* gene.

Erythrocyte antigens and erythrocyte chemokine receptors—Duffy (FY) blood group system (ISBT:008)

As we shall see, the Duffy blood group system represents the best example of evolution at play driving a particular blood group phenotype, Fy(a-b-). The Duffy glycoprotein is a promiscuous chemokine receptor that is expressed on a variety of cell types and not just erythrocytes, including high vein endothelial cells, epithelial linings of the kidney collecting ducts and lung alveoli, and also Purkinje cells of the cerebellum. It appears to function on erythrocytes to scavenge excess cytokines and chemokines from the peripheral circulation, and thus keep their actions local to the site of release. The Duffy antigen receptor for chemokines (DARC) binds many chemokines, including IL-8, RANTES (regulated on activation, normal T-expressed and secreted), MCP-1 (monocyte chemotactic protein 1), and MGSA (melanoma growth stimulatory activity). The *DARC* gene has recently been renamed *ACKR1* (atypical chemokine receptor 1).

The Fy^a/Fy^b blood group polymorphism is a SNP affecting codon 42, and induces an aspartic acid to glycine change. The mutation is balanced in the European population with the following frequencies: Fy(a+b-) 17%; Fy(a-b+) 34%; Fy(a+b+) 49%; the Fy(a-b-) phenotype is very rare. In Africans, by contrast, the Fy(a-b-) phenotype is common, and in parts of West Africa approaches 100% of the population. The majority of Fy(a-b-) phenotypes arise from a gene promotor mutation, -67T>C, which in Africans occurs on a *FY*B* genetic background, but also a *FY*A* background in Papua New Guinea. This T>C mutation destroys a GATA-1 transcription factor binding site, and abolishes the expression of the DARC protein on the erythrocytes of these individuals. The ACKR1 gene (like most genes) contains multiple transcription factor binding sites, and the destruction of the GATA-1 site has no effect on these, and ACKR1 expression in non-erythroid tissues remains normal. As a consequence, anti-Fy^b is rarely seen in

Fy(a-b-) individuals, as they express the Fy^b antigen on non-erythroid cells and do not recognize it as foreign when exposed to non-self erythrocytes.

So why the very high frequency of Fy(a-b-) in Africans, especially West Africans? ACKR1 is known to be a receptor, critical for invasion of erythrocytes by the malarial parasites *Plasmodium vivax* and *Plasmodium knowlesi*. Fy(a-b-) individuals are resistant to invasion by these parasites, and there is clear evidence that the GATA-1 mutation rapidly spread throughout the population where these parasites were once endemic. However, *P. vivax* is not found in Africa, but remains the leading cause of malaria in Asia and Latin America, and it was thus speculated that *P. vivax* was once endemic in Africa but became extinct due to the emergence of the Fy(a-b-) *P. vivax*-resistant erythrocytes. This theory has recently been reinforced by the fact that African apes are readily infected with a malaria parasite that is related to human *P. vivax*. Undoubtedly the South East Asian Fy(a-b-) phenotype arose due to the presence of *P. vivax* in that population.

Analogous to the weak D phenotypes, *FY(ACKR1)* weakening alleles have also been described. One at least is very common (approximately 3% in Europe) and weakens Fy^b antigen expression, named the FY*Bweak allele (commonly referred to as Fy^x or Fy$_{Mod}$). The mutation changes amino acid 89 (Arg>Cys) in the *ACKR1* protein (Figure 2.14), and clearly reduces the amount of the Fy^b-bearing protein in erythrocyte membranes. It is an issue clinically as some examples of anti-Fy^b are unable to detect the weakened Fy^b expression.

Key points

- Some blood groups are driven by evolution, for example in areas of the world where malaria is endemic. Examples include the West African Fy(a-b-) phenotype and Gerbich variants.

- Some erythrocyte membrane proteins function as enzymes (e.g. Kell) to process inactive precursors as soon as they reach the bloodstream, or to inactivate 'stray' bioactive molecules (e.g. acetylcholinesterase).

FIGURE 2.14
Protein structure and genomic organization of the Fy polypeptide and gene.
The seven-transmembrane topology and large extracellular chemokine binding N-terminal domain of the FY protein is depicted. The positions of the Fy^a/Fy^b polymorphic residue Gly42Asp, and the position of the weakening mutation Arg89Cys) (Fy^{bweak}) are shown (upper panel). The genomic configuration of the FY (*DARC*, now *ACKR1*) is also depicted, comprising a small two-exon gene located on 1q23.2. The T-67C GATA1 transcription factor mutation found in Fy(a-b-) individuals is also shown.

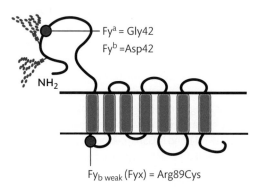

Fy^a = Gly42
Fy^b = Asp42

NH$_2$

Expressed on RBC (except Fy(a-b-)), high vein endothelial cells, colon, endothelium, lung, spleen, thyroid, thymus, kidney

Fy$_{b\ weak}$ (Fyx) = Arg89Cys

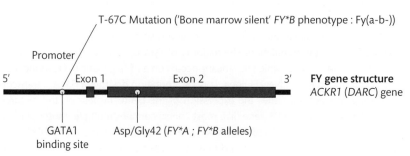

T-67C Mutation ('Bone marrow silent' *FY*B* phenotype : Fy(a-b-))

Promoter

5'   Exon 1   Exon 2   3'

FY gene structure
ACKR1 (*DARC*) gene

GATA1 binding site

Asp/Gly42 (*FY*A* ; *FY*B* alleles)

- Why are Kell system antigens depressed in the McLeod phenotype and Kx antigens elevated in the Kell null phenotype?

- Evolution has driven the emergence of rare blood group phenotypes in parts of the world— why is this and what are their genetic bases?

Antigens on erythrocyte complement control proteins

KN Knops, ISBT 022

Erythrocyte complement receptor CR1 (CD35), which is the receptor for C3b/C4b, expresses Knops (KN) system antigens—Knops (Kn^a), McCoy (McC^a and McC^b), Swain-Langley (Sl^a), and Villain (Vil/Sl(a-)) York (Yk^a) antigens. CR1 polymorphism takes three forms: (1) expression levels; (2) molecular size; (3) amino acid changes detailed here. CR1, along with CR2 (CD21), play an important role in the innate immune system, and also play important roles in the humoral immune response by retaining and allowing scanning of antigens during antigen presentation. CD35/CD21 also functions on B cells as a counter receptor for B-cell receptor (BCR) signalling. Depression of the levels of CR1 often gives rise to KN-negative/null pheno-types (e.g. Helgeson phenotype), estimated to be expressing between 20 and 100 copies of CR1 per erythrocyte; however, CR1 expression levels on erythrocytes is inherently low. One of these phenotypes, Sl(a-), has shown to be significant in West Africa where *Plasmodium falciparum* malaria is endemic. Sl(a-) erythrocytes do not form rosettes where *Plasmodium*-infected eryth-rocytes are able to bind uninfected cells and vascular endothelium. Interestingly, erythrocyte expression of the two complement control proteins CD35 (CR1) and DAF (CD55) are reduced during pregnancy, and have been proposed to be caused by an increase in immune complex formation and complement activation during pregnancy and resultant down-regulation of CD55/CD35 expression. Erythrocyte CR1 expression is also decreased in other pathological conditions, including HIV infection, systemic lupus erythematosus (SLE), haemolytic anaemia, and other conditions with high immune complex loads.

The CR1 protein comprises a cytoplasmic C-terminal, single membrane-spanning domain and 30 extracellular short consensus repeats, otherwise termed complement control protein mod-ules (CCPs). These CCPs are arranged as four long homologous regions (LHRs), which have arisen by the duplication of seven CCPs. CR1 has a size polymorphism which has arisen due to unequal crossing over between the four LHRs encoded by the *CD35* gene. These size polymor-phisms result in differences of CR1 isoforms by 30 KDa, with the largest form (CR1*4) having a molecular size of 280 KDa and the smallest (CR*1) being 180 KDa. Amino acid exchanges in the *CD35* gene that are responsible for KN system antigen expression have been identified. Amino acid exchanges within CCPs 24 and 25, encoded by exon 29 account for the Mc^a/Mc^b polymorphism (Lys1590Glu) and the Sl(a-) (Vil) →Sl(a+) phenotype (Arg1601Gly). Other KN system antigens have been localized to LHR-C and LHR-D.

CROM (Cromer) ISBT 021

The Cromer (CROM) blood group antigens are expressed on polymorphic forms of *CD55* (synonym: decay accelerating factor, DAF). DAFs function is to prevent the assembly and to accelerate the dissociation of C3 and C5 convertases of the classical and alternate complement pathways. Thus, DAF expression on erythrocyte surfaces prevents autolysis from activated complement. The DAF protein is 70 KDa in size, and on erythrocytes is GPI-linked (Figure 2.15). It has a 381-amino acid extracellular region that includes a leader sequence of 34 amino acids, which is post-translationally processed. It then has a membrane-proximal O-glycosidic-linked carbohydrate domain followed by four short consensus repeats (SCRs), which are 60 amino acids each in size. The SCRs are highly homologous to domains found in other complement binding proteins. CROM system blood group antigens have been mapped to the various SCRs of the DAF protein (see Figure 2.15). The Inab phenotype, which is extremely rare, lack all CROM antigens because they have a complete deficiency of DAF, but have other GPI-linked and non-GPI-linked complement control proteins. Inab phenotypes where the molecular basis is known are caused by nonsense mutations and mis-splicing.

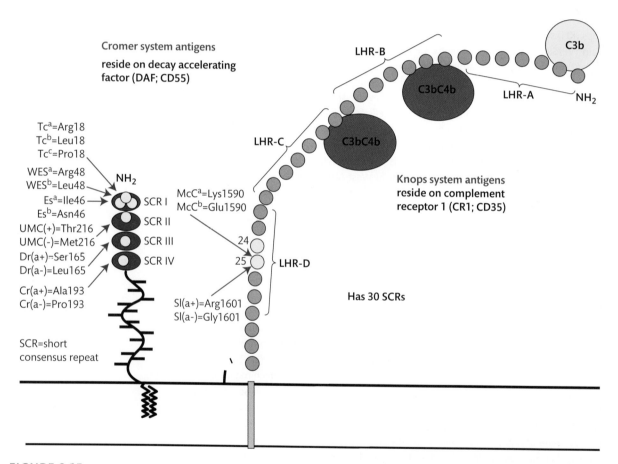

FIGURE 2.15

Erythrocyte antigen expression on complement control proteins.

The Cromer (CROM) and Knops (KN) system antigens are expressed by CD55 (decay accelerating factor) and CD35 (complement receptor 1), respectively. The figure depicts the glycophosphoinositol (GPI)-linked C-terminal tail of CD55, extensively O-glycosylated mid-region, and four short consensus repeat (SCRs) where all CROM antigens are located, of which a representative number are shown. CD55 functions to accelerate the dissociation of C3 and C5 convertases thereby inhibiting the action of complement. CD35 has 30 SCRs, and four (labelled A–D) long homologous regions, each of around 45 KDa in size. CD35 protrudes further from the erythrocyte surface and functions to bind C3C4 bound immune complexes (binding sites shown) and to block the formation of C3 convertase, thereby inhibiting the action of complement. The positions of the KN blood group polymorphisms on their respective SCRs are shown with the residue changes noted.

CD59 Membrane inhibitor of active lysis ISBT 035

CD59 has become the second most recently assigned blood group system. CD59 is a 20 KDa protein that inhibits the terminal attack complex of complement (C5a–9). The analysis of a CD59 deficient (CD59$_{null}$) patient showed that they had produced allo-anti-CD59, and they had mutated *CD59* genes (del 146A) inherited from heterozygous parents.

Chido-Rodgers (CH/RG) ISBT 017

CH/RG antigens are not expressed by erythrocyte complement control proteins but by C4d component of the complement cascade. In this process the complement component C4b is cleaved to inactivate it into two fragments, C4c and C4d. The C4d component remains membrane bound, and it is this protein fragment that expresses erythrocyte CH/RG determinants. Complement proteins are of course adsorbed onto the surface of erythrocytes from serum. Complement component C4 consists of two isoforms, C4A and C4B, and within these two isoforms there are 18 C4A variants and 21 C4B variants based on different electrophoretic mobilities. The polymorphic variation within these isotypes is largely confined to the C4d region, with C4A and C4B having 99% amino acid identity. The six Chido antigens Ch:1–Ch:6 are predominantly associated with the C4B isoform, whereas the two Rodgers antigens Rg:1 and Rg:2 are associated with C4A. The amino acid variation of C4d required for expression of the CH/RG epitopes has been defined.

Key points

- Complement control proteins exist on erythrocyte membranes to prevent lysis by activated complement, e.g. during infections.
- Complement-bound immunoglobulins are bound to erythroid CR1 (CD35) and are transported for processing by macrophages.

SELF-CHECK 2.6

- Why are PNHIII cells prone to complement-mediated lysis?
- Which blood group systems are polymorphic forms of complement components?

Antigens on erythrocyte adhesion molecules

Erythrocytes express on their surface a number of adhesion molecules, the functional significance of which is to interact with other cells during the erythroid life cycle. This includes the exit from the bone marrow compartment in the final stages of erythropoiesis, and enucleation of erythroblasts to form reticulocytes. Erythrocytes interact with endothelial cells of the vasculature, and this is especially apparent in vaso-occlusive crises in sickle cell anaemia. It is also known the erythrocytes and platelets interact during thrombotic events, and amplify signals to attract leucocytes to thrombotic plaques. At the end of the erythrocyte's life, it is removed from the circulation by a highly controlled process (referred to earlier) named *eryptosis* where effete erythrocytes are engulfed by splenic and liver-localized macrophages. Here the erythrocyte adhesion molecules that have been implicated in some of these life critical processes, and the blood group antigens they express are highlighted graphically in Figure 2.16.

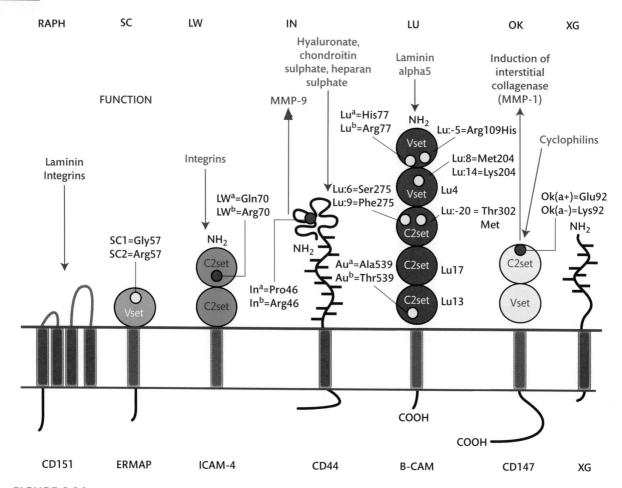

FIGURE 2.16

Erythrocyte antigen expression on cell adhesion molecules.

The identities of seven blood group systems carried by erythroid membrane proteins are shown. The predicted structures, including type of immunoglobulin superfamily domains they possess, are shown. The positions and identities of representative amino acid changes responsible for the blood group polymorphisms are depicted. All erythrocyte adhesion molecules have single membrane-spanning domains, with the exception of RAPH, which is a tetraspanin with four membrane passes. The known identities of binding ligands on other cell types is shown in blue, along with possible functional consequences of these interactions.

Lutheran glycoprotein (ISBT005)

Lutheran glycoprotein (basal cell adhesion molecule, CD239) (Eyler & Telen, 2006) is a receptor for laminin α5. The Lutheran glycoprotein and BCAM are products of the same gene, with alternate splicing producing two isoforms that differ in the length of their cytoplasmic tails and are of molecular weight 85 (Lutheran) and 78 KDa (BCAM), and both forms are found in erythrocyte membranes. Lu/BCAM are overexpressed on sickled erythrocytes, and thus thought to play a role in vasocclusion in the disease. Lu/BCAM expresses all LU system antigens, and these are shown on the molecule in Figure 2.16. The molecule comprises five IgSF domains (3 × C2 set, 2 × V set) and the precise locations of the antigens were initially mapped by expression of chimeric molecules *in vitro*. Clinically, antibodies to Lutheran system antigens are not especially significant. Mild HDFN requiring phototherapy and slightly raised bilirubin levels have been reported, as have mild delayed haemolytic transfusion reactions. The nulll phenotype (Lu(a-b-)) is rare, caused by mutations in the gene. However, the In(Lu) phenotype, which has absent or extremely weak Lutheran antigens and depressed CD44 glycoprotein, is caused by mutations in the *KLF-1* gene, an erythroid transcription factor (see later section on CD44).

LW (Landsteiner Wiener, ISBT 016)

The discovery of the LW blood group system is one of historical significance in transfusion medicine. In 1940 Landsteiner and Wiener described rabbit and guinea pig antibodies that were raised against *Macacus rhesus* erythrocytes. In this paper, they discussed that these antibodies were similar if not identical to those described in the Levine and Stetson 1939 paper, the first to describe the clinical significance of the Rh D antigen. It was this anti-rhesus (or, correctly termed, anti-Rh) that gave rise to the Rh blood group system, but this was actually a misnomer. By a process of elimination, it was found that the rabbit/guinea pig 'anti-Rh' did, in fact, bind to D-negative erythrocytes but did not agglutinate them. Subsequently, it was renamed anti-LW (Landsteiner-Wiener) after their discoverers, and although strictly incorrect it was decided to keep the Rh (for rhesus) name for the now rapidly accruing number of papers on the Rh system antibodies. The differential activity of the rabbit/guinea pig anti-LW was found to be due to the fact that D-positive erythrocytes express more LW antigens that D-negative erythrocytes.

LW antigens are expressed on erythrocyte adhesion molecule ICAM-4 (see Figure 2.16). Like all five known ICAMs, ICAM-4 binds to CD11a/CD18 integrins (LFA-1, $\alpha_L\beta_2$) expressed abundantly on lymphocytes, but has also been shown *in vitro* to bind CD11b/CD18 (Mac-1; $\alpha_M\beta_2$) and $\alpha_4\beta_1$ (LFA-4, CD49d/CD29), $\alpha_V\beta_1$ (CD51/CD29), and $\alpha_V\beta_5$ integrins.

The structure of the LW (ICAM-4, CD242) molecule has been modelled on the crystal structure of ICAM-2. LW^a→LW^b antigenicity is defined by a single amino acid exchange (Gln70Arg) located on β-strand E of the first (D1) domain of ICAM-4, but ICAM-4 lacks amino acids presumed to be critical (Glu34 and Gln73 of ICAM-1) for binding of LFA-1 to other ICAMs. ICAM-4 plays a critical role in stabilizing the interaction of erythroblastic islands the structures critical for maturation of erythrocytes from their progenitors in the bone marrow.

OK–EMMPRIN, (ISBT 024)

The Ok^a antigen is expressed on EMMPRIN (extracellular matrix metalloproteinase inducer, or Basigin) as are two other antigens, OKGV and OKVM. The protein is a 269 amino acid immunoglobulin superfamily (a C2 and V1 domain); all three antigens are high frequency and OK(a-), OKGV-, and OKVM–phenotype individuals are very rare. EMMPRIN (CD147) is required for the correct insertion of the erythrocyte monocarboxylate transporter MCT1.

IN (Indian) CD44 (ISBT 023)

Unsurprisingly, the Indian blood group is associated with the Indian subcontinent. The In^b antigen is of high incidence, and In^a of low frequency being present in the Indian subcontinent (~3%) but of higher frequency amongst Persians and Arabs with one report noting 10% amongst Iranians and 11.8% of people of Arabic descent in Bombay. The In^a/In^b polymorphism is a mutation in the *CD44* gene which encodes a single-pass adhesion molecule, associated with leucocyte homing but is ubiquitously expressed, the erythrocyte form CD44H comprising 248 amino acids of which Arg86Pro is the polymorphic change (incidentally, having other amino acid changes Tyr109Ser and Gly239Glu). Two high-frequency antigens have been identified, INFI and INJA; antibodies were made to these antigens in Moroccans (INFI; His85Gln) and Pakistanis (INJA; Thr163Lys). CD44 binds to the extracellular matrix primarily through the glycoaminoglycan hyaluronan, but also to collagen, fibronectin, and laminin. CD44 in non-erythroid cell types is critical in the adhesion of leucocytes to stromal cells (of the bone marrow), recruitment of leucocytes to sites of inflammation, and in metastasis of tumours. Its role in erythrocytes is unclear, but CD44-deficient erythrocytes have a novel form of congenital dyserythroblastic anaemia.

The antigen AnWj was initially thought to be transient, as anti-AnWj demonstrated this property. But in the 1990s AnWj-negative individuals were found, indicating a genetic origin, thought to be located on the CD44 molecule. Suppression of CD44 expression resulting in a In(a-b-) phenotype (and incidentally Lu (a-b-) phenotype, and depressed CO and LW antigens) is found in the In(Lu) phenotype. The erythroid transcription factor EKLF (erythroid Kruppel-like factor) is encoded by the gene *KLF1*. Mutations in *KLF1* have been to be causative of the In(Lu) phenotype.

XG (ISBT 012)

The XG blood group system was the first to be assigned to a sex chromosome and phenotypically related to the CD99 glycoprotein. XG expresses the Xg^a antigen, carried by a 180-amino acid heavily O-glycosylated membrane protein. The frequencies of Xg(a+) individuals were studied in over 2500 Northern European individuals and the following noted: Xg(a+) 66% male 89% female; Xg(a-) 34% male 11% female. The phenotypic relationship between XG and CD99 was noted in the 1980s; all Xg(a+) individuals express CD99 highly and Xg(a-) females are CD99 low expressers. However, in Xg(a-) males, 68% were CD99 high expressers and 32% low. CD99 encodes a homolog to XG, comprising 185 amino acids. The gene for XG is called *MIC2*, and is located at the pseudoautosomal boundary of both the X and Y chromosomes, although it is deleted to such an extent on the Y chromosome (it only possesses exons 1–3 of the 10 exon gene) it does not produce a viable protein. The pseudoautomsomal boundary is the region of both X and Y chromosomes where they diverge in sequence, and Y and X chromosome sequences lie downstream of *MIC2* (XG) which is at the boundary, called PAB1. CD99 lies within the autosomal region and is carried and expressed by both X and Y. Interestingly, both XG and CD99 escape the lyonization process (two of only 10 genes or so that do this) whereby one copy of each X-carried gene is silenced by the action of the *XIST* gene. Anti-CD99 has been detected in humans, albeit rarely (CD99 is a high-frequency antigen) and forms the second antigen of the XG system. The molecular basis of Xg(a-) has yet to be resolved, but a hypothetical regulator gene of both XG and CD99 called *XGR* has been proposed to control the expression of both *XG* and *CD99*. The function of XG is unknown, but it is related to CD99, which has cell adhesion properties and appears to be involved in T-cell activation on those cell types. Certain anti-CD99 block interactions of T cells with erythrocytes, and high levels of CD99 have been considered a tumour marker for Ewing's sarcoma.

Scianna (ERMAP) (ISBT 013)

The SC blood group system is expressed on the ERMAP (erythroid membrane-associated protein) IgSF molecule, which has a single membrane-spanning domain and a single IgV domain. There are two low-frequency antigens in the system (Sc2 and Rd (Radin)) and five high-frequency antigens (Sc1, Sc3, STAR, SCER, and SCAN), all of which are associated with SNPs changing amino acids in this IgV domain. Silencing mutations (two) have also been described ablating expression of all SC antigens and are caused by frameshift and nonsense mutations. Antibodies to Sc antigens are very rare and difficult to detect.

JMH (John Milton Hagen) ISBT 026

JMH antigen (John Milton Hagen) is expressed on erythrocyte CD108, otherwise known as semaphorin 7A (SEMA 7A), another example of a membrane protein that carries a GPI tail.

CD108 comprises a 80 KDa glycoprotein of 602 amino acids that carries five consensus N-glycan addition sites (the protein has a deglycosylated molecular weight of 68 KDa, and an RGD motif between residues 265 and 267, and a 500-amino acid sema domain, a hallmark of the semaphorin protein family). The Sema domain is followed by a single immunoglobulin superfamily domain. Semaphorins are important in neuronal development, providing attractive and repulsive stimuli during axonal guidance. They are also expressed on cells of the immune system, notably lymphoid and myeloid lineage cells (e.g. erythrocytes). CD108 does not induce cytokine production from B or T lymphocytes, but is a potent stimulator of monocytes, inducing both chemotaxis and pro-inflammatory cytokine production (IL-1β, tumour necrosis factor-alpha (TNF-α), IL-6, and IL-8). It has been postulated that immune cells are guided by semaphorin interactions to their appropriate targets.

The JMH system has six antigens—JMH, JMHK, JMHL, JMHG, JMHM, and JMHQ—all at high frequency and ablated by missense mutations in the *CD108* gene. There are no descriptions of adverse transfusion effects of individuals being negative for these antigens, save for reduced erythrocyte survival.

RAPH (MER-2) ISBT 025

A monoclonal antibody initially recognized an antigen named MER-2 that recognized erythrocytes. An alloantibody identical to MER-2 was described, and RAPH was designated a blood group in 1998 and named after the individual who made this antibody. RAPH was shown to be expressed by a tetraspanin molecule CD151 in 2004, which has cell-adhesive properties, interacting with both α and β integrins and laminin of the basement membrane. The MER2 antigen is silenced by missense mutations, and a null phenotype individuals lacking CD151 have been described, and had glomerulonephritis and sensorineural deafness. The original description of MER-2 had stated that 92% of the studied population were positive for the antigen. However, the vast majority of MER2–people do not make allo-anti-MER2, and most probably have low levels of CD151 on their erythrocytes.

VEL and SMIM1 ISBT 034

In 2013 two groups independently identified that small membrane protein 1 (SMIM1) is the carrier of the Vel blood group antigen. A small deletion of 17 nucleotides in the *SMIM1* gene resulted in no expression of Vel antigen on RBCs. Although described here as an adhesion molecule the function of SMIM1 is not known, and may serve as a regulator of RBC growth, as zebrafish SMIM1 knockdowns showed some reduction in RBC concentration, and a SNP that is associated with weakened Vel expression showed some reduction in haemoglobin concentrations within red cells in such individuals.

2.5 Non-polymorphic erythrocyte membrane proteins

A decreasing number of known erythrocyte membrane proteins are not known to be capable of eliciting and immune response when transfusion takes place with incompatible cells or transfusion into a null phenotype individual. The major erythrocyte component GLUT1 (SLC2A1), the erythrocyte critical for function glucose transporter, has over 100 variants that have changes to amino acids spread throughout the length of the protein when the 1000 genomes project for human variation was inspected (August 2016). Thus, the protein is polymorphic but presently has not be shown to generate immunological incompatibly (yet). Other well-characterized erythrocyte membrane proteins that fit this category include the erythrocyte Ca^{2+}/Mg^{2+} ATPase, the CD47 glycoprotein, the Na^+/K^+ ATPase. Perhaps immune responses to such 'mission critical' erythrocyte membrane components are incompatible with pregnancy and are in some way inhibited. Only time will tell if blood groups will be assigned to these interesting protein species in the future.

2.6 Blood group genotyping (BGG)

Following the establishment of the molecular basis of almost all blood group defining alleles, BGG emerged shortly following the definition of the most clinically significant (e.g. RhD and K). Initially, these polymerase chain reaction (PCR)-based assays were used to analyse DNA samples from fetuses (e.g. extracted from amniotic fluid) where it was far safer to sample DNA than to obtain erythrocytes that would need to be sampled from the umbilical cord. This soon evolved into directly diagnosing maternal plasma and is described in more detail in Chapter 3.

Genotyping an individual would not be possible without the successful design of the PCR in the mid-1980s. The PCR exploits the fact that DNA is double stranded and can be amplified *in vitro* using a mixture comprising synthetic oligonucleotides, the four deoxynucleoside triphosphates (dNTPs) Mg^{2+}, a DNA polymerase, and buffer salts. The oligonucleotides are of predefined DNA sequence, and are chosen to ensure the PCR product is of known and suitable size, and is stably amplified—certain sequences (e.g. GC-rich and repeat sequence regions) are more challenging to amplify and are avoided. PCR was developed using thermostable DNA polymerases isolated from thermophilic bacteria (e.g. *Thermus aquaticus* or *Taq*) so that the enzyme could withstand the high temperatures required to denature DNA—around 95°C. Repeated cycles of denaturation (95°C), annealing by cooling to a temperature that would allow the oligonucleotide primers to anneal to its target DNA on the template (normally 50–60°C, followed by elongation at a temperature close to the optimum polymerization.

PCR coupled with restriction fragment length polymorphism analysis (PCR-RFLP)

PCR-RFLP

The PCR amplifies a polymorphic sequence which is then recognized by a restriction endonuclease that cleaves on allele and the other intact. Normally detected by gel electrophoresis.

PCR-RFLP emerged as one of the first DNA-based tests for the analysis of blood group alleles, and its clinical use was first described in 1992. Briefly, it involved the PCR amplification of a region of genomic DNA flanking a blood group polymorphism followed by the digestion of the DNA by a restriction endonuclease, a large number of which are available commercially. The restriction endonuclease is chosen based on the changed nucleotide sequence resulting from the SNP that generates the bulk of blood group alleles. The digested PCR products are then separated by gel electrophoresis to visualize the fragmentation patterns and then to assign genotype. This method of testing is challenging for a number of reasons: (1) the SNP under investigation must create or destroy a restriction endonuclease site; (2) controls that confirm that the digestion has occurred are required for diagnostic use; (3) the availability of positive and negative controls; (4) and the method can only realistically be utilized in end-stage PCR reactions.

Allele-specific PCR

This method dispenses with the requirement for restriction endonucleases but does involve the design of a PCR assay to amplify a region of genomic DNA including the blood group-critical SNP. Most allele-specific amplification methods utilize the fact that there must be an almost perfect match to the genomic DNA at the 3′ end of each oligonucleotide primer; thus, by PCR design, one primer is matched perfectly to the blood group SNP at its 3′ end and if the PCR conditions optimized, will only amplify one allele and not the other. Many allele-specific PCR reactions can be combined into one tube, and this is termed multiplex PCR (a useful analogy is to think multiplex cinema). Allele-specific PCR has been at the mainstay of genetic diagnosis for several decades now, and the principles of the reaction have driven the development of higher throughput methods, such as real-time PCR, which utilizes allele-specific PCR in blood group genotyping diagnoses.

Real-time PCR (RT-PCR)

End-stage PCR reactions do not give an effective means of quantifying the amount of initial starting DNA (or cDNA) template, so methods were developed to detect PCR products in the reaction tube in real-time. Real-time PCR machines illuminate the reaction with white light, which excites fluorophores within the reaction mix to emit light at defined wavelengths. This can be done by the inclusion of intercalating dyes that bind to the major groove of DNA (e.g. SYBR-green) or the synthesis of specific probes, which are short segments of DNA to which fluorophores and quenchers are attached. The probe does not emit light as the fluorophore (termed a reporter) is in close proximity of a quencher. In the real-time PCR reaction, the *Taq* DNA polymerase, when progressing along the single-stranded DNA, removes the probe bound in front of it by the virtue of the fact that it has a 5′-exonuclease activity. The degradation of the probe physically separates the reporter dye from its quencher, and it diffuses away into the reaction mix, and will emit light at its fluorescence wavelength. Because the build up of PCR product can be monitored in real-time the assay is quantitative, and as such is sometimes referred to quantitative PCR or Q-PCR. By analysis of a standard curve of DNA samples at known concentrations, the amount of DNA in the sample can be accurately defined.

Commercially available real-time PCR platforms were ideally suited to blood group genotyping and other diagnostics in transfusion and transplantation science. They are high-throughput, and are closed systems and can be set up robotically. This minimizes the chances of contamination, a key requirement of diagnostic testing. The application of RT-PCR in transfusion and transplantation is widespread and forms a core component of virology nucleic acid testing (NAT) (see Chapter 5); for non-invasive prenatal blood grouping see Chapter 3.

DNA microarrays

For comprehensive blood group genotyping the previous methods, with the possible exception of RT-PCR, PCR-RFLP, and allele-specific PCR, the throughput of these preliminary methods was inadequate to simultaneously genotype for 100+ SNPs and combinations of SNPs required to assess all clinically significant blood groups. Two large studies based in New York, USA, and the European Union independently developed technical platforms for high-throughput genotyping, and are now commercially available. Both systems developed a series of probes bound to microspheres or glass arrays to which labelled PCR products, previously amplified from extracted DNA samples, are allowed to hybridize to. Positive reactions are then scored by computational analysis of the beads on a reader platform (e.g. Luminex) or by scanning the array to excite the fluorescently labelled PCR products followed by analysis of the array data using bespoke software. Despite the cost per test being relatively low (there are over 100 different SNPs analysed by one array platform), the assay costs remain comparatively high, and have not yet begun to become routine for testing blood donors.

Next-generation sequencing (NGS)

Several recent studies, including work performed in the author's laboratory, has shown the potential of NGS in BGG to support the clinical management of patients and blood donors. The technical approaches for NGS are beyond the scope of this book, but briefly 'first-generation' NGS entails the fragmentation of purified genomic DNA followed by ligation to adapters to produce a sequencing library. This is then processed by a variety of sequencing chemistries to produce sequences of 200–400 bp fragments that are then aligned by computer to the human genome sequence. Bioinformatic analysis then reveals the identities of blood group-specific SNPs, which can then be compared to reference sequences of each blood group allele under investigation.

Key points

- The PCR is a core technique in blood group genotyping, and can be adapted to make it allele-specific or to amplify segments of DNA for further analysis.

- Blood group genotyping is not yet widespread, but is highly effective when compared to serology and used to test multi-transfused patients.

SELF-CHECK 2.7

- What drives the specificity of the PCR?
- When is blood group genotyping preferred over serological phenotyping?

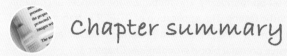

Chapter summary

- There are 36 blood group systems currently recognized by the ISBT.

- Blood group antigens are carbohydrate or protein in nature.

- Glycosyltransferases localized in the Golgi confer the genetic basis of carbohydrate antigens.

- Variations in protein backbone sequence confer the molecular basis of most blood group antigens.

- Exceptions to the above are null phenotypes where gene deletions (e.g. *RHD*) and silencing mutations (e.g. stop codons and splice site mutations) ablate the expression of that allele.

- The antigen carriers serve a wide variety of functions: membrane receptors, transporters, transporting immune complexes, inactivating complement, activation of pro-hormones, and removal of excess chemokines are some examples.

- A GATA-1 transcription factor binding site is mutated in the Fy(a-b-) phenotype, with the Duffy glycoprotein being expressed in non-erythroid tissues.

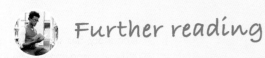 *Further reading*

- Avent ND. Human blood group antigen expression: Its molecular bases. *Br J Biomed Sci* 54 (1997), 16–37.

- BGMut (Blood group antigen gene mutation database)

  http://www.ncbi.nlm.nih.gov/gv/mhc/xslcgi.cgi?cmd=bgmut/home

- Daniels, GL. *Human Blood Groups*. 2nd edition. Blackwell Science Ltd, London (2002).

- Daniels, GL. Variants of RhD–Current testing and clinical consequences. *Br J f Haematol* 161 (2013), 461–470.

- Erythrogene: the search engine for blood group genes. http://www.erythrogene.com

- Eyler CE & Telen MJ. The Lutheran glycoprotein: a multifunctional adhesion receptor. *Transfusion* 46 (2006), 668–677.

- Leffler EM et al. Resistance to malaria through structural variation of red blood cell invasion receptors. *Science* DOI: 10.1126/science.aam6393

- Reid ME, Lomas-Francis C & Olsson ML. *The Blood Group Antigens Factsbook*. Academic Press, London, (2012).

- Rhesus base–a resource of all known Rh variants, curated by Dr Franz Wagner.

  http://www.rhesusbase.info

- Storry JR & Olsson ML. The ABO blood group system: a review and update. *Immunohematology* 25 (2009), 48–59.

- Storry JR & Peyrard T. The VEL blood group system; a review. *Immunohematology* 33 (2017), 56–59.

- Walker PS & Reid ME. The Gerbich blood group system: A review. *Immunohematology* 26 (2010), 60–65.

- Westhoff CM & Reis, ME. Review: the Kell, Duffy, and Kidd blood group systems. *Immunohematology* 20 (2004), 37–49.

3

Haemolytic Disease of the Fetus and Newborn

Neil D. Avent

Learning objectives

After studying this chapter your should be able to:

■ Understand the pathophysiology of haemolytic disease of the fetus and newborn (HDFN)— fetal and neonatal anaemia and alloimmunization events.

■ Understand the blood group incompatibilities that cause HDFN, including partial D antigens.

■ Comprehend the current clinical management of HDFN.

■ Demonstrate an understanding of the proposed mechanisms of action of prophylactic anti-D, and cellular assays to predict the severity of the disease.

■ Demonstrate an appreciation of the implementation of fetal blood group genotyping in the management of HDFN.

Introduction

Feto-maternal blood group incompatibility of both erythrocyte and platelet antigens can lead to alloimmunization events that produce maternal antibodies against paternally inherited fetal antigens. Incompatibility of platelet antigens (HPA) are described in Chapter 6. Where there are significant levels of IgG produced, a specific placental transport system delivers the maternal IgG into the fetal circulation and these antibodies attack fetal erythrocytes and platelets and in severe cases lead to fetal anaemia and thrombocytopaenia. These conditions, if not corrected *in utero* can lead to fetal death, in anaemia this causes the potentially fatal condition of *hydrops fetalis*. During the neonatal period the mother's role in the elimination of toxic products of erythrocyte breakdown (predominantly bilirubin) has obviously ceased, and the fetal biochemical pathways for bilirubin degradation start to become activated. When neonatal anaemia is severe the infant's system cannot cope, and excess bilirubin is deposited at the base of the brain, a condition known clinically as **kernicterus** which can cause brain damage and sometimes death if left untreated.

In fetal thrombocytopaenia, the shortage of platelets can lead to haemorrhage and fetal loss.

In both conditions, clinical management is stratified to identify high risk pregnancies as early as possible so that if necessary cordocentesis (fetal transfusion of erythrocytes or platelets) can be performed to alleviate the anaemia or thrombocytopaenia. The emphasis of identification of high-risk pregnancies has in the past 20 years shifted to non-invasive detection, including fetal genotyping and ultrasonography. This chapter describes both the immunology of maternal alloimmunization to paternally inherited fetal antigens, fetomaternal IgG trafficking, biochemistry of bilirubin detoxification, and clinical interventions and assessment by ultrasound.

Kernicterus
The highly pathogenic build up of bilirubin at the base of the fetal brain.

3.1 **Fetal alloimmunization**

In theory any blood group incompatibility between the fetus and its mother (by virtue of the inheritance of paternal alleles) can lead to alloimmunization events, but this is governed by several factors. First and obviously, the fetus must express the incompatible antigen during pregnancy (fetal development sometimes means that the antigen is expressed only late in pregnancy or in smaller amounts than on adult erythrocytes or platelets). Second, the blood group/platelet antigen is immunogenic. Third, there must be an alloimmunization event whereby fetal blood is exposed to the maternal immune system.

For HDFN the major causative blood group antigen is D of the Rh system. In Europe and North America between 15–20% of the population are D-negative, but in China and South East Asia only around 1%. Thus, the frequency of the D-negative phenotype in the pregnant population is a key factor as to the incidence of HDFN due to anti-D. In the UK, approximately 60% of pregnancies to D-negative mothers with D-positive fathers will be carrying D-positive infants, thus at potential risk. Prior to the introduction of the prophylactic anti-D programme in the late 1960s anti-D HDFN was a major cause of fetal death primarily because of the scale of numbers of D-positive fetuses in 15–20% of pregnancies.

It follows that where there are high frequencies of antigen negative mothers and high frequencies of antigen positive fathers then any incompatibility between mother and baby by virtue of the paternal inheritance of a blood group antigen could in theory lead to HDFN or neonatal alloimmune **thrombocytopenia** (NAITP). A list of blood group antigens that have been known to cause HDFN is shown in Table 3.1.

Thrombocytopenia
Low numbers of platelets in the circulation.

Feto-maternal IgG transport and HDFN pathology

Feto-maternal traffic of immunoglobulins (exclusively of the IgG isotype as we shall see later) is a critical component of the developing fetal immune system. At birth, virtually all the fetal circulatory immunoglobulins are maternally derived. Fetal IgG (maternally derived) levels are detected during the second trimester, but increase substantially during the third. So how do maternal IgG molecules get transported into the fetal circulation? Both the placental and newborn gut lining contain high levels of the protein **FcRN**. This molecule, as its name suggests binds the Fc portion of IgG and facilitates a pH-dependent movement of it across basolateral membranes (Figure 3.1). IgM is not actively transported, and as such does not play a role in the pathology of HDFN and NAITP. It has been hypothesized that as most anti-A and anti-B are IgM (although some are of IgG subclass) this is one reason why HDFN due to fetomaternal ABO incompatibility is not common.

TABLE 3.1 Erythrocyte antigens causing HDFN reported to date (August 2016).

Blood group antigen	Severity	Frequency	Notes
ABO system			
A	None to moderate	Rare	See Section 3.2 under heading *ABO HDFN*
B	None to moderate	Rare	
A, B	None to moderate	Rare	
RH system			
D (RH1)	Severe	Most common	D negatives and partial D HDFN
C (RH2)	Mild to severe	Rare	See Section 3.2 under heading *HDFN due to other RH system antibodies*
E (RH3)	Mild	Rare	
c (RH4)	Severe	Common	See Section 3.2 under heading *HDFN due to anti-c*
E (RH5)	Mild	Rare	
f (ce; RH6)	Mild	Rare	
Ce (RH7)	Mild	Rare	
C^W (RH8)	Mild/moderate	Rare	Latvians 9% C^W+
C^X (RH9)	Mild/moderate	Rare	
E^W (RH11)	Mild to severe	Rare	
G (RH12)	Mild to severe	Rare	
Hr0 (RH17)	None to severe	Rare	
D^W (RH23)	Moderate	Rare	
RH29	None to severe	Very rare	Associated with Rh_{null} (1 in 6 million)
Go^a (RH30)	Mild to severe	Rare	DIVa LFA
RH32	Mild to severe	Rare	R^N (RH32+phenotype) 1% in Africans
Be^a (RH36)	Moderate to severe	Rare	RH36 0.1%
Evans (RH37)	Mild to moderate	Very rare	Discontinuous epitope, see Chapter 2 DIVb and D.
Tar (RH40)	Moderate	Rare	DVII LFA (low-frequency antigen) see Section 3.2 under heading *Partial D phenotypes in HDFN*
RH42	Moderate	Very rare	2 reported
Riv (RH45)	Mild	Very rare	1 case reported
Sec (RH46)	None to severe	Rare	
STEM (RH49)	Mild	Rare	

Blood group antigen	Severity	Frequency	Notes
DAK (RH54)	Unknown but probable	Rare	Anti-DAK is often found in multispecific sera DIIIa LFA
LOCR (RH55)	Moderate	Rare	
Partial D phenotypes	Moderate to severe	Rare	
MNS blood group system			
S (MNS3)	None to severe	Rare	
s (MNS4)	None to severe	Rare	
U (MNS5)	Mild to severe	Rare	
Mi^a (MNS7)	Mild to severe	Rare	
Vw (MNS9)	None to severe	Rare	
Mur (MNS10)	None to severe	rare	
Mt^a (MNS14)	None to severe	rare	
Hut (MNS19)	None to moderate	Rare	
Hil (MNS20)	None to moderate	Rare	
M^v (MNS21)	None to moderate	Rare	
Far (MNS22)	Severe	Very rare	1 case reported
sD (MNS23)	None to severe	Rare	
En^a (MNS28)	None to severe	Rare	
Or (MNS31)	None to moderate	Very rare	
MUT (MNS35)	Moderate	Very rare	1 case reported
P1PK blood group system			
P^k (P1PK3)	None to severe	Rare	
Lutheran blood group system			
Lu^a (LU1)	None to mild	Rare	
Lu^b (LU2)	None to mild	Rare	
LU14	None to mild	Very rare	1 case reported
Kell blood group system			
K (KEL1)	Mild to severe	Common	Depresses erythropoeisis
k (KEL2)	Mild to severe	Rare	K+k- approx. 1:1000 in Europeans
Kp^a (KEL3)	Mild to severe	Very rare	

(Continued)

TABLE 3.1 Continued

Blood group antigen	Severity	Frequency	Notes
Kp^b (KEL4)	Mild to moderate	Very rare	Kp(a+) 2% in Caucasians Kp(a+b-) very rare
Ku (KEL5)	Mild to severe	Very rare	Anti-Ku made by K$_{null}$
Js^a (KEL6)	Mild to severe	Rare	More frequent in individuals of African descent
Js^b (KEL7)	Mild to severe	Rare	
Ul^a (KEL10)	None to moderate	Very rare	1 case reported, not strongly immunogenic
K11	None to mild	Very rare	
K14	None to mild	Very rare	1 case reported
K18	None to mild	Very rare	1 case reported
VONG (KEL28)	None to mild	Very rare	1 case reported
Duffy blood group system			
Fy^a (FY1)	Mild to severe	Rare	
Fy^b (FY2)	Mild	Rare	
FY3	Mild	Rare	
Kidd blood group system			
Jk^a (JK1)	Mild to moderate	Rare	
JK^b (JK2)	None to mild	Rare	
JK3	None to mild	Very rare	Maybe found in Jk$_{null}$ (Jk(a-b-) individuals)
Diego blood group system			
Di^a (DI1)	Mild to severe	Rare	Higher frequency in S. American Indians
Di^b (DI2)	Mild	Rare	
Wr^a (DI3)	Mild to severe	Rare	A relatively common antibody, but HDFN rare
WARR (DI7)	Mild	Very rare	
ELO (DI8)	Mild to severe	Very rare	
Scianna blood group system			
SC2	None to mild	Rare	
SC3	None to mild	Rare	
SC4	Mild to severe	Rare	
Colton blood group system			
Co^a (CO1)	Mild to severe	rare	
Co^b (CO2)	Mild	Rare	

Blood group antigen	Severity	Frequency	Notes
CO3	Severe	Very rare	Antibody made by Co$_{null}$ individuals
LW blood group system			
LW^a	None to mild	Very rare	
LW^b	None to mild	Very rare	
Gerbich blood group system			
GE3	Mild to severe	Rare	
Dh^a (GE8)	Severe	Very rare	1 case reported in 2016
Indian blood group system			
INFI (IN3)	Mild	Very rare	1 case reported
P blood group system			
P (P1)	None to mild		
RHAG blood group system			
RHAG4	Severe	Very rare	1 case reported
Junior blood group system			
Jr^a (JR1)	Severe	Very rare	Fatal in 1 reported case
Lan blood group system			
Lan	None to mild	Very rare	
VEL blood group system			
VEL	Severe	Rare	
Augustine (AUG) blood group system			
At^a	None to mild	Rare	Low frequency antigen

Bilirubin detoxification—neonatal period

During pregnancy, the maternal pathways to eliminate toxic breakdown products from fetal erythrocyte senescence (predominantly bilirubin and biliverdin) are predominant. In adults, effete (senescent) erythrocytes are removed by splenic macrophages, and the haem and globin are recycled. The haem is broken down to Fe^{2+} and bilirubin which then associates with serum albumin and is transported to the liver for detoxification. The liver contains a number of enzymes called UDP-glucoronosyltransferases (UGTs) at least one of which catalyses the glucoronidation of bilirubin to form a soluble conjugate. Conjugated bilirubin is then excreted into the gut as bile via the gall bladder. Bile is then broken down by gut flora to urobilinogen and stercobilinogen both of which are eventually excreted by reabsorption of urobilinogen via the kidney and disposal in urine and stercobilinogen in faeces which gives rise to its colour. Urobilinogen is

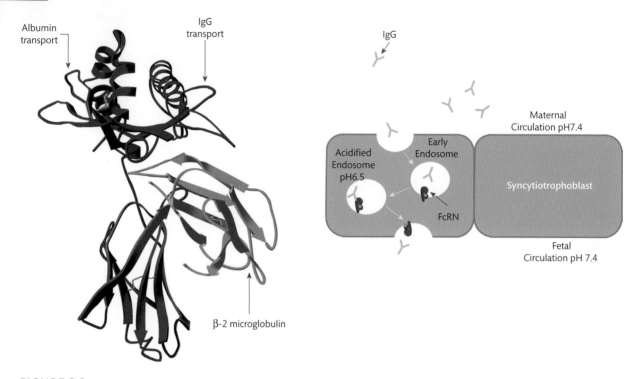

FIGURE 3.1
Three dimensional structure of the IgG transport molecule FcRN.
FcRN has a single membrane-spanning domain and two MHC class I-like extracellular domains, and like MHC-I binds a single β2-microglobulin molecule. FcRN binds IgG at acidic pH (binding site indicated) and also traffics albumin. In the right-hand panel FcRN binds IgG in acidic vesicles (pH 6.5), but is initially pinocytosed into endosomes by the placental syncytiotrophoblast, which becomes acidified, permitting IgG to bind to FcRN. The acidic endosome migrates to the fetal surface and IgG release is achieved when exposed to the fetal plasma at physiological pH.

colourless, but on exposure becomes oxidized and is an indicator of excessive bilirubin breakdown in the urine of anaemic individuals. After birth, fetal UGTs become active in the developing liver and then affect the bilirubin breakdown pathway in the infant. As the UGTs take several weeks to achieve maximal expression, the newborn can become jaundiced which is relatively common (termed physiological jaundice which occurs in 50–60% of newborns), but in HDFN cases this is much more exaggerated. As mentioned previously, excess unconjugated bilirubin is toxic due to its insolubility. It is deposited at the base of the brain causing kernicterus leading to neonatal brain damage. It was discovered in the late 1950s that bilirubin, when exposed to blue wavelength light is oxidized to soluble biliverdin, which does not cause kernicterus. Phototherapy is therefore a key treatment regime for newborns that have mild HDFN (see Section 3.5).

> **Key points**
>
> - HDFN and NAITP are diseases caused respectively by erythrocyte and platelet antigen incompatibility.
> - Incompatibility is caused by IgG which is transported by the FcRN transport system. IgM antibodies do not participate in alloimmune diseases.
> - The causes of HDFN are anaemia caused by fetal erythrocyte destruction, and by the build up of toxic waste products from haemoglobin break down.

- Why is the D antigen the most common cause of HDFN?
- Anti-A and anti-B are very common, why is therefore ABO HDFN not more frequent than it is?

3.2 Clinical management–laboratory investigations

Serological blood grouping and antibody detection

A timeline of antenatal management of HDFN is shown in Figure 3.2. At the first booking appointment during pregnancy, maternal blood grouping and the analysis of maternal serum for any blood group specific antibodies is performed. This process is a critical one for the **anti-D prophylaxis programme** which has been hugely successful in the large reduction in the incidence of HDFN. Where RhD negative mothers are identified, anti-D levels are monitored at subsequent antenatal tests. As mentioned in Chapter 2, D variant individuals, if exposed to D-positive erythrocytes, can make clinically significant anti-D. In the 'common' (its incidence is approximately 1:4000 individuals in the UK) DVI phenotype, there have been examples described in the literature where DVI phenotype mothers have made severe and clinically significant anti-D to the extent where there has been neonatal death due to HDFN. For this reason, DVI phenotype individuals are treated as D-negative patients during pregnancy, and the anti-D used for serological testing of mothers in the UK and other EC countries is selected to fail to react with DVI phenotype erythrocytes (it is an anti-epD6, RUM-1).

Prophylactic anti-D
A purified antibody preparation obtained from hyperimmunized male volunteers and given to RhD negative mothers to prevent alloimmunization.

Other blood group systems causing HDFN

Table 3.1 highlights that 17 of the 36 of the blood group systems have one or more antigens that have been reported as causing HDFN. It is important to stress though that in theory any antigenic variation between mother and fetus can result in alloimmunization and potentially IgG traffic to cause HDFN. As can be seen from Table 3.1 many have been reported as a single case, whilst HDFN due to anti-D, -K, and -c make up the bulk of the workload of obstetric departments managing alloimmunized mothers. It is, however, critical that the obstetric team in combination with the skilled immunohaematologist are able to detect rare maternal antibodies that could cause HDFN, and take appropriate clinical intervention as required.

Several additional factors must be considered when managing a pregnancy when antibody identification is needed. First certain antibodies are almost only found in certain ethnic groups—for example anti-Di^a is only found in South American Indians.

HDFN due to anti-K

9% of the UK population are K+k+, and thus anti-K can be made by K-k+ mothers. Anti-K is potentially very serious, and causes fetal anaemia by a different mechanism to that of anti-D. The Kell glycoprotein is expressed by early erythroid progenitors and also is present on fetal erythrocytes at an earlier stage of pregnancy (Rh antigens are not fully expressed until around 22 weeks' gestation). It is therefore believed that anti-K causes anaemia by disruption of fetal erythropoiesis rather than monocyte destruction and release of excess bilirubin

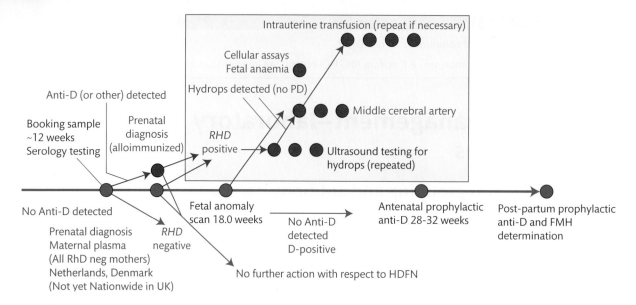

FIGURE 3.2

Antenatal management of HDFN.

The major clinical and laboratory investigations used currently (2016) in the management of fetal alloimmune anaemia caused by anti-D. The figure depicts the major diagnostic events during pregnancy (horizontal blue line) from booking (approximately 12 weeks). The blue line is not to scale as interventions and non-invasive diagnosis can be as early as 14 weeks depending on ultrasound results. At-risk activities are indicated in red, low risk in blue. The figure depicts the clinical and laboratory activities for the management of alloimmunized D-negative mothers that have made anti-D, but similar if not identical approaches are made for other detected antibodies, with the exception that prophylactic antibody treatment is not available.

in the fetal spleen as is seen in anti-D HDFN. K/k incompatible pregnancies are routinely referred for prenatal diagnosis at an early stage, and the treatment of anaemia is monitored and managed as per RhD HDFN.

HDFN due to anti-c

Anti-c is a major cause of HDFN, and like anti-K is a major concern as it accounts for a significant number of deaths (in the UK recent figures 46 deaths per 100,000 pregnancies) indicate approximately half of fetal and neonatal deaths are attributed to anti-D; the remaining further deaths are due to all other antibodies, the majority being anti-K and anti-c). In mothers that have made anti-c a significant proportion have severe HDFN requiring intrauterine or exchange transfusion. There is no prophylactic anti-c and non-invasive prenatal testing in Rh C+c- mothers is available.

HDFN due to other RH system antibodies

Table 3.1 lists RH system antibodies that have caused HDFN. Aside from anti-D and anti-c, anti-C, -E, -e, and G (an antigen expressed on C+D+ erythrocytes) is comparatively rare—the antibodies rarely cause HDFN—but when they do, it can be severe. However it is important that where an anaemic fetus has been determined as being D-negative by PCR, the presence of other RH system antibodies are defined, and the fetus genotyped (for example for RHCE.C or RHCE.E).

ABO HDFN

Despite the common occurrence of IgG anti-A and -B, HDFN due to these antibodies is rare, although obstetric interventions are not unknown. This may be due in part to the fact that A and B antigen expression in the developing fetus is comparatively weak, and that expression occurs on many tissues and in the plasma of the fetus. Fetal plasma is deficient in complement components, a key player in splenic haemolysis. Complement-mediated destruction of fetal erythrocytes by maternal IgG in the fetal spleen is a key pathology in HDFN. Most maternal anti-A and anti-B are of IgM subtype, and thus cannot transit across the placenta.

Partial D phenotypes in HDFN

As described in Chapter 2, partial D phenotype individuals can make anti-D when exposed to D-positive blood. This is because they have variant D polypeptides lacking D epitopes, which is variable depending on the mutation causing the phenotype. In the DVI phenotype (one of the most common in Europe) the most immunogenic D epitopes are missing from the erythrocytes (epD6/7). In pregnancy, therefore, a DVI phenotype mother can make anti-D if she carries a D-positive fetus with a normal *RHD* gene inherited from the father. In many countries DVI phenotype mothers are typed using anti-D that does not react with their erythrocytes; in other words, they are deliberately typed as D-negative (see earlier), and consequently will receive prophylactic anti-D. There have been reported cases of fetal death due to HDFN in DVI mothers. However, in the absence of maternal genotyping for *RHD*, other partial D phenotype mothers may be typed as D-positive and make potentially clinically significant anti-D. The partial D phenotypes DIIIc and DBT have been reported to cause severe HDFN, and there is a possibility that there are others. One aspect of partial D phenotypes already discussed in Chapter 2 is that novel structures arising from the genomic arrangements causing partial D phenotypes (e.g. hybrid RHD-RHCE polypeptides, point mutations causing externalized amino acid changes) creates a low-frequency antigen. For example, Tar (RH40) is associated with the DVII phenotype, and Go[a] (RH30) with the DIVa phenotype. In cases of D-negative mothers carrying partial D phenotype fetuses, these low-frequency antigens have caused severe HDFN (see Table 3.1).

Key points

■ The most severe causes of HDFN are due to anti-D, -K, and -c. They are therefore part of the routine maternal antibody screen.

■ Many other blood group antigens can cause HDFN, but they are not routinely screened for.

SELF-CHECK 3.2

- Why are partial DVI phenotype mothers deliberately serologically typed as D-negative?
- HDFN due to anti-K of the Kell system can often be very severe early in pregnancy—why is this the case?

Paternal zygosity testing

Using quantitative real-time PCR and other methods it is possible to define the zygosity status of the father, where paternity can be assumed. *RHD* genotypes are thus homozygous (e.g. CDe/CDe) or hemizygous (e.g. CDe/cde). If a father is homozygous of *RHD* the fetus will invariably be D-positive but has a 50% chance of being D-positive if the father is hemizygous.

3.3 **Prophylactic anti-D**

Since the late 1960s anti-D, prepared from D-negative hyperimmunized male volunteers, has been administered following the birth of a D-positive baby to a D-negative mother. It is a highly effective treatment and prevents alloimmunization in the vast majority of mothers, but is not 100% efficient. The *post-partum* administration (the norm until the last decade) was the main cause of failure to prevent alloimmunization due to the fact that there are small fetal haemorrhages into the maternal circulation during the latter stages of pregnancy. In the past decade, most countries have switched to the administration of prophylactic anti-D during the third trimester (normally given at 28–32 weeks), and has resulted in the reduction of alloimmunization events. This treatment is recommended by NICE in the UK.

Fetal prophylaxis—possible immunological mechanisms

In most countries with high proportions of D-negative women of childbearing age, there is a routine screening programme in place to prevent alloimmunization to the D antigen. This programme arose through pioneering work in the late 1960s by a number of UK-and Canadian-based researchers. They had hypothesized that the rapid elimination of fetal D-positive blood from the D-negative maternal circulation could prevent alloimmunization. It appears most likely that this is due to the fact that splenic macrophages routinely remove senescent erythrocytes during routine blood circulation, and thus any antibody-coated erythrocyte would be rapidly removed in the spleen before any peripheral blood memory B lymphocytes are primed to induce an immune response. However, recent work has tended to suggest that rapid removal of fetal erythrocytes, coated with prophylactic antibody is not the immunologic mechanism of anti-D prophylaxis. This work quite rightly notes that engulfment by macrophages usually elicits release of pro-inflammatory cytokines, and thus accelerating an immune response and B and T cell activation.

In immunological terms, it is not entirely clear how prophylactic anti-D works. There are three proposed models, as presented in Figure 3.3. A probable mechanism is that the prophylactic anti-D blocks the cross linking of the B cell receptor (BCR) and thereby preventing its activation, which is driven by immunoreceptor tyrosine activation motifs (ITAMs) carried by the α and β chains of CD79 that form a multimeric complex with the BCR. ITAMs induce cell signalling pathways when their tyrosine residues become phosphorylated as a direct result of external ligation of the BCR with antigen. The B cell then becomes activated, and matures to form a plasma cell producing antibody and memory B cells. In turn immunoreceptor tyrosine inhibitor motifs (ITIMs) are stimulated when prophylactic anti-D IgG molecules bind to FcγRII

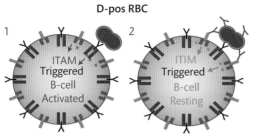

1. B cell activation via ITAM activation of BCR (no prophylactic anti-D)
2. Inhibition of BCR cross linking and trigger of FcγRII ITIM

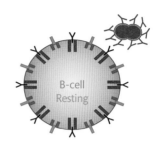

3. Masking of D antigen by prophylactic anti-D

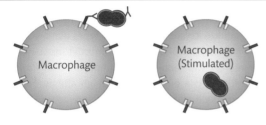

4. Rapid macrophage RBC engulfment

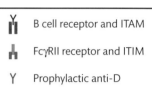

	B cell receptor and ITAM
	FcγRII receptor and ITIM
Y	Prophylactic anti-D
	FcγRI & FcγRIII and ITAM

FIGURE 3.3
Possible immunological mechanisms of action of prophylactic anti-D.
The immune cells involved in the humoral response to the D are depicted (T cells not shown). The major immune regulatory molecules that bind IgG are also shown, including the B cell receptor (BCR) and the Fcγ receptors RI (macrophage), RII (B-cell), and RIII (macrophage). 1. Normal immune response on exposure of maternal B cells to fetal D-positive blood. The BCR immunoreceptor tyrosine activation motif (ITAM) becomes phosphorylated when the BCR specific to the D antigen binds fetal D antigen, and is cross-linked by the erythrocyte to at least one other BCR. This activates the B cell to become a plasma cell producing initially IgM and in a secondary immune response the pathogenic IgG anti-D. A proportion of the B cells will become memory B cells that participate in the secondary response. 2. Prophylactic anti-D is bound to the fetal D-positive erythrocyte, and prevents cross-linking of two BCRs, and also binds to FcγRII, which possesses immunoreceptor tyrosine inhibitor motifs (ITIMs). This leads to no B cell activation. 3. Saturation of fetal D antigen sites, blocking cross-linking of BCRs, probably unlikely as very high levels of anti-D would be required to saturate fetal D antigen sites. 4. Rapid removal of sensitized D-positive fetal cells by maternal macrophages before B cells are activated. Again unlikely as macrophage FcγRI and FcγRIII receptors possess ITAMs, and thus recruitment of both B and Th cells.

receptors on the surface of the B lymphocyte. Interestingly, macrophages possess both FcγRI and FcγRIII that have ITAM motifs, and a model for the mechanism of prophylactic anti-D has proposed that the rapid engulfment of sensitized erythrocytes (and before B cells bind the D-positive fetal erythrocytes) by macrophages inhibits the humoral response. This is at odds with the well-known responses of macrophages in recruiting both B and Th cells when engulfing foreign bodies.

Cellular assays to predict the severity of HDFN

The utilization of cellular-based assays has declined since their peak in the early 1990s, and were then used frequently in the management of HDFN. Their use in particular the UK is much reduced, but some countries (e.g. the Netherlands) still use them as part of a routine screening programme of alloimmunized women. For this reason, and the fact that it readily demonstrates the cellular responses involved in fetal erythrocyte destruction, they are described here.

Antibody titres measured manually or by autoanalyser are used to quantify the level of anti-D in maternal serum. However, this measure is not on its own sufficient to predict the possible occurrence of severe HDFN. It is rare for mothers with anti-D levels of 4 IU/ml (0.8 μg/ml) or less to have severely affected fetuses, but this level cannot be used as a threshold value. Several instances in the literature have shown no sign of HDFN in mothers with titres of 6 IU/ml or more. This variance in response reflects the fact that there are significant differences between the biological and functional characteristics of anti-D between alloimmunized mothers. Furthermore, in up to a third of all cases of alloimmunization, almost all IgG subclass is IgG1, and in the remainder a mixture of IgG1 and IgG 3.

A number of cellular-based assays have been developed since the 1960s to predict the severity of HDFN (see Figure 3.4). All assays utilize isolated immune cell types that are involved in the pathogenesis of HDFN, namely K (killer)-lymphocytes and (mostly) monocytes. These cells bear IgG (FcR)receptors that interact with anti-D; K-lymphocytes bear FcγRIIIa and monocytes FcγRIa, FcRγIIa, and FcRγIIIa. FcRγIa binds IgG with high affinity, FcRγIIa with low affinity, and FcRγIIIa with an intermediate affinity. The FcR-IgG interaction involves the

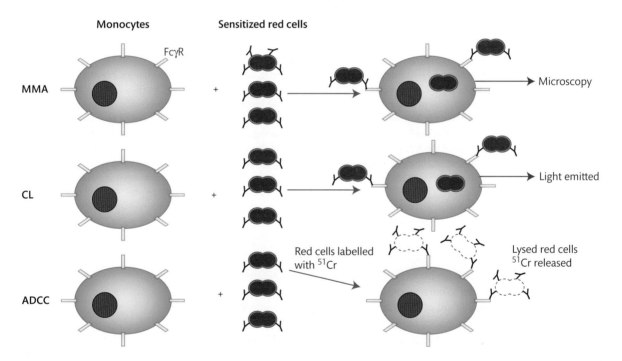

FIGURE 3.4
Cellular assays to predict the severity of HDFN.
MMA: monocyte monolayer assay. Monocytes derived from peripheral blood are incubated with D-positive erythrocytes and maternal derived anti-D. The level of monocyte binding of erythrocytes is then monitored by microscopy.
CL: chemiluminescence test. Monocytes are as above incubated with D-positive erythrocytes and maternally derived anti-D. Monocyte metabolic responses are proportional to their immune activity, and incubation with a chemiluminescent substrate leads to release of light and reflects this level of metabolic activity.
ADCC: antibody -dependent cellular cytotoxicity. Monocytes are incubated with ^{51}Cr labelled erythrocytes which have been sensitized with maternal anti-D. The release of ^{51}Cr from lysed erythrocytes that bind to monocytes is directly proportional to their immune activity.

N-glycosylated residue Asn-297 (of IgG) to which is attached a branched carbohydrate moiety. These carbohydrates can have varying levels of fucosylation, with low fucose content having higher affinity for the FcγR. To further complicate issues, the Fcγ receptors exhibit polymorphisms that affect their binding to IgG. In response to these inter-individual variations, a number of cellular-based assays have been developed to predict the severity of HDFN by assay of the interaction of maternal anti-D with effector cells (K-lymphocytes or monocytes).

Antibody-dependent cellular cytotoxicity assay (ADCC)

ADCC has been developed to use either K-lymphocytes (K-ADCC) or monocytes (M-ADCC) to predict HDFN severity, these cells are sourced from normal blood donors. Most diagnostically utilized assays are M-ADCC based, and the purified monocytes and maternal serum are mixed with ^{51}Cr-labelled D-positive erythrocytes. The levels of erythrocyte lysis are then measured by counting ^{51}Cr-release into the assay supernatant. In some countries (e.g. the Netherlands) the M-ADCC is used on all alloimmunized pregnancies, and a threshold level then indicates where further obstetric management is required.

Monocyte monolayer assay (MMA) and chemiluminescence test (CLT)

In the MMA, isolated monocytes (purified by density centrifugation) are plated onto culture plates as a monolayer and are incubated with sensitized D-positive erythrocytes—using maternal anti-D from serum. The antibody-coated erythrocytes are then engulfed or adhere to the macrophage surface, which is visualized through a microscope. By utilizing the fact that monocytes undergo metabolic changes, an adaptation of this test is to use a chemiluminescent substrate which gives off light. The reaction is then monitored in a luminometer and the extent of erythrocyte adherence/engulfment is directly proportional to the light emitted.

Fetomaternal haemorrhage (FMH) determination

After delivery a sample of maternal blood from D-negative women is analysed by the Kleihauer-Betke test. This is performed in order to detect any excessive bleed during childbirth that may diminish the effectiveness of the administered prophylactic anti-D. This is also performed if there are any potential sensitizing events after 20 weeks of pregnancy (e.g. a fall, miscarriage, amniocentesis, ectopic pregnancy, etc.). This is a cytological stain prepared from a maternal peripheral blood smear, which is washed with an acid buffer and stained with haematoxylin. Adult haemoglobin is predominantly $\alpha2\beta2$, and is acid soluble whilst fetal haemoglobin is predominantly $\alpha2\gamma2$ and is not acid soluble, and forms the basis of the test. Fetal erythrocytes are readily stained, whilst the majority adult erythrocytes are not and appear as 'ghosts'. Based on the count of fetal erythrocytes, and using various calculations in the literature, an estimate of the fetal leakage into the maternal circulation is made. If the fetal leak is >2 ml then flow cytometric analysis of maternal blood is performed. Here the flow cytometer is able to count the number of (fetal) D-positive erythrocytes amongst tens of thousands of maternal (D-negative) cells. The flow cytometer detects fluorescently labelled erythrocytes—the maternal blood being previously incubated with a dye-labelled anti-D. Normally the dye used is fluorescein isothiocyanate (FITC). Based on the level of FMH, an additional dose of anti-D is then administered calculated on the basis of 125 IU per ml of fetal leaked cells when administered intramuscularly. The normal administered dose of 500 IU is thought to give protection of a fetal leak of up to 4 ml.

3.4 Neonatal alloimmune thrombocytopaenia (NAITP)

NAITP can be considered an analogous disease to HDFN, but with a markedly different pathology due to the cellular components being very different, namely alloimmunization leading to a shortage of fetal platelets rather than erythrocytes. As described in Chapter 6 almost all platelet antigens are caused by single nucleotide polymorphisms (SNPs) in a number of platelet expressed genes, most notably located on integrins in the platelet membrane. The reader is referred to Chapter 6 for more details on platelet antigens, but also to Chapter 9, as HLA molecules are also present on the platelet membrane and thus anti-HLA antibodies can sometimes lead to platelet destruction.

Key points

- Prophylactic anti-D has been a major triumph of twentieth- century medicine, dramatically reducing the incidence of anti-D HDFN, once a common cause of fetal mortality.

- The mechanism of the action of prophylactic anti-D remains unknown, but it may be due to the rapid removal of fetal D-positive erythrocytes by macrophages or negative feedback mechanisms imposed on B cells.

SELF-CHECK 3.3

- Why is there a requirement to monitor the levels of fetal erythrocytes leaked into the maternal circulation? How is it performed?

- What are the similarities and differences between HDFN and NAITP (see Chapter 6 before answering this!)

Fetal genotyping
The process of defining fetal blood group using DNA-based methods. This now has switched from the analysis of amniotic fluid to the analysis of maternal plasma at no risk to the fetus.

3.5 Fetal genotyping

Once the main culprits that cause HDFN and NAITP were identified at the molecular level, DNA-based tests were developed to define fetal blood group using initially invasively sampled material (mainly amniocytes obtained following amniocentesis, but sometimes chorionic villus sampled material was used) and were published and pressed into clinical use. This was first described in 1993. The tests exploited DNA extraction of fetal cells that were usually discarded during Liley curve investigations, which was a mainstream technique in the clinical management of HDFN since the 1950s to estimate bilirubin levels (now largely obsolete, see Section 3.6). In the period 1993–1999 techniques to genotype alleles that predicted fetal blood group RhD, c, E, K1, and Fy^a were published and implemented into routine clinical use. For most blood group alleles requiring detection using DNA-based methods this was a relatively simple procedure to use a PCR-based test, but for RHD it was realized that due to the fact that multiple alleles caused D-negative phenotypes and that certain partial D phenotypes had hybrid *RHD–RHCE* genes, at least two regions of the *RHD* gene should be analysed by a multiplex PCR. A summary of the technical aspects of the diagnostic PCR assays used is described in Chapter 2.

In 1997 there was a significant breakthrough in the field of prenatal diagnostics. Professor Dennis Lo, at the time working at the Radcliffe Infirmary in Oxford, had discovered that there were very significant amounts of **free fetal DNA** (ffDNA) found in the maternal circulation. He had surmised correctly that because the placenta was undergoing rapid growth, free DNA, discovered just a few years earlier by analysis of tumours, would be present in the maternal circulation. Lo et al., followed by others, used maternal plasma from D-negative mothers to test the applicability of this phenomena in a diagnostic test to define fetal RhD blood group status to great effect. The key benefit of switching from DNA extraction from amniocytes to ffDNA in maternal plasma was that amniocentesis, an invasive and risky procedure, was not required. Amniocentesis is generally regarded as having a risk of 1% spontaneous miscarriage, which, compounded with the fact that there is often significant risk of fetal haemorrhage, potentially exacerbates the alloimmunization event. High-risk HDFN pregnancies have been for over a decade tested using non-invasive methods of sampling fetal DNA using maternal plasma. Some countries including the Netherlands and Denmark have introduced mass-scale prenatal *RHD* genotyping using maternal plasma. This identifies RhD-positive fetuses and thus directs the efficient use of antenatal prophylactic anti-D to only these pregnancies. Mothers with RhD-negative fetuses do not require such treatment (which is approximately 40% of cases), and is thus useful economically and avoids the unnecessary use of a human-derived product.

> **Free fetal DNA (ffDNA)**
> Placentally derived DNA found in maternal blood that is >150 bp and used now extensively in the non-invasive prenatal diagnosis of blood groups.

3.6 Clinical management—obstetrics

Ultrasonagraphy

Part of the routine investigation performed on the developing fetus is to screen for signs of hydrops or hepatosplenomegaly when immune antibodies have been detected. This is done by ultrasound (see Figure 3.5). In the past, where hydrops was detected, amniocentesis was performed and the levels of bilirubin measured by determining the absorbance of the supernatant fraction at 450 nm. The absorbance was then compared to a Liley curve which was able

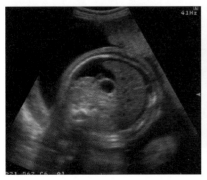
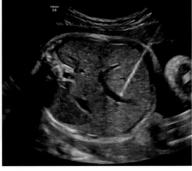

FIGURE 3.5

Ultrasound monitoring and intrauterine transfusion.

The left photograph shows a fetus demonstrating fetal liver ascites, whilst the right hand photograph shows a fetus undergoing intrauterine transfusion into the intrahepatic vein. There is a thin rim of ascites where the needle is inserted into the fetus. Photo courtesy Dr Tim Overton, St Michael's Hospital, Bristol.

to predict the severity of HDFN in the fetus. Liley curves were first published in 1961, when the management of HDFN (then termed HDN as most clinical management was in the newborn period) was of newborns and in the third trimester of pregnancy. As obstetrics advanced, management of the second trimester became the norm. As Liley curves proved to be inaccurate when extrapolated back to the second trimester, John Queenan and colleagues in 1993 published improved curves (hence called Queenan curves) for predicting severity of HDFN from as early as 14 weeks' gestation. These techniques have largely become historical and replaced by middle cerebral artery assessment.

Middle cerebral artery (MCA) measurement

Doppler ultrasonagraphy
A method of ultrasound that measures the blood flow in vessels non-invasively (see middle cerebral artery)

MCA **Doppler ultrasonagraphy** has replaced the use of amniocentesis followed by OD_{450} prediction of HDFN risk. MCA Doppler measures the velocity of fetal blood flow in the fetal middle cerebral artery, and can predict the severity of anaemia based on the fact that anaemic fetuses will have higher blood velocities than normal. This technique was first described in the mid-1990s (Mari et al., 2000), and is now a routine technique used by obstetricians (see Figure 3.6). Based on MCA measurements or other means to predict fetal anaemia different clinical decisions are then made to manage the pregnancy. Fetal blood sampling (FBS) is still performed, and of course is an invasive procedure where fetal blood is sampled via a needle under ultrasound guidance. This is often performed in conjunction with cordocentesis where anaemia has been shown to be severe.

Severe risk of HDFN

Cordocentesis (or intrauterine transfusion) is performed in severely affected fetuses under ultrasound guidance. In all cases of HDFN due to anti-D, D-negative erythrocyte units are used, and are specially prepared. All fetal transfusions are performed with O-negative (unless fetal ABO type known) K-negative, plasma-depleted (haemocrit of 0.7–0.85), leucodepleted, CMV antibody-negative, sickle-negative, and five days or less in age erythrocyte units. The units

FIGURE 3.6
Middle cerebral artery (MCA) Doppler ultrasonagraphy.
Photograph shows a fetus undergoing MCA assessment. The fetal blood flow velocity in the middle cerebral artery is measured by Doppler ultrasonography. High velocities compared to the normal range are proportional to the level of fetal anaemia. The MCA is clearly shown in this photograph in red. This analysis has almost completely replaced the measurement of fetal anaemia by amniocentesis and OD_{450} measurement of the amniotic fluid to estimate fetal bilirubin levels. Photo courtesy Dr Tim Overton, St Michael's Hospital, Bristol.

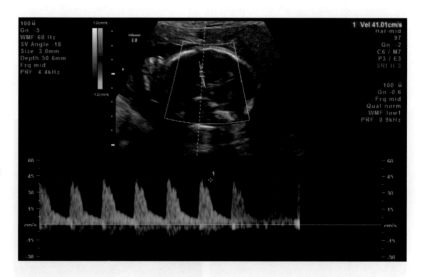

use citrate phosphate dextrose as **anticoagulant** to avoid problems using other anticoagulants, and are gamma irradiated to destroy any residual leucocytes that may cause transfusion associated graft versus host disease. A cross match of the to be transfused cells and maternal serum is performed to confirm compatibility, and the unit is prewarmed to 37°C prior to transfusion. Cordocentesis is normally performed between 14 and 34 weeks of pregnancy, and repeated if signs of anaemia are still apparent.

Anticoagulant
A substance which when it is added to the blood inhibits clotting.

Severe to moderate HDFN—exchange transfusion

Exchange transfusion is performed in the neonatal period on severely anaemic newborns that have either demonstrated heart failure or have severe hyperbilirubinaemia. As discussed earlier in the chapter, once born, the neonatal UDP-glucoronyltransferases that conjugate bilirubin take several weeks to become fully expressed. In this period, therefore, the neonate is susceptible to kernicterus where there are high levels of bilirubin, as it no longer utilizes the maternal disposal systems to eliminate this toxic by-product of erythrocyte breakdown. Constant assessment of neonatal bilirubin levels are performed (every 3–4 hours), and levels of 100 µmol/L or greater (or rapidly rising) indicate exchange transfusion is necessary, or indeed cord blood haemoglobin levels of less than 8 g/dL. Identical requirements of the transfused erythrocytes used for cordocentesis are applied. There are action tables utilized as clinical intervention depends on other variable such as neonatal age, weight, and degree of premature birth.

Moderate to mild HDFN—phototherapy

Where any sign of anaemia exists, phototherapy (blue green light, 460–490 nm) is conducted on the newborn if rapid rises in levels of bilirubin have been observed. The bilirubin molecule (termed 4Z, 15Z-bilirubin which is lipophilic) absorbs light and is converted into two structural isomers: 4Z, 15E bilirubin, and Z-lumirubin, both of which are less lipophilic and can be excreted into bile without the need for enzymic glucoronidation. Some bilirubin is also photooxidized, and generates a colourless product that can be excreted in urine.

Key points

■ HDFN clinical management has moved towards non-invasive monitoring, hence the renaming of the disease from HDN to HDFN because much of the clinical management is now in the antenatal period.

■ High-risk pregnancies are identified at an early stage due to well stratified screening and focused obstetric care.

SELF-CHECK 3.4

• Why is maternal plasma based fetal genotyping preferred in the management of HDFN?

• Why has the analysis of amniotic fluid largely been abandoned in the management of HDFN and how has it been replaced?

3.7 **Concluding comments**

HDFN was originally termed 'HDN', haemolytic disease of the newborn, but the addition of 'fetus' was made to reflect the fact that clinical management of the disease had moved on significantly in the past 20 years to managing the fetus rather than the newborn. There has been great advance in the management of the disease, which accounted for over 1:1000 fetal and neonatal deaths in the 1950s; now there are fewer than 25 deaths due to RhD HDFN per annum in the UK (approximately 640,000 pregnancies per annum). The introduction of prophylactic anti-D is the most significant treatment to cause this huge reduction, and is widely heralded as one of the best advances in medicine in the twentieth century. HDFN clinical and laboratory management is a constantly evolving area, with some techniques becoming obsolete—in fact, non-invasive prenatal *RHD* genotyping was the first mass scale application of maternal plasma-based testing, a very significant advance. The reduction in invasive amniocentesis to manage HDFN has also been a significant medical advance, and a key driver in the eventual consignment of this technique to the history books.

 Chapter summary

■ Prevention of HDFN is now due to mass-scale screening of all pregnancies to identify those at risk (i.e. RhD-negative mothers, antibody screen).

■ The most common antibodies causing HDFN are anti-D, -K, -c, -E, and -Fy^a.

■ A large number of other blood group antigens can cause HDFN but are uncommon.

■ FcRN is a protein that mediates the transport of IgG; IgM is not transported.

■ Tests that can monitor the severity of antibodies formed are available but are not used in all countries.

■ Monitoring of at-risk pregnancies is now largely non-invasive and is done by ultrasonography (e.g. middle cerebral artery Doppler) or by fetal genotyping, utilizing free fetal DNA in maternal plasma.

 Further reading

● Avent ND. Prenatal testing for haemolytic disease of the newborn and fetal neonatal alloimmune thrombocytopenia—current status. *Expert Rev Hematol* 7 (2014), 741–745.

● Hadley A & Soothill PW. *Alloimmune Disorders of Pregnancy.* Cambridge University Press, Cambridge (2002).

● Kim YA & Makar RS Detection of fetomaternal hemorrhage. *Am J Hematol* 87 (2012), 417– 423. http://onlinelibrary.wiley.com/doi/10.1002/ajh.22255/full

- Mari G, Deter RL, Carpenter RL, Rahman F, Zimmerman R, Moise KJ Jr, Dorman KF, Ludomirsky A, Gonzalez R, Gomez R, Oz U, Detti L, Copel JA, Bahado-Singh R, Berry S, Martinez-Poyer J & Blackwell SC. Noninvasive diagnosis by Doppler ultrasonography of fetal anemia due to maternal red-cell alloimmunization. Collaborative Group for Doppler Assessment of the Blood Velocity in Anemic Fetuses. *N Engl J Med* 342 (2000), 9–14.

- Roopenian DC, Akilesh S. FcRN: The neonatal Fc receptor comes of age. *Nature Immunol* 7 (2007), 715–725.

- White J, Qureshi H, Massey E, Needs M, Byrne G, Daniels G & Allard S. Guideline for blood grouping and erythrocyte antibody testing in pregnancy. *Transfusion Med* 26 (2016), 246–263. http://onlinelibrary.wiley.com/doi/10.1111/tme.12299/epdf

Answers to the questions in this chapter are provided on the book's accompanying website:

Go to www.oup.com/uk/avent2e

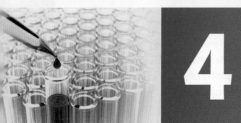

4

Clinical Use of Blood Components

Lionel Mohabir

Learning objectives

After studying this chapter you should be able to:

- Understand basic circulatory physiology and the structure and function of the components of blood.
- Understand the normal physiological response to anaemia and/or bleeding and how different patient groups may respond.
- Understand the coagulation cascade.
- Describe the different blood components available and their appropriate and inappropriate use based on best practice national guidelines.
- Understand the preparation of plasma products by fractionation and recombinant technology.
- Understand the benefits of transfusion therapy and the alternatives available to using allogeneic blood.
- Outline how best to manage the use of the precious resource—blood.
- Understand how good communication, standards, audit, and review of product use will aid appropriate use of blood components.
- Outline national initiatives designed to facilitate the appropriate use of blood.

Introduction

This chapter covers the function of blood *in vivo* and the body's response to anaemia and bleeding. Having gained an understanding of what blood component is needed for within the body, the reader can then consider how to best support patients by choosing the most appropriate treatment therapies. This chapter does not contain detailed information about blood components themselves, their manufacture, preparation for use, or the appropriate groups to be issued. However, there is an overview of the coagulation cascade, plasma fractionation, and recombinant technology. This chapter also considers the alternatives available to traditional transfusion therapies based on donor (allogeneic) blood.

4.1 Structure and function of blood

It is important to understand the function of the individual components *in vivo* before considering the therapeutic use of the blood components currently available. Blood is a complex fluid which is essential for life, carrying oxygen, nutrients, chemical messages, and waste products to and from the tissues and organs of the body, and playing a significant role in regulating the body's temperature and preventing disease and blood loss. The arteries transport blood away from the heart towards tissues and organs, the thin walled capillaries allow exchange between the tissues and the circulating blood. The veins return the blood back to the heart. The different organs of the body have different circulatory requirements, with cardiac output being adjusted depending on individual needs. For example, when exercising the usually high requirement of the digestive systems and the kidneys is diverted to skeletal muscle.

When blood is removed from the body and mixed with an anticoagulant it will slowly separate into three distinct layers. This process can be accelerated by centrifugation. The layers are:

- Erythrocytes (red cells) are at the bottom; these cells transport gases. An adult will have over 20 trillion red cells, each with a lifespan of about 120 days. Red cell production is triggered by a reduction in oxygen delivery to the kidneys, which secrete the hormone erythropoietin. Erythropoietin stimulates the bone marrow into producing more red cells whose primary function is the transport of oxygen.

- **Buffy coat**, containing leucocytes (white cells) and **thrombocytes** (platelets) forms the middle layer. Leucocytes defend the body against invasion by microorganisms and foreign antigens. Thrombocytes are fragments of larger cells, megakaryocytes, and play a major role in the formation of blood clots following injury.

- Plasma is the top layer. Plasma contains salts and proteins (albumin, globulins, and clotting factors) dissolved in water, and carries nutrients, wastes, and hormones. Albumin is a large, 'sticky' protein which cannot easily cross the capillary walls. Albumin molecules bind salts, bilirubin, and some drugs for transportation around the circulation, but also play a significant role in maintaining the osmotic pressure of the vessels, by pulling in or repelling water. Globulins are proteins that are involved with transporting ions and vitamins and gamma globulins, the body's defences.

The volume of blood present depends on the size and weight of the individual, but in an adult is usually around four to six litres, of which approximately 55% will be plasma and 45% red cells.

Buffy coat
The layer of leucocytes and platelets sitting on top of the red cell layer after centrifugation.

Thrombocytes
Alternative term for platelets (especially in Europe).

4.2 Normal physiological response to anaemia and/or bleeding

Oxygen is delivered to the tissues by the haemoglobin (Hb) inside the red cells. The oxygen transport system normally operates to maintain constant oxygen consumption (although this will vary depending on the individual needs of each tissue/organ). Oxygen delivery is the product of cardiac output and the oxygen content of the arterial blood. When oxygen delivery to the tissues decreases, oxygen extraction from the lungs increases. The oxygen dissociation curve is a graphical plot that shows the proportion of saturated haemoglobin against the oxygen tension. This determines how readily haemoglobin will release the oxygen molecules to the tissues. When this compensation cannot occur, hypoxia (low oxygen) results and this can cause tissue damage and even, in extreme conditions, organ death. Whilst a patient's haemoglobin level is helpful when deciding whether a patient needs transfusion, the individual's vascular system, cardiac, lung, and bone marrow function will greatly affect the decision whether or not to transfuse.

Other factors that affect oxygen delivery include body temperature, acid base status, 2,3-diphosphoglycerate (2,3 DPG) levels, and the structure of the haemoglobin molecule itself (i.e. anything other than the 'normal' Hb AA can affect oxygen carrying and delivery).

In a patient, transfusion of red cells may be considered because a fall in the number of red cells (drop in haemoglobin) has been observed. The drop in haemoglobin may be caused by loss (bleeding), decreased survival time (increased destruction), or decrease in production (bone marrow failure). Acute blood loss is not always visible as blood can accumulate in body cavities and can be very difficult to identify clinically, particularly in children.

In summary, it is important to consider each patient individually, taking into account all of the above factors, when deciding whether to transfuse.

Key points

Maintaining the supply of oxygen to the tissues by red cells is vital as hypoxia can lead to tissue damage.

4.3 **Blood coagulation**

Haemostasis is the process where blood coagulates following vascular injury and the dissolution of the clot after the damaged tissue is repaired. Platelets are attracted to the injury site and form a plug. Clotting factors become activated resulting in the formation of fibrin network over the platelet plug to form a solid clot over the injury site. Most of the clotting factors circulate in inactive forms as precursors of proteolytic enzymes.

The primary response to blood vessel damage is the formation of a platelet plug to stop the bleeding. Platelets are attracted to the wound and are activated by thrombin. von Willebrand factor (vWF) forms a bridge between platelets and collagen by binding to platelet glycoprotein GP1b and collagen. There is morphological change in the shape of the platelets, affecting the size, shape, and growing pseudopods resulting in an increase in the surface area. Platelets contain two types of granules:

- α granules contain fibrinogen, factor V, factor VIII, platelet factor IV, P-selectin, fibronectin, platelet growth factor, and tumour growth factor α.
- δ (dense) granules contain ADP, ATP, Ca^{2+}, serotonin, epinephrine, and histamine.

Degranulation of the platelets occurs following adhesion to the injury site. ADP released from δ granules increase platelets aggregation. It also causes conformational change of platelet glycoprotein GPIIb/IIIa causing deposition of fibrinogen on the platelet surface.

Two coagulation pathways result in the formation of fibrin clots (see Figure 4.1):

- **Intrinsic pathway**—this is initiated by abnormal physiology such as hyperlipidaemia and bacterial infection. It requires prekallikrein (PK) and high molecular weight kininogen (HMWK) together with calcium ions and phospholipids which are released from platelets. Contact with plasma with a negatively charged surface results in the binding of factor XII (FXII) which auto-activates to FXIIa. FXIIa activates PK to kallikrein which cleaves HMWK to produce bradykinin, which is a potent vasodilator. Kallikrein further activates FXII resulting in amplification of the system. FXIIa also activates factor XI (FXI) to FXIa which, in the presence of Ca^{2+}, converts factor IX (FIX) to FIXa. The next step in this cascade is the activation of factor X (FX) to FXa, which requires a tenase complex on the surface of activated platelets. The tenase complex consists of FVIIIa, FIXa, FX, and Ca^{2+}. FVIIIa is a cofactor in this process and is formed by activation of FVIII by minute quantities of thrombin. Higher concentrations of thrombin will inactivate FVIIIa.

- **Extrinsic pathway**—this is initiated as a result of vascular injury. After vascular damage, sub-endothelial tissue containing collagen is exposed and von Willebrand factor (vWF), tissue factor (factor III), and other proteins are released. Factor III activates prothrombin to form thrombin. One of the proteins causes constriction of the blood vessel to reduce or stem the flow of blood. In this pathway, factor VII is activated to FVIIa by thrombin and also by FXa. FVIIa forms a complex with tissue factor (TF) which activates FX to FXa. From this point both

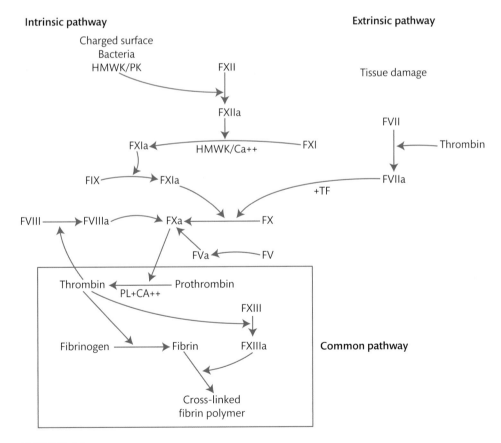

FIGURE 4.1

Coagulation cascade showing the interaction between the intrinsic, extrinsic, and common pathways.

the intrinsic and extrinsic pathways have a common cascade leading to fibrin clot formation. FXa together with phospholipid (PL) and Ca^{2+} activates prothrombin to thrombin. As shown in Figure 4.1, thrombin can activate FV, FVII, and can also activate FX. It also activates fibrinogen to fibrin monomers and FXIII to FXIIIa. Fibrin monomers spontaneously aggregate to form fibrin polymers and result in a weak clot formation. FXIIIa, a transglutaminase, cross-links the fibrin polymers to form a solid clot.

Control of coagulation

The coagulation process is controlled by several inhibitors that limit clot formation. Platelets would not normally adhere to the blood vessel walls unless there is vascular damage, abnormal physiology, or bacterial contamination. Platelet membranes have receptors which interact with effector molecules to regulate activation. Prostacyclin, which is released from the endothelium, inhibits platelet aggregation. This together with thromboxane A2 (which is a vasoconstrictor and induces platelet aggregation) limits the size of clot formation to the site of injury.

Thrombin also plays a regulatory role by combining with thrombomodulin (which is present on the endothelial cell surface) to form a complex which activates protein C. Activated protein C degrades FVa and FVIIIa which limits their effect on the coagulation cascade. There are four specific inhibitors of thrombin, the most important of which is antithrombin III, which also inhibits the activities of FIXa, FXa, FXia, FXIIa, plasmin, and kallikrein. The activity of antithrombin III is enhanced by heparin.

Dissolution of the clots is potentiated by plasmin, a serine protease. Plasmin is the activated form of plasminogen which can bind to fibrinogen and fibrin. Tissue plasminogen activator which is released from the endothelial tissue following injury and urokinase converts plasminogen to plasmin. Plasmin digests fibrin to form a soluble product. There are inhibitors of plasmin and plasminogen, and activated tissue plasminogen activator.

4.4 Blood components available and their appropriate use

Blood products should only be given when it will benefit the patient and the decision to transfuse should be based on clinical guidelines, although it is sometimes necessary to modify the guidance according to individual patient needs. It is important that the reason for giving the blood product is recorded on the request form and clearly documented in the patient's clinical notes. All blood components in the UK (with the exception of granulocyte preparations) are leucodepleted, i.e. the majority of white cells are removed by filtration.

Red cells

The majority of red cell products produced in the UK meet the following criteria:

- Red cells (leucocyte depleted, i.e. less than 1×10^6 leucocytes/unit) in additive solution
- Volume of 280 ± 60 ml
- Greater than or equal to 40 g Hb per unit
- Haemolysis <0.8% of red cell mass
- Haematocrit 0.55–0.75

- Thirty-five-day shelf-life
- Storage temperature 2–6°C
- Transfusion over a maximum of 4 hours from removal from controlled storage.

See Figure 4.2.

The usual reason for transfusing red blood cells is to increase the patient's oxygen carrying capacity, which may have decreased either due to loss or lack of production of the patient's own red cells. The clinical reason for transfusion may be due to the primary diagnosis such as haemoglobinopathy, cancer, anaemia of chronic disease (i.e. ineffective production of red cells), or bleeding (i.e. increased loss of red cells). Prior to the decision to transfuse, the level of bone marrow function and the need for the patient to maintain an appropriate activity level must be considered. In accordance with the British Society of Haematology (BSH) guidelines, an adult patient should not be transfused if the Hb is above 100 g/l, but there is a strong indication for transfusion if the Hb is below 70 g/l, and transfusion will usually become essential when the Hb falls to below 50 g/l. It is thought that an Hb between 80 and 100 g/l is a safe level even for those patients with significant cardiorespiratory disease, although transfusion may need to be considered when a patient is symptomatic (is short of breath, suffers from angina, is weak, or very tired). However, these triggers can vary greatly, depending on the primary reason for the anaemia, for example a thalassaemia patient may require a maintenance Hb of >100 g/l in order to suppress the bone marrow and a patient with sickle cell disease (Hb SS) may be symptom free with an Hb of 70 g/l. It is difficult to state a formula for the volume of red cells to be transfused in a non-bleeding patient. The BSH guidelines recommend that depending on the starting haemoglobin (Hb) one or two units should be transfused and then the patient's Hb and symptoms should be reassessed to see if more red cells are required. The age of the component, the weight of the patient, and the volume of red cells transfused will all affect the incremental rise in haemoglobin. However, as a rough guide, one unit of red cells

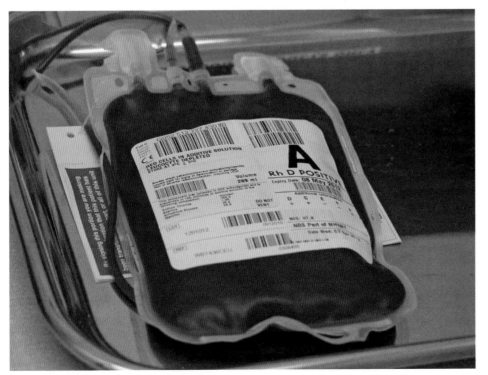

FIGURE 4.2
A unit of red blood cells (in additive, leucocyte depleted). The unit number is displayed on the top left of the label, below which is the product and storage conditions. The ABO and Rh D group of the blood component is displayed on the top right of the label, below which is the expiry date and below that is additional information on red cell phenotypes and high titre anti-A/B (HT) status. Cytomegalovirus (CMV) status when known is also printed in this location.

will give an incremental rise of approximately 10 g/l in a 70-kg adult. In patients who are bleeding, prompt action and good communication are key, with the maintenance of tissue perfusion being vital to prevent shock. As above, it is rarely necessary to use red cell components where the patient's haemoglobin is above 100 g/l, but where possible the aim should be to maintain the haemoglobin above 80 g/l.

Whilst most of the concepts of red cell transfusion considered above apply equally to the treatment of both adults and children, the component chosen for administration can be different as there are a number of small volume paediatric and neonatal red cell components available.

Key points

The main reason for transfusing red cells is to maintain or increase the oxygen carrying capacity of the blood. However, not all individuals need to have the same Hb level to prevent hypoxia; an Hb of >80 g/l is usually sufficient.

SELF-CHECK 4.1

Name three factors that may affect the expected haemoglobin rise (10 g/l) post-transfusion of one unit of blood to a patient who is not bleeding.

Fresh frozen plasma (FFP) and cryoprecipitate (cryo)

Fresh frozen plasma (FFP) is comprised of 90% water, and 8% proteins and carbohydrates. It is prepared from anticoagulated whole blood before refrigeration and where the donation time does not exceed 15 minutes. It contains high levels of all coagulation proteins, including the labile factors V and VIII. FFP is made, where possible, from male donors as female donors with a history of pregnancy may have **human leucocyte antigens (HLA)** or human neutrophil antigens (HNA) antibodies in their plasma, which has been shown to increase the incidence of transfusion-related acute lung injury (TRALI). See Figures 4.3 and 4.4.

Human leucocyte antigen (HLA)

The highly polymorphic class 1 and class 2 HLA molecules give rise to the prime cause of organ rejection.

FFP for neonatal use is treated with methylene blue in order to reduce the risk of transmission of pathogens. Currently the product is recommended for use in children born after 1996.

Each 150–300 ml pack of FFP contains 2–5 mg/ml fibrinogen, >0.7 iu/ml Factor VIII, and other clotting factors. Cryoprecipitate (cryo) is made by thawing FFP slowly at 2–6°C, centrifuging, and re-suspending the precipitate in 10–20 ml of plasma and contains >140 mg of fibrinogen and >70 iu of Factor VIII per pack. The possible adverse effects of using FFP include allergic reactions, fluid overload, TRALI, and immune suppression. When it is decided to use FFP, giving the patient an adequate dose is really important. Usually 12–15 ml/kg is the accepted starting dose, depending on the clinical situation. Therefore, a therapeutic dose in a 60 kg woman will be approximately 900 ml and in an 80 kg male 1200 ml. Where requests for FFP are made for an adult below 900 ml, the weight of the patient should be queried with the requesting clinician. Packs with a smaller volume of FFP are available for infants and children.

Clinical situations where FFP has been shown not to be of benefit are in formula replacement (for example giving one unit of FFP for every two units of red cells). However, in a patient suffering from massive haemorrhage it is accepted that additional clotting factors will be required when the patient has had the equivalent of one body volume replaced by donor blood. In this instance clotting tests, to determine the extent of the coagulopathy, may take too long and FFP

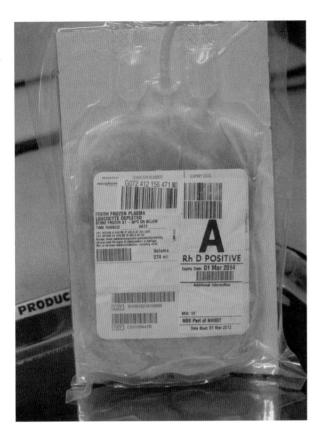

FIGURE 4.3
A unit of FFP, the volume of the unit indicated in the middle of the label is 274 ml.

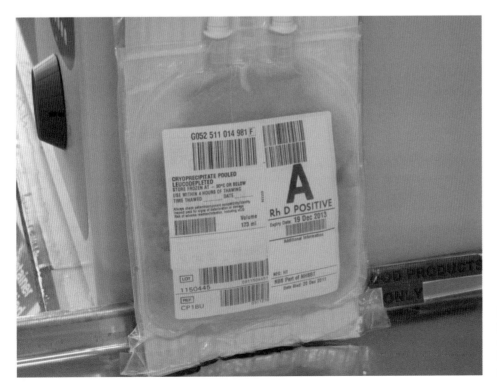

FIGURE 4.4
Example of a unit of cryoprecipitate pooled leucocyte depleted depleted plasma.

should be given as soon as possible. Also, in the treatment of hypovolaemia (low fluid volume) crystalloids or colloids are more suitable, and where bleeding is significant, red cells should be given. In accordance with the BSH guidelines, FFP should not be used for the reversal of warfarin overdose in the presence of bleeding where an alternative prothrombin complex is available. A patient with a moderately prolonged international normalized ratio (INR) in the absence of bleeding should be corrected by giving intravenous vitamin K at a dose between 0.5 and 2 mg. In patients with disseminated intravascular coagulation (DIC) treatment should be directed at the cause. However, FFP is recommended where there is haemorrhage and an abnormality of coagulation.

In massive transfusion, there is no evidence that prophylactic replacement prevents the onset of abnormal bleeding but where the prothrombin time (PT) >19.5 and/or activated partial thromboplastin time (APTT) >48 seconds, FFP is recommended, starting at a dose of 15 ml/kg. In patients where the fibrinogen level is less than 1.0 g/l cryoprecipitate is indicated.

In adults, cryoprecipitate is usually given as one therapeutic dose (two pooled packs) and then the fibrinogen level repeated to ensure that the patient's fibrinogen is >1.0 g/l. When the patient is having a massive transfusion it is important to repeat haematological and biochemical tests regularly in order to monitor the patient's progress and assess the need for blood components. In liver disease the risk of bleeding may be increased due to thrombocytopenia and increased levels of tissue plasminogen activation. Fresh frozen plasma may be indicated if the patient is bleeding or where surgery is proposed. However, complete correction is virtually impossible. In summary, therefore, FFP and cryoprecipitate should only be used having considered both the clinical and laboratory findings.

The supernatant left when producing cryoprecipitate (cryoprecipitate depleted frozen plasma) is used for plasma exchange during the treatment for thrombotic thrombocytopenic purpura (TTP).

SELF-CHECK 4.2

According to the BSH guidelines, what is the recommended dose for an adult requiring FFP?

Platelets

Apheresis

Collection of different blood cells using a machine.

A platelet concentrate may be produced either from several whole blood donations or by **apheresis** of a single donor. Apart from exposing the patient to fewer donors, the apheresis donation has the same specification as pooled platelet and offers no additional advantage. After production, platelets are stored for up to 5 or 7 days at 20–24°C in plastic packs designed for gaseous exchange, and on equipment designed to continuously agitate the component. The shelf life of the platelets depends on the time of sampling for bacterial testing. If the sample is taken on day 1, the shelf life is 5 days but this can be increased to 7 days if the sample is taken after 36 hours. One adult 'pack/dose' is provided in 150–300 ml plasma containing >240 $\times 10^9$ platelets. See Figure 4.5.

Adverse effects of transfusing platelets include a slightly higher risk of bacterial contamination than red cells, due to their being stored at 22°C (but this is reduced by bacterial testing), and the possible risk of alloimmunization due to the presence of a small number of red cell fragments.

In patients with a low platelet count, the cause of thrombocytopenia should be established prior to transfusion. In accordance with the BSH guidelines, the transfusion of platelets is indicated to prevent and treat haemorrhage in patients with thrombocytopenia or platelet

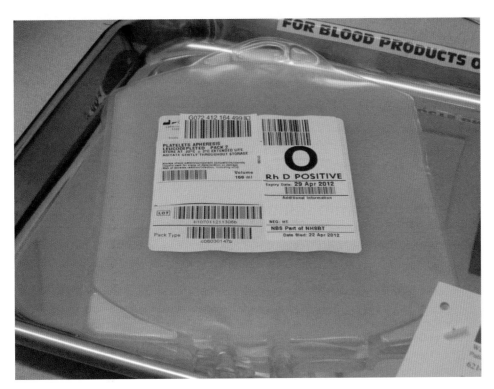

FIGURE 4.5
Example of a unit leucocyte depleted apheresis platelets.
As part of the storage information (below the unit number on the left hand side of the label) it is stated that the product requires gentle agitation on storage.

function defects. This component is not usually indicated in idiopathic thrombocytopenia (ITP) and is contraindicated in thrombotic thrombocytopenic purpura (TTP). In patients with bone marrow failure, prophylactic platelet transfusions have been shown to decrease morbidity and in such patients the platelet count should be maintained above 10×10^9/l to reduce the risk of haemorrhage. Where the patient is haemorrhaging and receiving a massive blood transfusion, the platelet count should be maintained above 75×10^9/l. In patients with disseminated intravascular coagulation (DIC), platelets are indicated where bleeding is associated with thrombocytopenia. The more controversial area of platelet transfusion is where thrombocytopenic patients require a surgical procedure. The guidelines state that biopsy may be performed, provided adequate surface pressure is applied, in patients with severe thrombocytopenia without platelet support. For more invasive surgical procedures the platelet count should be raised to 100×10^9/l for operations in critical sites such as the brain or eyes, and to at least 50×10^9/l for other procedures. Dosage will depend on the required incremental rise, with one adult dose of platelets expected to raise the platelet count by 20×10^9/l.

Granulocyte preparations

Granulocyte component is prepared from pooled buffy coats suspended in plasma and platelet additive solution. This component should be prepared as soon as possible after preparation or stored at 20–24°C. Transfusion should start before midnight after the day of collection. The total granulocyte count should be $>5 \times 10^9$/unit. The granulocyte components should be irradiated prior to issue for transfusion. While there are no good data to show that transfusing white cells is clinically effective, some clinicians will use granulocyte preparations for patients with very low neutrophil counts who have an overwhelming infection that is not responding to drug therapy.

> *Key points*
>
> All blood components should only be transfused if there is a clinical indication. Fresh frozen plasma is not to be used as a plasma expander. Platelets should be used to correct a low platelet count in cases of bone marrow suppression or failure, but not for cases of ITP or TTP.

4.5 Blood products

Human albumin solutions

Human albumin solutions (HAS) were first produced in the Second World War as a resuscitation fluid. There is a lot of debate as to their clinical effectiveness. Human albumin solutions were produced from large quantities of pooled plasma which was then fractionated and heat treated. These products have an excellent safety record. Human albumin solutions are usually available as 20, 4.5, or 5% solutions in various volumes. Whilst there is debate regarding the clinical effectiveness of this product, with the recommendation that alternatives (crystalloid or artificial colloid) should be used whenever possible, HASs are still used in resuscitation, management of renal disease, replacement fluid in severe hypovolemia, draining of significant ascites, and in burns (although not in the first 24 hours). Whether HAS or artificial colloids should be used will depend on the patient's renal function, sodium/potassium levels, and the risk of oedema.

Factor concentrates

These include Factor VIII, IX; Factor II, VII, IX, and X; prothrombin complex concentrate (PCC) and recombinant Factor VIIa. These products are usually recombinant licensed pharmaceutical products used in the treatment of patients with inherited coagulation deficiencies. PCC and recombinant VIIa may also be used in life-threatening bleeds.

Human immunoglobulins

Immunoglobulins are produced from normal pooled plasma, either to produce a specific immunoglobulin such as anti-D (see 'Anti-D immunoglobulin') or non-specific, which can be used to replace immunoglobulins in patients with antibody disorders. Pooled immunoglobulins are provided in intravenous (IVIg) and subcuteanous (SCIg) formats, with the dose being monitored to achieve the required levels of immunoglobulin (IgG) in the patient's serum.

Anti-D immunoglobulin

Anti-D immunoglobulin (Ig) is prepared from human donors with high levels of alloimmune anti-D antibodies. Preparations are available from a number of companies and in a number of different doses. As the use of this product is very specific, the manufacturer's instructions must be followed within the guidance given in the BSH guidelines on the use of anti-D immunoglobulin. The BSH guidelines recommend the following for Rh D-negative patients:

- <12 weeks' gestation—a minimum of 250 iu anti-D Ig prophylaxis should be administered within 72 hours for ectopic and molar pregnancy, therapeutic termination, and in some cases of unusually heavy bleeding or associated with abdominal pain. There is no requirement to test for fetal-maternal haemorrhage (FMH).

- Between 12 and 20 weeks gestation—at least 250 iu anti-D should be given within 72 hours of the sensitizing event without the need for an FMH test.

- After 20 weeks' gestation'—a minimum of 500 iu anti-D Ig should be administered with in 72 hours of a potentially sensitizing event. A test for FMH is needed to determine the requirement for further anti-D Ig.

- Routine antenatal anti-D prophylaxis (RAADP)—a single dose of 1500 iu anti-D Ig should be administered between 28 and 30 weeks or a minimum of 500 iu anti-D Ig given at 28 and 34 weeks.

- Following delivery—determine the ABO and Rh D blood group on the cord blood. A minimum dose 500 iu anti-D Ig should be administered to previously non-sensitized Rh D negative women if the baby's Rh D type is positive. This should be done as soon as possible but within 72 hours of delivery. A test for FMH is required to determine the need for further administration of anti-D Ig.

4.6 **Special requirements**

Irradiated blood components

Cellular blood components potentially contain T lymphocytes and require **irradiation** prior to administration to patients who may be immunocompromised, in order to prevent transfusion-associated graft versus host disease. Patients with inherited or acquired immune disorders (Hodgkin's disease), patients who have received treatment with purine analogues, individuals who have had a bone marrow/stem cell transplant, unborn babies, and babies requiring exchange transfusion should all receive irradiated cellular products. For more detailed guidance the reader may refer to the relevant BSH guidelines.

Irradiation

A process for inactivating donor lymphocytes using gamma (or X-ray) irradiation to prevent transfusionassociated graft versus host disease (TA-GVHD), a rare but potentially fatal consequence of blood transfusion.

Cytomegalovirus (CMV)-negative products

The transfusion of cellular blood components containing lymphocytes has been shown to transmit CMV. Whilst CMV infection tends to be asymptomatic in most individuals it can lead to severe morbidity and mortality in immunocompromised individuals. Although the risk of CMV transmission is now very low due to the majority of cellular products being leucocyte depleted, it is recommended that components indicated as being CMV negative are transfused to vulnerable patients such as pregnant women, neonates, and transplant patients whose CMV status is unknown or who are CMV negative.

4.7 **Plasma fractionation**

Plasma contains approximately 60 g/l of proteins of which 57 g are used to make therapeutic products. Often these are the only options available to clinicians to treat, manage, or prevent life-threatening conditions such as congenital plasma protein deficiency (Factor VIII and IX), infections, immunological disorders, and trauma. The separation of the therapeutic products from plasma is achieved by the cold fractionation process developed by Cohn and colleagues in the 1940s where human serum albumin was the main product. This was followed by intramuscular immunoglobulin and in 1981 by intravenous immunoglobulin.

Plasma is either collected by apheresis or recovered from whole blood donations. More than 80% of the plasma used for fractionation is collected by commercial companies by apheresis from paid donors. The plasma is tested for various virological markers and frozen.

The Cohn cold ethanol fractionation process has five stages to separate the plasma proteins. After each stage, the precipitate or fraction is removed and the supernatant is subjected to further processing by adjusting the ethanol concentration, pH or ionic strength. The following plasma proteins are separated from each fraction:

- Fraction I: Factor VIII, fibrinogen, and complement proteins
- Fraction II and III: IgG, IgM, IgA, coagulation factors, and globulins
- Fraction IV.I: antitrypsin, antithrombin III, and globulins
- Fraction IV.4: ceruloplasmin, transferin, haptoglobin, and globulins
- Fraction V: albumin and globulins.

The current technology in use is still based on the cold ethanol fractionation process but with the introduction of chromatography to enable increased capture of labile proteins and increased purity. There is also a **pathogen inactivation**/reduction step incorporated into the process to increase the safety of these products. More than 20 plasma therapeutics are prepared from human plasma. A simplified version of a current fractionation process is shown at Figure 4.6.

A new development is the use of affinity chromatography without the need for cryoprecipitation to separate plasma proteins. This process produces factor VII/von Willibrand complex, plasminogen, fibrinogen, IgG, and albumin, as well as other drugs. Further purifications steps are required.

Pathogen reduction steps that are current available are:

- Solvent/detergent (S/D)—tri-(n-butyl)-phosphate (TNBP) an organic solvent and Triton X-100 a non-ionic detergent is the most commonly used S/D. The plasma product is treated with the S/D for 1–6 hours at 20–37°C after which the chemicals need to be removed. It is effective against enveloped viruses.
- Low pH—the plasma product is treated at pH 4 and 37°C for 20-30 hours and is effective against enveloped viruses.
- Pasteurization—plasma proteins in solution are heated to 60°C for 10 hours. There is possible protein alteration by this process. It is effective against enveloped and most non-enveloped viruses.
- Dry heat—the product is heated to 60–68°C for up to 4 days or 96°C for 30 minutes or three days at 80°C. As with pasteurization, protein stabilizers are generally required. It is usually used as a secondary viral reduction step for both enveloped and non-enveloped viruses.
- Caprylic acid—the product is incubated with caprylic acid at a pH of less than 6 and is effective against enveloped viruses. It is used only for pathogen activation of immunoglobulins.
- Nanofiltration—products are filtered through membranes with a porosity of <35 nm and is effective against both enveloped and non-enveloped viruses.

Pathogen inactivation

A process for removal of infectious agents in blood components/products through chemical or heat treatment and filtration.

Pathogen reduction

Process for reducing or eliminating most infectious agents in blood components/products.

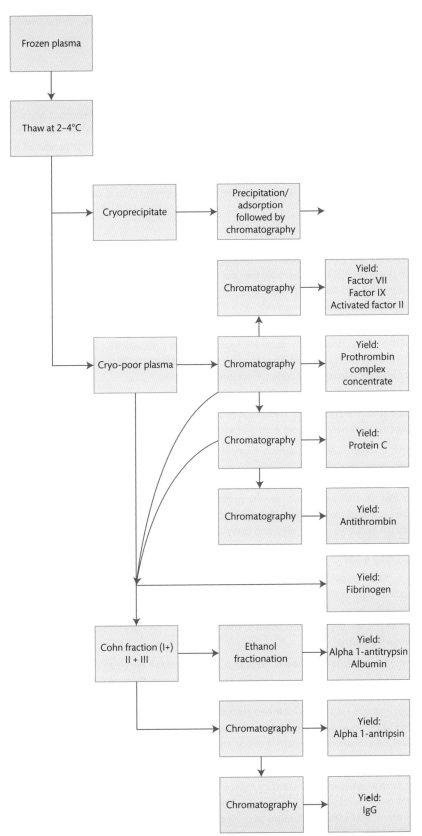

FIGURF 4.6
Flowchart for the Cohn ethanol fractionation of plasma.

Two or more pathogen reduction steps are usually used to ensure the safety of the plasma products with nanofiltration increasingly being used as one of those steps.

Recombinant plasma proteins

The inability to meet the demand for plasma proteins from recovered and sourced plasma, risks of pathogen (including prion) transmission, and high production costs has fuelled the research and development of recombinant proteins. Human insulin was first produced in recombinant bacteria in the early 1980s. Since then, there has been varying success in producing human blood proteins in transgenic species. Recombinant blood products currently available include: Factors VIIa, VIII, IX, thrombin, activated protein C, and antithrombin.

Expression systems available to produce recombinant proteins are:

- *Escherichia coli (E. coli)*—this bacterium has been used successfully to produce recombinant insulin and human growth factor, but the production of complex functional glycoproteins has been unsuccessful. This is because the post translation modification required for protein folding and formation of disulphide bonds is lacking. The proteins produced are less stable and clinically less effective.

- Yeasts—these can potentially synthesize and excrete large amounts of recombinant proteins intracellularly or secreted. Early-stage N-glycosylations are possible but terminal sialyation has only recently been achieved. They have been used for large-scale production of albumin but were unable to fold and secrete monoclonal antibodies.

- Insects cells harbouring baculovirus-Sf9 expression vector systems have been used to produce small amounts of proteins. These cells do not survive the infection, requiring the repeat of the process with new cells and virus preparation.

- Transgenic animals—Chinese hamster ovary (CHO) has been used successfully to produce transgenic post-translationally modified proteins secreted into the culture medium. The amount of recombinant proteins obtained from cell culture medium is low with high production cost. In transgenic animals, the protein of interest is secreted into the milk and has to be separated and purified. The yield from the milk of transgenic mice is low. Other animals such as rabbits, goats, pigs, and cows secrete higher levels of recombinant proteins into their milk. Recombinant proteins have also been produced in the egg white of chickens. A drawback of these production systems is that the recombinant protein produced may be species or tissue specific and elicit immune response in the transfused patients. Also, it may be difficult to separate the human protein from that of the animal. There is a risk of human viral pathogens being present in the protein preparations. This can be overcome by careful selection of the animal. It is also possible that the protein produced may have an adverse reaction on the animal.

- Transgenic plants—enzymes used for research and diagnosis have been produced in transgenic plants but to date no plasma protein has been licensed. Proteins produced are capable of post translational folding but lack terminal sialic aid and contain xylose which may induce an immune response. Unlimited amounts of proteins can be produced in the leaves and seeds of plants and the production costs are low. Unlike animal cells, transgenic plants are unlikely to contain human pathogens or prions. Therapeutic monoclonal antibodies are under development in transgenic plants.

Transgenic farm animals are generated by microinjection of DNA into embryo pronuclei using transposons or lentiviral vectors. The transgene injected must contain a promoter, enhancers, isolators, introns, and a transcript terminator. The promoter used must be from the promoter genes from where the transgenic protein will be expressed. For example, the promoters from milk protein genes are used for the expression in milk.

Recombinant coagulation factors

Factor VIIa (FVIIa)

Intravenous administration of FVIIa is one of the treatment options available for patients with haemophilia A who developed anti-FVIII inhibitors. It works by enhancing thrombin generation on the platelet surface at the site of injury which is independent of the presence of FVIII/FIX and results in the formation of a tight fibrin haemostatic plug. Recombinant FVII is secreted from baby hamster kidney (BHK) cells and is identical to the plasma derived product and is clinically effective. It is licensed for FVII congenital deficiency, acquired haemophilia and Glanzmann's thrombasthenia. One of the side effects of this treatment is thromboembolism.

Factor VIII (FVIII)

The incidence of FVIII deficiency or haemophilia A is between 1/5000 and 1/10,000 male births (X chromosome linked) and requires lifelong treatment. Recombinant FVIII was first developed in CHO and BHK cells by transfecting the full sequence of the human FVIII cDNA into the expression vector. The yield of the protein in CHO cell was low. This was increased 20-fold by deleting the B-domain from the cDNA sequence inserted into the expression vector. The procoagulant activity of the FVIII produced was unaffected. Full-length and B domain deleted recombinant FVIII is commercially available with and without plasma-derived albumin.

Factor IX (FIX)

The incidence of FIX or haemophilia B deficiency is 1/30,000 of male births. Most patients with haemophilia B receive treatment when bleeding occurs. However, those with severe haemophilia B receive prophylactic treatment of FIX to prevent bleeding. The FIX gene was the first coagulation factor to be cloned. Recombinant FIX is produced from BHK cells. The yield can be increased to about 30 times that of plasma-derived FIX by using specific strains and optimizing the growth conditions. The growth medium is serum free, making purification easier. Recombinant FIX has a similar half life to that of the plasma-derived product. However, there is a 30% reduction in recovery leading to the infusion of higher doses. Expression of the recombinant FIX in the mammary glands of transgenic mice and the fruits of tomato plants is being explored.

Factor XIII (FXIII)

Plasma-derived FXIII is available. A recombinant FXIII was developed in yeast (*Saccharomyces cerevisiae*) and has a mean half life of 8.5 days. Normal function was demonstrated in healthy volunteers and FXIII-deficient patients.

von Willebrand factor (VWF)

von Willebrand disease is caused by a deficiency or defect of vWF which plays a critical role in normal blood clotting. A recombinant vWF was developed in CHO with the large multimeric protein secreted into a protein-free medium. The product is purified by chromatography and exhibits a prolonged half life compared to that derived from plasma. Safety and efficacy was demonstrated for on demand and control of bleeding episodes. A recombinant vWF was developed in swine. The product is secreted into the milk at a concentration of 28 to 56 times that of human circulation vWF.

Fibrinogen

Plasma-derived fibrinogen is extracted from cryoprecipitate or Cohn fraction 1 at the expense of FVIII. Low levels of recombinant fibrinogen can be obtained from engineered CHO and BHK cells. It is also expressed in the milk of transgenic mice, goats, and cows with improved yield.

Thrombin

Plasma-derived prothrombin from prothrombin concentrate complex (or as a by-product of FIX) is chemically activated using $CaCl_2$ to produce thrombin. The concentrate is available as fibrin sealant. Recombinant thrombin is obtained from CHO cell culture medium.

Antithrombin

This product is prepared from cryo-poor plasma or Cohn fraction IV-1 by immobilized heparin affinity chromatography. Recombinant antithrombin is expressed in CHO cells and the milk of transgenic goats. The yield from transgenic goats can exceed 10 times that of the plasma derived product with over 50% recovery.

C1-inhibitor

This is obtained from cryo-poor plasma by anion exchange chromatography. Recombinant C1-inhibitor has been secreted into the milk of transgenic rabbits.

Activated protein C

A plasma-derived product is not available from fractionation. Human embryonic kidney 293 (HEK293) cells have been used to produce recombinant activated protein C which was shown to significantly reduced mortality in patients with severe sepsis.

Albumin

Albumin is produced in Cohn fraction V of ethanol fractionation with a purity of about 98%. Commercial recombinant albumin is prepared in the fermentation processes of yeasts *Saccharomyces cerevisiae* and *Pichia pastoris*. High purity albumin to a concentration of 1.4 g/l was obtained from this process compared to 23–27 g/l from the fractionation process. Production of recombinant albumin from transgenic cows with a yield of up to 40 g/l has been reported.

4.8 Decision making, who needs a transfusion, risks and benefits

Whilst transfusion can be essential for some patients, blood components are sometimes transfused without understanding the exact clinical benefit. It is important that the normal physiological response to anaemia and/or bleeding, along with the body's ability to produce the cells quickly if necessary, are considered in the decision to transfuse. Although transfusion is very safe, particularly in comparison to other risks during a hospital stay, it is not risk free. Therefore, it is very important that a critical approach is taken to prescribing blood components. Where possible, patients must be informed about the benefits, risks, and alternative choices available to them. There is also the issue of managing a valuable, precious, and potentially scarce resource. Blood components and products must be used wisely to ensure sufficient availability for those patients that have life-threatening problems. There are risks to being transfused as highlighted in the annual **Serious Hazards Of Transfusion (SHOT)** adverse incident reporting scheme reports. Transfusion

Serious Hazards Of Transfusion (SHOT)
The UK haemovigilance scheme.

transmitted infections, acute or delayed reactions due to serological incompatibilities, or receiving blood intended for someone else, as a result of human error, are amongst the risks discussed in these reports. Allogeneic blood components should only be used when there are good reasons to believe that the benefits will outweigh the risks. It is important that there is some clinical benefit to the patient, improving their condition and/or quality of life. Decisions also need to be made about whether suitable alternatives (autologous or pharmacological) are available that may have the same beneficial outcome without exposing the patient to the risks of allogeneic transfusion, as even when blood is considered safe by current standards, it may contain unknown pathogens.

When the patient is bleeding it is very difficult to quantify how much blood is being lost. Blood may be spilt onto bed sheets, curtains, the floor, doctors, and nurses, as well as into drains and suction devices often along with other bodily fluids. It is essential that there are good policies and procedures (both clinical and within the laboratory) to manage such patients appropriately and quickly. When significant blood loss occurs, the fall in oxygen carrying capacity, together with the reduction in blood volume, causes a fall in oxygen delivery. If intravenous therapy (crystalloid or colloid) maintains a normal blood volume, an increase in cardiac output may occur, enabling adequate oxygenation of the tissues. The resultant haemodilution reduces the viscosity of the blood, improving capillary flow and enhancing the supply of oxygen to the tissues. However, when the haemoglobin falls below 7 g/dl, it is unlikely that increased cardiac output alone will maintain adequate oxygenation of all tissues. In patients who are haemorrhaging, the decision to transfuse should be based on the clinical condition of the patient (in particular their heart and lung function) and their ability to compensate for a reduction in oxygen supply. However, in surgical patients the duration of the bleeding/anaemia is generally short, with the haemoglobin (number of red cells) expected to rise rapidly in the post-operative period. In medical patients, anaemia may be expected to remain for months or even permanently. It should be clear that blood component selection, and transfusion triggers and transfusion regimes will be very different in different patient groups as well as within individual patients within the same patient group.

An example of poor decision making is shown in Table 4.1.

Table 4.1 shows the results of two patients under the care of the gynaecology department. They were both in for elective surgery, one for a myomectomy and one for a hysterectomy. Blood taken at a pre-admission clinic 4 weeks before the operation showed that both patients had a haemoglobin level below 10 and both were iron deficient. The patients were transfused intra-operatively and both were discharged with a haemoglobin level higher than it was pre-operatively. These two patients should have received iron therapy prior to their admission for such an elective procedure. It could also be argued that they should not have had a higher haemoglobin post-operatively than they started with, and that the transfusion intra-operatively was unnecessary.

TABLE 4.1 Poor decision making

Pre-op Hb	MCV	Fe deficient?	Operation	Red cells txed	Post-op Hb
9.2 g/dl	66.4	Yes	Myomectomy	1 unit	10.4 g/dl
9.3 g/dl	65.6	Yes	Total abdominal hysterectomy	2 units	11.1 g/dl

Reducing the need for transfusion

It is important to understand how good communication, adherence to standards, audit, and review of product use will aid the appropriate use of blood components and thus manage this precious resource. Improving practice requires a planned, consistent approach. Unless there is local dissemination and implementation with supportive education a change in practice will not be achieved. So how can inappropriate transfusions be prevented? There are a number of national and local initiatives:

- Adherence to national guidelines when introducing local policies and procedures to ensure appropriate use of the blood products.

- The use of hospital transfusion teams (which include the blood bank manager, a transfusion practitioner, and a medical consultant lead) to give guidance, implement policy, provide an educational and training resource, and audit/review performance.

- The investigation and reporting of errors and near misses both locally and nationally provides data and information which can be used to improve practice. It is a requirement of the Blood Safety and Quality Regulations that all errors and incidents are appropriately reported, with all incidents involving laboratory errors or errors resulting in patient potential or actual harm being reported externally to the Medicines and Health care products Regulatory Agency (MHRA).

- Audit is a valuable tool to ensure that the predefined standard of care is met and that blood component use is appropriate. Audits may be local, regional, or national. Local audits may be used to ensure compliance to local guidelines, whereas participation in national audits allows comparison to other similar establishments. Audits of practice compared to a 'standard' provide clinical staff with relevant information and can aid in education, understanding, and subsequently modifying behaviour.

- It is important that, where possible, patients are well informed of both the risks and the benefits of the treatment they are to receive. It is equally important that they are advised of any alternative treatment options that may be available so that an informed choice may be made about whether they wish to receive a blood transfusion.

- The use of performance indicators, such as those provided by the Blood Stocks Management Scheme (BSMS), allows transfusion teams to monitor blood component use and wastage. Whilst this in itself may not reduce the number of patients receiving blood, it does provide valuable information on hospital stock levels and wastage, which can be compared to 'national averages', ensuring that individual sites control stocks effectively.

Key points

There are many risks associated with transfusions and these have to be taken into account when deciding whether to transfuse, or use suitable alternatives.

SELF-CHECK 4.3

Suggest four local/national initiatives which help to ensure the appropriate use of blood and blood products.

4.9 **Alternatives to donor blood**

Appropriately used donor blood is essential for many medical treatments and can save lives. However, donated blood is a limited resource and the potential impact of variant Creutzfeldt–Jakob disease (vCJD) and a decreasing donor population is affecting the blood supply. The health service circulars *Better Blood Transfusion* encourage hospitals to ensure blood transfusion is an integral part of patients' care and that the use of effective alternatives to donor blood and where appropriate, the use of autologous blood is offered to patients. Autologous blood is an individual's own blood, whereas allogeneic blood is blood or components from another individual.

The emergence of HIV/AIDS in the 1980s highlighted the need for better screening and made the public more aware of the risks of receiving an allogeneic blood transfusion. However, the development of 'auto transfusion' came from the USA in the early 1970s mainly in response to the growth of coronary artery and other surgeries, leading to an ever-increasing demand for blood. It is possible that oxygen carrying resuscitation fluids may become available within the next few years; however, 'artificial blood' is probably many years away. With a decreasing blood supply (due to the elderly population, new and re-emerging blood transmissible infections, and vCJD), there is an urgent need for successful blood conservation strategies in order to maintain a healthy blood supply for those patients where autologous transfusion is not an option.

Conservation strategies

Some of the strategies for blood conservation in surgical and/or bleeding patients are considered below. Conservation in medical patients is not considered, as strategies are limited and vary greatly depending on the clinical diagnosis and the type of transfusion required.

Early assessment (pre-admissions)

An early full blood count assessment and advice on good diet or supplements in the months prior to planned surgery can ensure that when the patient attends for surgery their haemoglobin is at a good level. In patients where iron or B12/folate deficiency is identified, the patient should be sent for assessment and treatment prior to admittance for surgery. Oral haematinics (oral iron or B12/folate supplements) take time to have an effect but are cheap, safe, and effective. The higher the haemoglobin prior to surgery the lower the chance of requiring transfusion of donor red cells. Also required is a planned approach to surgery, for example not taking aspirin or non-steroidal anti-inflammatories, and where possible stopping warfarin.

Near patient haemostatic assessment

The provision of timely biochemistry and haematology results can play a big role in the management of a surgical or bleeding patient. Timely and appropriate transfusion treatment where blood components are ordered and transfused based on real time results reduces unnecessary transfusion and aids positive clinical outcome. Instruments such as those in Figures 4.7 and 4.8 can be used to measure Hb and coagulation in the operating theatre.

Surgical and anaesthetic technique

The patient's position, body temperature, type of anaesthesia, surgical technique, and pain management can make a big difference to the amount of blood shed during the surgery.

Fibrin sealants

Fibrin sealants are topical biological adhesives which mimic the final stage of coagulation. These agents, made from human cryoprecipitate, convert fibrinogen to fibrin. The 'kit' consists of concentrated fibrinogen which is activated at the surgical bleeding site by adding thrombin and calcium chloride, and then sprayed onto the site of the bleed, ensuring local haemostasis.

Pre-operative autologous blood donation (PAD)

Although not now used in the UK, this is a system whereby a patient has a standard donation of blood collected every week for up to 4 weeks before a planned operation. The donations are labelled with the patient's details, tested in the same way as any donor blood, and stored

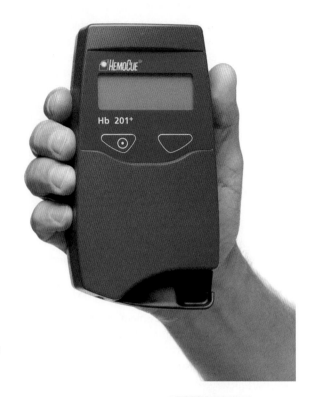

FIGURE 4.7
Picture of a hand-held
'HemoCue'® machine, used for
quick haemoglobin assessment
close to the patient. (© www.
hemocue.com.)

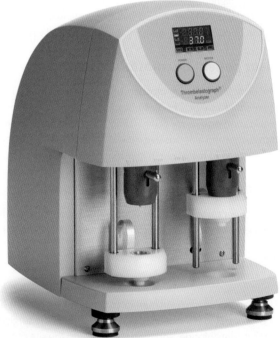

FIGURE 4.8
Picture of a TEG® 500
Thrombelastograph Analyser
(Haemonetics). (© www.
haemoscope.com.)

at 2–6°C. If the patient requires blood during or after their operation then these units can be transfused. Although this sounds an attractive proposition, in practice it was difficult to operate and its effect on the supply of allogeneic blood was minimal. It has therefore been abandoned except for patients who might have blood of a very rare phenotype and even for these their blood is usually collected on a regular basis and stored in the National Frozen Blood Bank.

Autologous salvage

Collecting the patient's own blood for return to them during the surgery has advantages in terms of the oxygen carrying capacity of the red cells, reduced risk of transfusion transmitted infections, alloimmunization, and immunosuppresion. There are a variety of ways of collecting the patient's own blood, some of which are outlined below. A combination of these techniques gives the biggest advantage in terms of reducing the need for allogeneic transfusion.

Acute normovolaemic haemodilution (ANH) This is collection of the patient's whole blood immediately prior to anaesthesia/surgery, followed by infusion of colloid or crystalloid. Moderate isovolaemia means that the patient bleeds a lower haemoglobin/haematocrit during the surgery. In patients with normal cardiac function the decrease in blood viscosity means that oxygen delivery is well maintained. The collected units are kept by the patient at room temperature and are re-infused towards the end of the procedure when blood loss is minimal. It has the advantage that no testing is required and the risk of bacterial contamination and/or the wrong blood being given back to the patient is reduced. This technique is considered to complement intra-operative salvage as the units collected have functional clotting factors and platelets. Acute normovolaemic haemodilution can be considered in patients without cardiac impairment, where the surgery is likely to result in significant loss (greater than 20% of the patient's blood volume) and the patient's starting haemoglobin is above 100 g/l. Some Jehovah's Witness patients may accept ANH, particularly if the collection and re-administration sets can be set up as a continuous loop, but this would be a matter of personal choice.

Intra-operative salvage (IOS) This system is useful in reducing or eliminating the need to use donor red cells. It is the process whereby shed blood lost during surgery is mixed with anticoagulant and collected into a reservoir. The patient's collected blood is then processed and returned to them. The decision to use IOS will be based on a number of factors, including the risk of the patient bleeding, the anticipated blood loss, the site of the surgical field, and whether IOS is acceptable to the patient. This technique is usually used in surgical procedures where the blood loss is expected to be greater than 1 litre. Patients with religious beliefs where treatment cannot include the transfusion of donor blood (for example Jehovah's Witnesses) may often accept IOS. It should not be used in circumstances where the patient's shed blood may be contaminated, such as where there is a risk of bowel contents, infection, gastric, or pancreatic secretions, or any pharmacological substances entering the system and being re-infused into the patient. In patients undergoing surgery for malignant disease, in obstetrics, or in patients with sickle cell disease careful consideration needs to be given due to the potential risk of malignant cells, foetal contaminants/amniotic fluid being re-infused, or causing a sickle cell crisis. It must also be remembered that where massive bleeding occurs, the re-infused product does not contain any clotting factors or platelets. See Figure 4.9.

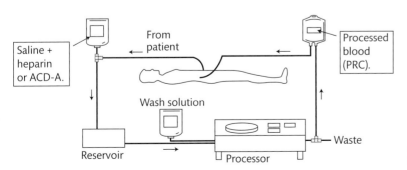

FIGURE 4.9

A diagrammatic representation of the setup for intra-operative cell salvage.

Post-operative salvage (POS) This is a relatively simple adaptation of existing wound drains. The wound drains are attached to a reservoir and the blood is collected directly into a blood bag within a closed system. When over 400 ml is collected, the bag can be detached from the system and the blood re-infused. This system is useful in patients where there is anticipated, clean post-operative blood loss. The system is of particular use in orthopaedic surgery traditionally for knee replacements. Collected blood must be reinfused within six hours of collection. Contraindications with this system are similar to IOS, such as a contaminated collection site, untrained staff using the system, patients with sickle cell disease, malignancy, and the potential risk of re-infusing activated white blood cells. See Figure 4.10.

Pharmacological approaches to reduce blood loss

Erythropoietin (EPO) Under normal conditions the production of red cells matches the natural loss. This process (erythropoiesis) is regulated by erythropoietin, a natural hormone produced by the kidney. An artificially made EPO (originally used in patients with renal failure) has been used in some patients to increase red cell production, usually either prior to or after surgery.

Intravenous iron (iv Fe) Serious iron deficiency, or where the patient is not responding, or is intolerant to oral iron, may be treated with intravenous iron solutions. Intravenous solutions are often used in combination with EPO to maximize an increase in the haemoglobin.

Recombinant Factor VIIa Recombinant Factor VIIa works by activating coagulation and platelet adhesion. The product is normally used for the treatment of severe haemophilia (see Recombinant coagulation factors).

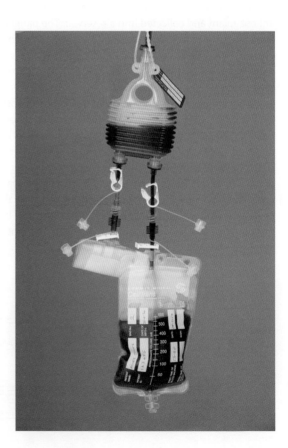

FIGURE 4.10
An example of post-operative salvage, where blood shed after the operation is collected into a blood bag for reinfusion. Picture courtesy of CellTrans™ Summit Medical.

Desmopressin (DDAVP) This drug can promote haemostasis by improving platelet function and release of coagulation factors. It may reduce the need for transfusion although it may have a limited effect if the patient has already lost a significant amount of blood.

Lysine analogues (tranexamic acid)/anti-fibrinolytics These act by attaching to plasminogen and inhibiting the activation of fibrinolysis.

Key points

Various blood conservation strategies are available for a bleeding or surgical patient and these include autologous blood salvage, such as acute normovolaemic haemodilution (ANH), intra-operative salvage (IOS), and post-operative salvage (POS).

SELF-CHECK 4.4

Name four contraindications when considering using intra-operative cell salvage.

4.10 Case history examples

The following case histories have been included as examples of poor practice. Some are based on examples cited in SHOT reports and others have been adapted from real cases from the author's place of work. They have been included to allow the reader to think about where things go wrong.

Inappropriate use of red cells

A pre-dialysis full blood count (FBC) result on a 20-year-old female patient attending for routine renal dialysis due to kidney failure showed her haemoglobin (Hb) was 43 g/l and her haematocrit 13.1%. No comment was made on the results and the patient received two units of red cells. At the following dialysis session 2 days later, the pre-dialysis FBC results showed an Hb 112 g/l and haematocrit 29.5%. Review of previous results showed that this young patient's haematocrit usually ran between 24% and 28%. It was likely that the FBC sample showing an Hb of 43 g/l was diluted, probably being taken from the same arm used for a saline drip. This example shows the need to review previous results before making a decision about transfusion and not basing that decision on just one result.

Timely transfusion and good communication

A 47-year-old male, with a history of non-Hodgkin's lymphoma, presented in the accident and emergency department. Initial bloods showed his haemoglobin as 37 g/l, a reticulocyte count 12.8%, his DAT was positive, and the blood film and blood group serology suggested warm type autoimmune hemolytic anaemia. It was suspected that the patient had suffered a CVA (stroke) and due to the profound anaemia four units of red cells were requested. Over 5 hours later the patient had still not received any blood. On investigation it was established that the laboratory had referred the sample to the reference laboratory as they were not able to find compatible blood and were waiting for that 'compatible' blood to arrive. Given the clinical condition of the patient and the need for an immediate transfusion, this was one instance when 'least incompatible', ABO, Rh, and Kell matched units should have been issued, rather than waiting for lengthy investigations to have been completed.

Importance of correctly calculating the dose

A 110 kg, 56-year-old male patient was brought into the accident and emergency department with liver failure and suffering from acute melaena. He had a history of alcohol and drug abuse. His haemoglobin was 79 g/l, platelet count was 90×10^9/l, PT 21 seconds, APTT 48 seconds, and fibrinogen 0.6. A request for two units of red cells and one unit of cryoprecipitate was made by the attending clinicians and issued by the laboratory. Whilst the request for cryoprecipitate (fibrinogen of <1) was appropriate, the amount requested, particularly in a man of this size, would not have been sufficient.

A 4-year-old, 12-kg female patient with neuroblastoma and persistent thrombocytopenia was due to receive chemotherapy. One adult dose of platelets was requested, issued, and all of the pack was transfused. The platelet pack contained 310 ml, which was twice the volume required by someone of that weight.

Calculating the amount or volume of a blood component that the patient should receive is very important. Larger patients require large volumes, and smaller patients will require smaller volumes. This is true of all blood components. As well as wasting resources and exposing the patient to unnecessary risks, consideration must be given to maintaining normovolaemia as overtransfusion and undertransfusion can be detrimental to the patient.

Examples of overtransfusion (adapted from data taken from the SHOT reports)

An 80-year-old female patient, with expressive dysphasia, had been to theatre for repair of a fractured neck of femur. Her pre-operative Hb was 95 g/l and there had been little intra-operative blood loss. Eight hours following surgery the patient was noted to be restless, hypotensive, and tachycardic; a repeat full blood count gave an Hb result of 39 g/l. A junior doctor diagnosed hypovolaemia and prescribed six units of red cells, all of which were administered over a 16-hour period. The post-transfusion Hb was 182 g/l; the patient subsequently died from cardiac failure. Investigation revealed that the pre-transfusion sample had been taken from an arm that had an intravenous infusion of saline running and that it was in fact diluted. Again, previous results should have been considered rather than basing the decision on just one result.

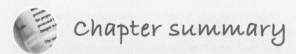

Chapter summary

- Having considered the basic composition and function of blood, particularly the red cells and platelets, it is clear why these blood components are needed for transfusion: red cells to maintain or increase the oxygen carrying capacity of the blood, and platelets to prevent bleeding.

- Other clotting factors can be replaced either by using fresh frozen plasma (FFP) or cryoprecipitate which is rich in fibrinogen and Factor VIII.

- However, transfusion is not without risks, which have to be considered before deciding to transfuse.

- Allogeneic, or donor, blood can, in some surgical operations, be replaced by autologous blood salvaging techniques, such as by collecting blood from the patient either before or during the operation and re-infusing it afterwards.

- There are also some pharmacological approaches to reducing blood loss.

- Blood can be a life-saver but it is not a panacea.

 # Further reading

- Contreras M (ed.) *ABC of Transfusion*. 3rd edition. BMJ Books, London (1998).

- Maniatis A, Linden PV, & Hardy J-F (eds) *Alternatives to Blood Transfusion in Transfusion Medicine*. 2nd edition. Wiley-Blackwell, Oxford (2010).

- McClelland DBL (ed.) *Handbook of Transfusion Medicine*. 5th edition. The Stationery Office, Norwich (2013).

  www.transfusionguidelines.org/transfusion-handbook

- Murphy M & Pamphilon D (eds) *Practical Transfusion Medicine*. Wiley-Blackwell, Oxford (2017).

- Thomas D, Thompson J & Ridler B (eds) *A Manual for Blood Conservation*. TFM Publishing, Shrewsbury (2016).

  Blood transfusion is highly regulated with both statutory regulations and professional guidelines. These are constantly being reviewed and for the most up-to-date versions visit the following websites:

- BSH Guidelines covering many aspects of blood banking and transfusion: http://www.b-s-h.org.uk/guidelines/.

- *Handbook of Transfusion Medicine, Guidelines for the Blood Transfusion Services in the United Kingdom*. Other guidelines, useful information and links: www.transfusion-guidelines.org.uk.

- MHRA guidance for reporting incidents (SABRE): www.mhra.gov.uk/Safetyinformation/Reportingsafetyproblems/Blood/index.htm.

- Serious Hazards Of Transfusion (SHOT) annual reports: www.shotuk.org.

- Network for Advancement of Transfusion Alternatives (NATA): www.nataonline.com.

- NHS Blood and Transplant (NHSBT) Blood Matters is a regular publication with up-to-the-minute articles on all aspects of transfusion and transplantation: http://hospital.blood.co.uk/customer-service/blood-and-transplant-matters/.

- Blood Stocks Management Scheme, monitors the usage of blood and components in hospitals: www.bloodstocks.co.uk.

- British Blood Transfusion Society (BBTS) has information and links to other relevant professional bodies: www.bbts.org.uk.

Answers to the questions in this chapter are provided on the book's accompanying website:

 Go to www.oup.com/uk/avent2e

5

Microbiological Testing of Blood Donations

Catherine Hyland, John Barbara, and Lionel Mohabir

Learning objectives

After studying this chapter you should be able to:

- List the mandatory microbial testing requirements for blood donations.
- Describe the aetiology (i.e. how the disease condition is caused) for the transfusion transmitted viral infections—hepatitis B (HBV), hepatitis C (HCV), and human immunodeficiency virus (HIV).
- Describe the principle and key steps for a chemiluminescent immunoassay, an enzyme-linked immunosorbent sandwich assay (ELISA), and nucleic acid tests (NAT).
- Explain the algorithms for microbiology testing and donor re-instatement.
- Define three ways to reduce bacterial contamination of blood and components.
- Explain the aetiology of the transfusion transmitted parasite infection—malaria.
- Understand the elements associated with blood screening for transfusion-transmissible infections (TTIs) that ensure the overall safety of the blood supply.

Introduction

Microbes are single cell organisms and can be viral, bacterial, fungal, or protozoan parasites. There are many tens to hundreds of thousands of microbes. This chapter considers viral, bacterial, and parasitic agents which are TTIs and of major concern for blood safety. No fungal transmissions from transfusion have been reported. However, non-cellular protein, defined as prions, have been linked to TTIs in rare situations.

This chapter will commence with the biology and life cycle for viral pathogens after they have infected the human host. The knowledge from this basic research science has been used to design screening systems to test blood donations for the presence of viral markers. These systems screen either directly for viral antigen markers or indirectly for antibody markers made by the human immune system in response to the infection. Additional systems test directly for the viral genetic material using nucleic acid testing technologies (NAT).

The first part of the chapter will discuss:

- Screening strategies for TTIs that are mandatory (required under legal jurisdiction and/ or by health or regulatory authorities) for all donations and critical for patient and public safety.
- Selected testing of products for 'common' viral agents that pose a risk to immunocompromised patients such as stem cell transplant patients or low birth weight neonates.
- Bacterial testing for blood components stored at 22°C (e.g. platelets) which can enhance bacterial multiplication.

This century has seen the re-emergence of agents such as West Nile virus and dengue fever virus that are insect borne, and hepatitis E virus which is transmitted by untreated water or via porcine (from pig) contamination. The second part of this chapter will consider:

- Emerging issues for blood safety.
- Insect and animal borne pathogens: including the malaria parasite–long an enemy to man–as well as the re-emerging viral agents.
- Management strategies for the future.

5.1 Requirements for microbiological testing of blood donations

It is mandatory to screen all blood donations for the viruses that cause hepatitis B, acquired immune deficiency syndrome (AIDS), and hepatitis C. Donations are also screened for human T cell leukaemia virus and for the bacteria responsible for syphilis. These microorganisms are all transmissible by transfusion and exhibit predisposing properties.

The shared properties for these TTIs include a long incubation period before the infected person may show any symptom after infection (asymptomatic).

Other causes of inapparent infection are:

- carrier states (e.g. for HBsAg in hepatitis B) where expressed viral antigens and virions may be present in the blood and persist for several years, and
- latency where viral nucleic acid is incorporated into host cell DNA.

Both a carrier state and latency may occur with HIV. This results in inapparent infection although the individual expresses a viral carrier state with or without cell-associated latency (i.e. the virus lies in a dormant state).

The shared properties also include the ability for the virus to be transmitted by blood products to the patient and be pathogenic to the recipient. Table 5.1 shows the shared properties amongst TTIs of most concern to blood safety.

TABLE 5.1 Predisposing properties shared amongst micro organisms transmitted by transfusion and mandated for blood donor screening.

Property	Comment
Present in blood for lengthy period/ high viral load (high titre)	All agents mandated for testing exhibit these properties
Persists for long incubation periods	
Infection not apparent—asymptomatic	
Expressed carrier state	
Cell associated latency state	Characteristic of HIV-1 and 2, HTLV-I and II CMV*
Stability in stored blood	Viruses mandated for testing are stable The bacterium causing syphilis is not stable
Transmission of infection occurs by transfusion and results in a pathological condition in a proportion of cases	All agents

*Requirement for CMV testing is not mandatory but dependent on patient and blood product—see Section 5.5

5.2 **The virus life cycle: basic biology**

Once a virus enters the blood stream and infection occurs in host cells, the virus replicates within the host and can reach a high viral load (i.e. referred to as viral titre) before there is an **immune response**. The speed of replication, or doubling time, and the viral load reached varies with the different infectious agents. The formation of IgM antibodies followed by IgG results in a decline in the viral load, often to below the level of detection. The antibodies persist in the patients for varying times depending on the virus and the host immune competence. In several TTIs the virus may not be eliminated by these antibodies.

The period between inoculation and detection of the infection using laboratory tests is termed the **window period** (WP) (Figure 5.1 and Table 5.2). This is normally measured in days or weeks and would depend on the test used and the test **sensitivity**:

- NATs detect the DNA or RNA of the virus whilst it is replicating and has the shortest window phase.
- Antigen assays will become positive later in the infection.
- Antibody assays become positive after there is an immune response. If this is the only test used, then the window period may be longer and some infectious donations will not be detected.

During the NAT window period there is an eclipse phase when the donation is not infective. At the end of the eclipse phase, just before the NAT test becomes positive, the donation may be infectious but the risk is extremely low.

SELF-CHECK 5.1

What is the window period?

Immune response

The body's ability to recognize and defend itself against substances that appear foreign and harmful such as bacteria and viruses.

Window period

This is the period between the onset of the infection and the appearance of the detectable infectious agent or antibodies to it. For a virus, the window period is shorter for the detection of the viral RNA/ DNA than antibodies which are produced later in the infection.

Sensitivity

This can be simply described as the ability of a test to detect a marker as early as possible. The most sensitive tests detect the marker earliest.

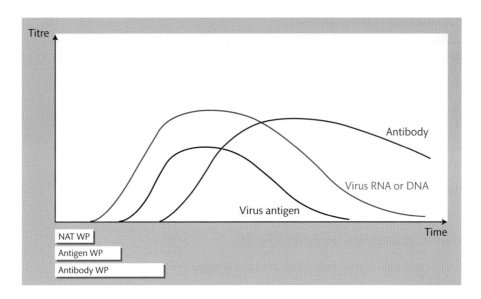

FIGURE 5.1

Generalized time course after infection showing when viral related markers can be detected in the blood: the time course is indicative only and not to scale. The window period (WP) is shortest for NAT based assays which detect viral RNA or DNA markers. During the window period there is an eclipse phase when the donation is not infective. At the end of the eclipse, just before the NAT or viral marker test becomes positive, the donation may be infectious.

Viral antigens are detected later followed by detection of antibodies that are produced by the immune system. Different specific antibodies become detectable at different times; e.g. with HBV, the appearance of anti-HBc precedes anti-HBs (and HBsAg). IgM antibodies are the first to be detectable followed by IgG antibodies.

TABLE 5.2   Window period (WP) for serology tests compared to NAT tests for disease markers: note the reduction in the window period using NAT.

Disease marker	WP for serology test	WP for NAT
HBV	36 days	15 days for ID NAT 28 days for mini-pools of 8 samples
HCV	65 days	5 days for ID NAT 5 days for mini-pools of 8 samples
HIV	15 days for anti-HIV 11 days for combined antibody/antigen test	5 days for ID NAT 7 days for mini-pools of 8 samples
HTLV	45 days	Not available

5.3 Epidemiology for hepatitis B and C and for HIV (AIDS)

Modes of transmission

Modes of transmission occur by direct entry of the virus into the blood circulation. For hepatitis B, for example, such entry can occur from contaminated blood in a needle, from splashes of

TABLE 5.3 Documented routes of transmission for TTIs.

Transmission route of infection	HBV	HCV	HIV	HTLV
Blood transfusion*	√	√	√	√**
Sexual contact with infected person; unprotected sex with infected person	√	√	√	√
Infants born to infected mothers (maternofetal route); perinatal from mother to baby	√	√	√#	√
Acupuncture, tattooing, and body piercing using infected needles	√	√	?	?
Intravenous drug users; through sharing needles and syringes	√	√	√	√
Occupational contact in healthcare professionals; needle stick injury	√	√	√	?
Haemodialysis patients if the equipment is not properly sterilized	√	√	?	?
Household contacts of infected individuals; sharing objects such as toothbrush, razor contaminated with blood	√	√	√	?
Institutionalized individuals such as prisoners and psychiatric in-patients	√	?	?	?
From mother to baby during breast feeding	?	?	?	√##

? Evidence for transmission by this route is not clear.

* Transmission by blood transfusion is very rare in countries where screening (including NAT) is mandatory.

** HTLV transmission occurs through blood transfusion of whole blood or cellular components as the virus is present in the host immune T cells. Transmission for HTLV is rare by plasma transfusion and leucodepletion to remove white cells (including T cells) has decreased the transmission of this virus. The use of an antibody test has significantly reduced transmission through this route.

An estimated 15–30% of HIV-infected mothers will transmit the infection to their babies during pregnancy or at delivery in the absence of any intervention. Latent HIV transmission is rare in patients on anti-retroviral prophylaxis and elective Caesarian delivery.

HTLV 1 is transmitted from infected mother to baby mostly through breastfeeding. This is because the virus infects the host immune T cells which are present in breast milk. One in four babies born to an infected mother acquires the infection this way.

contaminated material into the mucosal membranes (such as eye membrane) or from mother to baby before or at the time of birth (referred to as vertical transmission). Importantly TTIs are not generally transmitted by the oral-faecal route as the viruses are not resistant to the acidic conditions of the stomach. Exceptions are the occasionally transfusion-transmitted cases of hepatitis A virus, HAV, and hepatitis E virus, HEV. Documented modes of transmission routes are summarized in Table 5.3 for the different TTIs.

Hepatitis B (HBV)

Australia antigen was discovered by Blumberg in 1965 in the serum of an indigenous Australian, when the serum formed precipitin lines in an immunodiffusion assay with serum from a multi-transfused haemophiliac patient. It was subsequently called hepatitis B surface antigen (HBsAg). In 1970, Dane and co-workers identified the infectious agent of HBV (Dane particle) using electron microscopy. More than 257 million people in the world are infected with HBV, with the highest prevalence of between 8–20% in South-East Asia, China, and Africa.

HBV belongs to the hepadnavirus family. The Dane particle is the complete virion and contains the DNA which is enclosed in the nucleocapsid. A large excess of envelope material in the form of small spheres and rods of average width of 22 nm is produced as a result of HBV infection.

These small particles lack DNA and are not infectious. The Dane particle is 42 nm in diameter and consists of:

- An outer lipid layer which contains embedded proteins responsible for binding and entry into liver cells. These surface proteins express the antigen referred to as hepatitis B surface antigen (HBsAg). The HBsAg is also present on the excess 22 nm particles just referred to above. This excess production is a 'gift' for screening as it facilitates detection of the viral infection.

- An inner nucleocapsid core—hepatitis B core antigen (HBcAg). The nucleocapsid is composed of protein and encloses the partially double-stranded circular viral DNA and DNA polymerase.

- The partially double stranded circular viral DNA of approximately 3200 base pairs codes for four genes called C, P, S, and X.

Response to viral infections

Once in the blood stream the hepatitis B virus infects the hepatocytes of liver but does not usually cause direct damage to these cells. Following infection the host may respond by producing antibodies to the hepatitis core antigen, called anti-HBc, and to the hepatitis B surface antigen, called anti-HBs.

This host cellular immune response to HBV producing anti-HBs is the cause of liver damage—the more vigorous the immune response, the greater the resulting damage. This can lead to complete viral clearance and the development of anti-HBs to prevent re-infection. However, due to inadequate immune response and host factors, the infection may persist in some individuals.

Clinical course of infection

The onset of HBV infection is usually insidious:

- There is an incubation period of 60–90 days but this can be as long as 180 days. This is dependent on the viral dose, route of infection, and host factors, including immune response factors. The different routes of infection documented for hepatitis B are shown in Table 5.3.

- There is a period of acute infection during which HBsAg and HBeAg (derived from the core gene, modified and exported from the liver) are detectable. Patients may present with symptoms such as mild fever, fatigue, nausea, anorexia, vomiting, dark urine, and skin rashes, and abdominal, muscle, and joint pains. Jaundice is found in 30–50% of individuals who are infected when over five years of age, but in less than 10% of those infected under the age of five.

- Most HBV infected adults will recover and develop immunity. Anti-HBs, anti-HBc, and anti-HBe can be detected. Some individuals with HBV will develop chronic infection which is age related. The risk of progression to chronic infection is approximately 90% for neonates and children under one year, 30% for children aged 1–5 years, and 2% for those over five years old.

Genotypes and mutants

Eight genotypes have been identified (genotypes A–H). In addition, there are several sub types of HBV.

HBV replicates by the use of reverse transcriptase (RT) to form an RNA intermediate. Reverse transcriptase lacks proof-reading capability and therefore error in transcription is not detected and corrected. This can lead to mutant strains of HBV which, if the conditions are right, can result in its survival along with the wild-type or replace it. Mutant strains can also spontaneously evolve. HBV escape mutants are increasingly being seen in individuals who have been vaccinated and have high levels of anti-HBs.

Tests

Sensitive enzyme–linked immunosorbent assays (ELISA) and chemiluminescence assays for the detection of hepatitis B surface antigens (HBsAg) are available for blood donation screening. A multiplex NAT for HBV, HCV, and HIV has been introduced for blood donation screening. The current consensus is that both the serological antigen tests and the viral NAT tests are required to screen donors as different viral markers may be present at different stages.

Tests on serial samples for anti-HBs, HBeAg, and anti-HBe from HBsAg–positive patients are useful as an indication of the chronicity or infectivity and the stage of the infection.

- The presence of HBsAg for more than six months would indicate a chronic infection.
- Seroconversion from HBsAg to anti-HBs suggests a resolution of the disease and establishment of immunity.
- HBeAg positivity indicates infectivity.
- Seroconversion from HBeAg to anti-HBe indicates progression to a reduced level of infectivity.

Discretionary testing for anti-HBc is performed on samples from donors who have body piercing/tattoos, acupunctures, and endoscopy at least four months after the procedure or the donors are suspended for 12 months (six months for endoscopy).

Key points

HBV is a partially double-stranded DNA virus which infects the hepatocytes of the liver. The damage to the infected cells is due to the host cellular immune response. Many genotypes, sub types, and mutants have been described.

Hepatitis C (HCV)

Hepatitis C (HCV) was the first virus to be identified by molecular cloning methods by Choo and co-workers in 1989. It was previously referred to as non-A non-B hepatitis virus. HCV infects only humans and chimpanzees, and is a member of the *Flaviviridae* family. It is a small, lipid enveloped virus with a single positive–stranded RNA.

According to the World Health Organization (WHO), approximately 1% of the world population, that is, more than 71 million people are infected with HCV. The prevalence of HCV infection in the developed world ranges from 0.5–2%, with 6.5% in parts of Equatorial Africa and up to 20% in Egypt. There are six main HCV genotypes (genotypes 1–6) with geographical associations.

The modes of HCV transmission are similar to HBV, see Table 5.3.

Clinical course of infection

The onset of infection with HCV usually goes unnoticed: 60–70% of infected people are asymptomatic, with only 10–20% developing non-specific symptoms such as malaise, fatigue, and abdominal pain. The average incubation period is 6–7 weeks, but can vary from 2–26 weeks or more. In 10–30% of infected individuals, the infection is self-limiting, leading to recovery. The remainder will develop chronic hepatitis, with 10–20% developing cirrhosis. Between 1–5% of the chronically infected patients will develop hepatocellular carcinoma over a period of 20–30 years.

The liver is the major site for HCV infection, where it multiplies rapidly, with up to 10^{12} viruses produced daily. There is evidence of HCV reservoirs outside the liver in the peripheral blood lymphocytes, epithelial cells in the gut, and the central nervous system.

Key points

HCV is a small single-stranded RNA virus which mainly infects the liver cells. Approximately 3% of the world population is infected with this virus. Approximately 1% of the world population is infected with this virus.

Tests

An antibody test for HCV was first introduced in the UK for blood donation screening in 1991. This has resulted in a significant reduction in transmission of this virus by blood transfusion. The assay (ELISA and chemiluminescence) has since been enhanced to marginally increase the sensitivity and **specificity**. Any samples which are repeatedly reactive are confirmed by testing with an alternative ELISA and recombinant immunoblot assays (RIBA). Nucleic acid testing for HCV (and HBV and HIV-1) is performed on all donor samples.

Specificity
This is the proportion of people who are correctly identified by a screening test as negative for the disease/infection.

Human immunodeficiency virus (HIV)

In 1981, the Center for Disease Control in Atlanta, USA, reported cases of homosexual patients suffering from previously rare conditions such as pneumocystis pneumonia and Kaposi's sarcoma. This condition, called acquired immunodeficiency syndrome (AIDS), was shown in 1983 to be caused by a newly recognized human immunodeficiency virus (HIV-1). HIV-2 was later reported in West African patients as another cause of AIDS.

There are more that 40 million HIV-infected individuals worldwide, with nearly equal numbers of infected men and women. The majority of these are in countries in Sub-Saharan Africa, Asia, and South America.

Three HIV-1 groups have been known for some time: M (for main), O (outlier), and N. A rare fourth HIV-1 group, P, has been identified in Cameroonians living in Paris. Groups O and N are rare and are found predominantly in Cameroon in Central Africa. Nine sub types have been recognized in group M. They are A, B, C, D, F, G, H, J, and K. In addition, there are the recombinant forms which are the results of recombinations of two or more group M sub types. Genotype B is the main one found in the developed countries but genotype C is prevalent in most of the world.

HIV has two copies of positive single-stranded RNA which codes for the virus's nine genes. It is amongst the most variable of all human pathogens. The variability arises because:

- The RNA has to be transcribed into DNA using an enzyme reverse transcriptase (RT) which lacks proof reading. As a result, errors are introduced at an average rate of one substitution per genome per replication round.

- The virus replicates rapidly *in vivo*, generating approximately 10^{10} virions per day.
- During recombination, RT copies the two viral RNA molecules which are packaged together in a virion. As a result of 7–30 cross overs per replication round, mosaic genomes are produced.

The main routes of HIV transmission are similar to that for HBV and HCV, see Table 5.3. Modes of transmission include unprotected sex with an infected individual; the risk increases with repetitive sexual contacts. The risk of infection also increases in the presence of other sexually transmitted disease.

Clinical course of infection

HIV-1 is an RNA retrovirus belonging to the lentivirus family. These viruses typically have a long period of clinical latency during which there is virus replication and central nervous system involvement. Following HIV infection, the virus targets the CD4+ T cells where it enters the cells and multiplies. This is the acute phase of infection and can last up to eight weeks, during which:

- The infected individuals may be asymptomatic or display flu-like symptoms. Symptoms resembling infectious mononucleosis have also been described. The symptoms last for 7–10 days but rarely more than 14 days.
- As a result of intense replication, viral loads of 100 million copies of HIV-1 RNA/ml can be reached.
- There is seeding of virus into a range of tissue reservoirs, particularly in the lymphoid tissues of the gut.
- There is destruction of CD4+ T cells leading to a decline in counts, sometimes to levels that allow development of opportunistic infections.

Following the host immune response and antibody production, referred to as seroconversion, there is a rapid decline in the viral load and the CD4+ T cell count starts to rise but never reaches the pre-infection levels.

Equilibrium between viral replication and the host immune response or viral setpoint is reached, which is a strong predictor of long-term disease progression. This chronic phase or period of clinical latency can last for 8–10 years or longer. During this period, there is a high turnover of virus, with the resultant destruction and decline of CD4+ T cells.

Host factors mainly determine how rapidly the decline into AIDS occurs. A CD4+ T cell count of less than 200 increases the risks of AIDS defining illnesses such as opportunistic infections.

Tests

Early detection of HIV infection will enable the patient to benefit from appropriate therapeutic treatment and prevent transmission of infection. Fourth–generation ELISA and chemiluminescent immunoassay (CLIA) screening tests will detect antibodies to HIV-1, including most sub-types, and HIV-2 and will also detect p24 antigen of the virus particle, thus reducing the window period. Many countries now screen donors by single testing of each donated blood using multiplex HBV, HCV, and HIV NAT.

Donated blood in the UK is also tested in pools of 24 samples by multiplex HBV, HCV, and HIV NAT.

> **Key points**
>
> HIV has two positive single strands of RNA and it infects CD4+ T cells. Destruction of the infected CD4+ T cells can lead to opportunistic infections. The progression from infection to AIDS is dependent on host factors as well as response to treatment.

Syphilis

Syphilis is caused by a spirochete bacterium, *Treponema pallidum*. It is estimated that worldwide, there are 10–12 million new infections each year. Penicillin is very effective at treating this infection, although other treatments are available. If untreated, the course of infection is classified into the following stages:

- Primary syphilis—usually a painless lesion (chancre) develops at the site of infection after around 9–90 days (usually 2–3 weeks) with local, tender lymphadenopathy. Occasionally multiple painful lesions develop. The lesion(s) spontaneously heal after 4–5 weeks.

- Secondary syphilis—this usually occurs 4–8 weeks after primary syphilis. The symptoms include fever, malaise, generalized lymphadenopathy, and a diffuse rash, typically on the palms, soles, and scalp. There may be other clinical presentations and complications in a small percentage of patients. These patients spontaneously improve, but a quarter may relapse into secondary syphilis. These relapses are rare after one year.

- Early latent syphilis—this is less than two years' duration and the patients are asymptomatic but still infectious.

- Late latent syphilis—this is an asymptomatic, non-infectious stage of more than two years' duration.

- Tertiary syphilis—this occurs 3–20 years after exposure. About 35% of untreated patients will develop tertiary syphilis. Three main manifestations are neurosyphilis, cardiovascular syphilis, and gummatous syphilis.

Syphilis can also be transmitted transplacentally from infected mother to baby. This happens mostly during the first two years of infection, although there have been cases of transmission during late latent syphilis. A third of the pregnancies will result in miscarriage or stillbirth, and a third with congenital syphilis. The remaining third of babies will be born without infection. There is a two to five-fold increase in risk of acquiring HIV infection in individuals who are infected with syphilis. This is because the genital sores provide an entry point for the HIV virus during sexual contact.

The immune response to syphilis involves a 'non-specific' antibody response to a broad range of antigens such as cardiolipin, and specific anti-treponemal antibodies. Specific anti-treponemal IgM antibodies are developed towards the end of the second week of infection and become undetectable 3–9 months after treatment of early syphilis. Anti-treponemal IgG antibodies appear at about four weeks.

Tests

Serological tests for syphilis are classified into:

- Non-treponemal (non-specific) for cardiolipin antibodies—for example Venereal Diseases Research Laboratory (VDRL) and Rapid Plasma Reagin (RPR) tests. Sensitivity of these tests is estimated to be 78–86% for primary infections and 95–100% for secondary and latent infections with specificity of 85–99%.

- Treponemal (specific) for antibodies—for example *Treponema pallidum* haemagglutination assay (TPHA) and *Treponema pallidum* particle agglutination assay (TPPA). Other examples include fluorescent and enzyme immunoassays. Fluorescent treponemal antibody-absorbed (FTA-abs) has a specificity of 96% and a sensitivity of 84% for detecting primary syphilis and 100% for the other stages of infection. Enzyme immunoassay (EIA) is rapidly becoming the screening test of choice because of the high sensitivity (98.5–100%) and specificity (97–100%) and can be automated.

Key points

Syphilis is caused by the *Treponema pallidum* spirochetes. If left untreated, patients can develop tertiary syphilis which manifests as neurosyphilis, cardiovascular syphilis, and/or gummatous syphilis. The risk of being infected with HIV is increased in individuals with syphilis.

Human T cell lymphotropic virus

Human T cell lymphotropic virus type I (HTLV-I) is a retrovirus which infects T cells. The virus was first isolated in a patient with cutaneous T cell lymphoma in 1980. The infection is asymptomatic in the majority of individuals, but they are infectious for life.

Human T cell lymphotropic virus type I is endemic in Japan, the Caribbean, Africa, and South America. It is also found in southern India, northern Iran, and indigenous populations of northern Australia. There are an estimated 10–20 million people worldwide who are infected with this virus. In Europe and North America HTLV-I is found predominantly in migrants from endemic areas and intravenous drug users.

Human T cell lymphotropic virus type I is the causative agent of adult T cell lymphoma (ATL), which is a very aggressive T cell malignancy. The mean age at diagnosis is 60 years in Japan but 40 years in the Caribbean and Brazil. For ATL, men are more commonly affected, with an M:F ratio of 1.5:1.

Human T cell lymphotropic virus type I also causes a variety of chronic inflammatory syndromes such as HTLV-I associated myelopathy (HAM) or tropical spastic paraparesis (TSP). This is an inflammation of the nerves in the spinal cord and causes stiffness, weakness in the legs, low back pain, incontinence, and constipation, though all the symptoms may not be present in the same patient. The mean age at onset for HAM/TSP is 40 years and women are two to three times more likely to be affected than men.

Human T cell lymphotropic virus type II was identified in the 1980s. It is not definitively linked with any disease but has been associated with several cases of HAM/TSP.

leucodepletion

A process for removal of white blood cells from blood components to less that 5×10^6 per unit through an in-line filter.

The routes of transmission include transmission from infected mother to baby mostly through breastfeeding. Table 5.3 lists the known routes of transmission. One in four babies born to an infected mother acquires the infection this way. Transmission occurs through blood transfusion of whole blood and cellular components. Because it is cell-associated, **leucodepletion** has decreased the transmission of this virus. The use of an antibody test has also significantly reduced transmission through this route.

Tests

Enzyme immunoassay (EIA) is used to screen for HTLV-I and HTLV-II infections on all donations and immunoblot for confirmation. The EIA tests are performed on pools of 24 samples in the UK blood services.

Key points

HTLV-I is a retrovirus which is endemic in Japan, Africa, the Caribbean, and South America. It can cause T cell lymphoma, HTLV-I associated myelopathy, and tropical spastic paraparesis.

5.4 Screening strategy for mandatory viral tests

Pre-donation screening prior to blood donation is an essential step in reducing the number of potentially infective donations collected. Blood services screen millions of blood donations each year. Testing is usually performed on automated equipment with online data/result transfer to the host computer. Testing is performed within a quality controlled and quality management system in blood establishments. The laboratories are also subjected to audits by regulatory agencies.

The *Guidelines for the Blood Transfusion Services in the United Kingdom* states that all blood components must be tested for the following disease markers and satisfactory results obtained before blood and blood components can be released from quarantine for use:

- HBsAg.
- Anti-HIV.
- Anti-HCV.
- Anti-syphilis.
- Nucleic acid testing for HCV RNA and HIV RNA*.
- Nucleic acid testing for Hepatitis B DNA.
- Anti-HTLV*.

* In some countries these tests can be performed using a pool of plasma from several donations, whereas all the other tests are performed on individual donations. However, there is a progression toward testing all donations individually to achieve maximum sensitivity in the ability to detect low levels of virus. See Table 5.4 which sets out microbial testing requirements for blood donations.

An effective and almost universal strategy for blood donor screening is to retest all initially reactive samples, in duplicate, using the original assay, and determine the status of the donation from the repeat results. (Two or three reactive test results out of three tests are considered reactive). This strategy may improve specificity as any non-specific initial reactive result may not be repeatable.

TABLE 5.4 Microbial testing requirements for blood donations.

Requirement	Virus/bacteria/parasite	Screening test*
Mandatory	Hepatitis B virus (HBV)	Hepatitis B surface antigen (HBsAg) HBV DNA
Mandatory	Human immunodeficiency virus (HIV 1 and HIV 2)	Anti- HIV 1 & 2 (HIV p24 antigen is combined with the HIV antibody test) HIV RNA
Mandatory	Hepatitis C virus (HCV)	Anti-HCV HCV RNA
Mandatory in some regions	Human T cell lymphotropic virus (HTLV-1)	Anti-HTLV I
Mandatory	Syphilis bacteria	Anti-*T. pallidum*
Dependent on patient and blood product	Cytomegalovirus	Anti-CMV
Surveillance by travel history	Malaria	Anti-*P. falciparum* after a defined period of travel

* Antibody tests (anti-) are indirect tests for the host immune response to the viral infection

Serological tests for antigen and antibody markers

Two test systems are used within the UK blood services and many other services:

- Abbott PRISM for HIV (antibody or combination antigen antibody test), anti-HCV, and HBsAg detection. The tests are performed in dedicated channels for HIV, HCV, HBsAg, anti-HBc (if performed), and anti-HTLV. There is a sixth channel which is used as a backup in case of failure of any of the dedicated channels. A chemiluminescent immunoassay (CLIA) is used for the detection of the test markers or analytes.

- Ortho Summit is also used for HIV (antibody or combination antigen antibody test), anti-HCV, and HBsAg detection. The tests are performed in microplates using enzyme–linked immunosorbent assay (ELISA).

Antibodies to syphilis are mostly tested for using a *Treponema pallidum* haemagglutination assay (TPHA) or *Treponema pallidum* particle assay (TPPA) on the Beckman Coulter blood testing analyser. ELISA test for anti-syphilis is sometimes used in routine blood donation screening. Anti-HTLV ELISA testing is performed in pools of 24 samples. Recently the English Blood Services have restricted anti-HTLV testing to new donors and to those donations being used to produce non-leucodepleted components. In general, leucodepletion greatly reduces the risk of transmitting cell-associated agents.

SELF-CHECK 5.2

What serological tests are performed for detection of HBV, HCV, and HIV contamination of blood donation?

METHOD Chemiluminescent immunoassay (CLIA) methods

Three methods used on the Abbott PRISM are three-step sandwich assay, two-step sandwich, and two-step competitive assay. The tests are performed on microparticles in specially designed black reaction trays which each have two sets of eight wells. The microparticles are coated with antigens and/or antibodies, depending on the analyte being detected. The tests are incubated at 37°C in heated channels of the PRISM.

Three-step sandwich assay

- The first step of the assay is the incubation of the sample and microparticles in the incubation well of the reaction tray. Analyte(s) in the sample will bind to the corresponding antigen and/or antibody on the microparticles.

- The incubation mixture is washed into a reaction well where the microparticles with or without bound analytes are trapped on a glass fibre matrix. Any unbound material is washed through to an absorbent material contained in the reaction tray.

- Further reactions take place on the microparticles on the glass fibre matrix.

- A biotinylated probe is added to the reaction well and incubated. The probe will bind to the free arm of antibody (from sample or control) attached to the microparticles. Unbound probe is washed away.

- Acridinium labelled conjugate is added to the reaction well and after incubation unbound conjugate is washed away.

- A background reading is taken, and then activator is added to the reaction well. The activator will cause acridinium to emit light (photons) which is measured. This reading is corrected for the background and compared with the cut-off to determine if the reaction is positive or negative.

Two-step sandwich assay

This is the same as the three-step sandwich assay but the step involving the incubation with a biotinylated probe is omitted.

Two-step competitive/blocking assay

This is same as the two-step sandwich assay but the conjugate attaches to any binding site on the microparticles that are not occupied by antigens or antibody from the sample.

METHOD ELISA methods

Two-step sandwich assay

ELISA is usually performed in 96–well microplates. Antigens and/or antibodies are coated to the bottom of the microplate well. Incubation temperatures vary with assay types.

- Sample is added to the microplate well and incubated, allowing the analyte to bind to the coated microplate well. Unbound sample is washed away, usually using an automated plate washer.

- Conjugate (usually an antibody to the analyte conjugated to an enzyme such as horseradish peroxidase or alkaline phosphatase) is added to the well and incubated. The conjugate will bind to any bound analyte from the sample. Unbound conjugate is washed away.

- A substrate is added which will be cleaved by the enzyme on the conjugate (if present) to a coloured substance. The reaction is stopped with an acid after a fixed time, usually resulting in a change in colour, the optical density of which can be measured in a microplate reader. The colour change indicates a positive reaction.

Competitive ELISA method

- Sample and conjugate are added to the microplate well and incubated. The conjugate is the analyte conjugated to an enzyme such as horseradish peroxidase or alkaline phosphatase and will compete with the analyte being tested for to bind to the coated microplate well. Unbound sample and conjugate is washed away.

- The substrate is added and after a period of incubation, the reaction is stopped with an acid and the microplate read.

- A negative reaction is indicated by a high optical density as in the absence of the analyte from the sample, the conjugate will bind to the coated wells.

Because there are only two incubation steps, the assay is quicker to perform than the sandwich assay.

Key points

Serological tests were first introduced to detect antibodies and antigens from infectious agents. Introduction of NAT further reduced the risk of transmission of infectious agents through blood transfusions.

Nucleic acid testing for viral DNA or RNA genes

Nucleic acid testing (NAT)

Following the transmission of HCV through a commercial intravenous immunoglobulin (IVIg) preparation, the European Committee for Proprietary Medicinal Products recommended that from 1999 HCV RNA–negative plasma is used for intravenous immunoglobulin (IVIg) preparation if there is not a viral inactivation step. HCV RNA (HCV NAT) test using **polymerase chain reaction** (PCR) was introduced in the UK. The test was initially performed on pools of 96 plasma samples and then subsequently on pools of 48 samples. Cross-pools were prepared and tested on positive pools to identify the infected donation(s).

Hepatitis C NAT has now been extended to include **all** blood components. Release of products with a shelf-life of less than 24 hours without the NAT result may be permitted in rare emergency situations where there is a justified clinical imperative. Fully automated NAT for HBV, HCV, and HIV has been implemented either by testing in a single donation format or, as in the UK, by testing in mini-pools of 24 samples, increasing further the safety of the blood supply. For a positive mini-pool, sub-pools are prepared to identify the infected donation. The use of mini-pools can be justified in countries where the prevalence of the tested virus is low. However, in countries where there is a high prevalence of the tested virus (such as HIV) it would be prudent to perform individual donation NAT (ID NAT). The reduction of the window period for microbiology serology and NAT is shown in Table 5.2.

The principle of NAT is:

- Concentration, extraction, and purification of the nucleic acid (DNA and RNA). In some cases the sample is centrifuged at high speed to concentrate the viral cells and increase the sensitivity of the test. The samples are mixed with a lysis buffer to disrupt the viral cell wall and release the nucleic acid. The nucleic acid is then captured on a solid phase such as silica or using sequence specific probes. After washing away the impurities, the nucleic acid is re-suspended.

- Amplification of the nucleic acid to increase the number of copies and hence, the sensitivity of the test.

- Detection of the specific component of the DNA or RNA.

An internal control is included in each pool of samples (or each sample for ID NAT) to ensure that the extraction, amplification, and detection have taken place. The internal control must be positive for the test to be valid.

A fully automated commercial NAT system, Roche cobas s201 is in use in the UK Blood Services for the detection of HBV, HCV, and HIV. This system uses real-time PCR, where the products of amplification are measured during the reaction. The sample with added internal control is pre-treated in the sample preparation unit (SPU) to lyse the viral envelope and the released RNA or DNA bind to the positively charged silica surface of magnetic glass particles. The magnetic glass particles (with or without captured nucleic acid) are transferred into bar-code labelled sample input tubes (S tubes) for genome amplification and detection and the end result is the emission of light for a positive reaction which is measurable.

An alternative commercial NAT system is the fully automated Chiron Tigris which uses a pat-ented transcription mediated amplification technology (TMA) for multiplex HBV, HCV, and HIV-1 detection. The viral genome capture, amplification, and detection take place in a single tube at the same temperature as described below:

- Samples (or pools) with internal control are lysed to release the RNA/DNA in a multi-tube unit (MTU). Capture probes hybridize to targeted nucleic acid which then attach to magnetic particles by their tail sequence. Any unbound material is washed away.

- Amplification reagent containing a reverse transcriptase, RNA polymerase, and primers is added to the MTU. The primers bind to targeted RNA/DNA and are used by the reverse transcriptase to create DNA copies of viral RNA. A second complementary copy of DNA is produced to form a double–stranded DNA duplex. The RNA polymerase makes multi-ple copies of RNA amplicons from the DNA template. The reaction continues until all the reagents are used up, resulting in billions of copies in one hour.

- A single-stranded nucleic acid probe labelled with acridinium ester is added to the mixture and hybridizes to the complementary amplicon. Unhybridized probes are inactivated to reduce background noise. Hybridized probes produce a chemiluminescent signal which is measured in a luminometer.

 METHOD *Basic PCR method*

1. PCR can amplify and detect DNA sequences directly. However, for RNA viruses such as HCV, a reverse tran-scription step using the enzyme reverse transcriptase is necessary to produce complementary DNA (cDNA) which can be used as a template for PCR.

2. The purified DNA (or cDNA) is mixed with a thermostable DNA polymerase (taq polymerase), two oligonucleotide primers, deoxynucleotide triphosphate (dNTPs), reaction buffer, and magnesium. Other additives may be included. The following reactions take place in a thermocycler which automatically changes the temperature for preset times.

3. The reaction mixture is heated to 95°C to denature the DNA, causing each double strand to separate into two single strands (sense and antisense).

4. The temperature is lowered to 50–65°C to allow the oligonucleotide primers to bind to the complementary sequence of the DNA.

5. The temperature is then raised to 72°C for the Taq pol-ymerase to cause the primers to 'grow' or 'extend' the primer sequence by reading along the single–stranded DNA template chain to produce two amplicons (and two double-stranded DNAs).

6. The reaction cycle is repeated many times by alternating the temperature to 95°C, then 50–65°C, and then 72°C to produce millions or billions of copies of DNA. The high power of this amplification process creates the exquisite sensitivity of PCR-based assays.

7. The end product can be visualized using a stable and environmentally safe fluorescent dye after gel electro-phoresis of the PCR amplicon products.

A diagram of this process is shown in Figure 5.2.

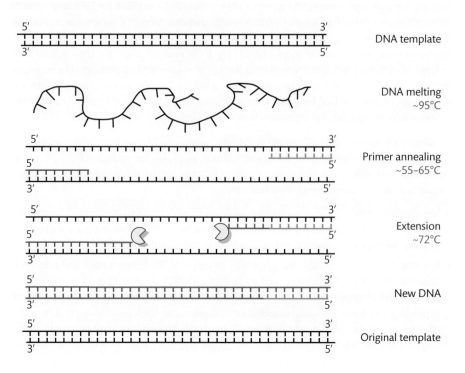

FIGURE 5.2

Diagrammatic representation of the basic PCR method. (© The Biomedical Scientist, 2007, Step Publishing.) The three key steps comprise melting or **denaturing** the DNA at high temperatures; lowering the temperature to permit **annealing** of primers to DNA strands and **extension** of the primer sequences. The primer extension is achieved using enzymes that are resistant to heat denaturation. This permits repeating the cycles resulting in over a million-fold amplification of the target sequence.

Confirmatory testing

Donations which are negative for the mandatory tests and the required additional markers can be released to stock if all the required blood group serology tests are satisfactory. Donor samples which are reactive for any microbiology marker ('initial reactive' samples) are retested in duplicate as stated above. All blood and components derived from that donation must be quarantined to prevent inadvertent issue. The duplicate test must be performed using the same assay which was used in the original test. Thus:

- If the duplicate repeat results are non-reactive (negative), all components prepared from the donation can be released to stock if the blood group serology tests are satisfactory.
- If one or both of the repeat tests are repeat reactive (positive):
  - All components prepared from the donation must be labelled 'Not for transfusion' and discarded.

    For a 'repeat reactive' donation, any components from the previous donation(s) which are still in stock (e.g. fresh frozen plasma or cryoprecipitate) should be quarantined until the infectious nature of the current donation is determined. This is a precautionary measure as it is possible, but unlikely, for the previous donation to be in the 'window phase' and therefore possible it could transmit the infection even though the screening tests for the mandatory microbiology markers were negative at the time.

  - The donor record must be flagged for confirmatory testing. Sample(s) from the donation testing as repeat reactive must be referred to a reference centre for confirmatory testing. The reference centre should be independent of the microbiology screening laboratory. The assays used for confirmatory testing should (where possible) be at least as sensitive as the screening assay. The confirmatory testing is necessary because all microbiology test kits have a small percentage of false positive reactions. By testing with different test kits/assays or additional tests for that marker, the true infectivity of the sample can be determined.

- If the reference centre confirms the result as positive, the donor must be *permanently excluded* from further donation. The donor should be offered counselling and an additional sample taken to confirm the infection.

  As an important public health measure it is critical to ensure prompt *donor notification* to provide for medical treatment and to contain further transmission of the virus within the community.

- If the reference centre result is negative or indeterminate, the donor record should be flagged for repeat testing after 12 weeks (see re-instatement algorithm).

Re-instatement algorithm for reference centre negative or indeterminate results

Samples should be taken from the donor at least 12 weeks after the previous donation was found to be repeatedly reactive. This is to allow any infection in the 'window period' or early seroconversion to reach a detectable level. The 12-week follow-up sample is tested at the blood service screening laboratory and the reference centre and if the results are:

- Non-reactive for that microbiology marker at both the screening laboratory and reference centre, the donor can be returned to the active donor panel. The next donation can be used if all mandatory and additional tests are satisfactory.

- Non-reactive at the screening laboratory for that microbiology marker but reactive or indeterminate at the reference centre and considered to be a false positive reaction, the donor can be returned to the active donor panel. The next donation can be used if all mandatory and additional tests are satisfactory.

- Still reactive for that microbiology marker by the current screening assay but non-reactive by an alternative assay of equivalent sensitivity at the blood service but non-reactive or indeterminate at the reference centre and considered to be a false positive reaction, it can be retested using an alternative screening assay. The next donation can be used if all mandatory and additional tests are satisfactory. Procedures must be in place at the blood service to ensure that the donor sample is tested using the alternative screening assay for the offending infectious disease marker.

- If the use of an alternative is not feasible, the donor must be deferred from further donations and a letter sent to explain the false reactivity.

SELF-CHECK 5.3

Why was nucleic acid test (NAT) introduced?

5.5 Testing strategy to protect immunocompromised patients

Cytomegalovirus

Cytomegalovirus (CMV) is a member of the herpes group of viruses. The virus has a double-stranded DNA, 160–180 nm in diameter and replicates in leucocytes and other **haemopoietic**

Haemopoietic
Blood cells produced in the bone marrow.

cells. In healthy individuals CMV infection may not be apparent or they may exhibit mild flu-like symptoms. However, in immunologically compromised or immunosuppressed patients (low birth weight infants, pregnant women, transplant recipients, and AIDS patients) it can be a life-threatening condition.

After primary infection, there is an incubation period of 22–40 days during which IgM and then IgG antibodies are formed. Among blood donors, between 50–70% have antibodies to CMV. Following infection, the CMV DNA becomes integrated into the human host genome, where it remains latent. During the latency period, the individual is normally free of infectious virus. The virus can be activated when the immune system is compromised, for example as a result of pregnancy and immunosuppressive therapy.

The routes of CMV transmission are:

- Pre-natal (congenital) where the sources of infections are semen, maternal cell bound viraemia, and ascending genital infection. This is determined by the presence of CMV in urine by cell culture during the first week of life.
- Perinatal infection during delivery, possibly from cervical secretions or during breastfeeding. Cytomegalovirus is not isolated from the urine during the first week of life but can be detected in the urine and/or saliva from two weeks to six months after delivery.
- Sexual contact.
- Blood transfusion.

Testing

In the UK, all blood components are leucodepleted. Because CMV resides in the white cells, there is reduction in the risk of transmission by blood transfusion. However, the risk reduction may not be sufficient to remove the need for CMV testing. Thus, blood components for intra-uterine transfusions, neonates up to 28 days post–expected date of delivery, pregnant women, and for granulocyte transfusions are screened for antibodies to CMV usually using an ELISA test and those tested as CMV antibody negative are considered 'safe' from latent CMV. In practice, blood services will flag CMV antibody reactive donors on their computerized records and will not retest further donations.

Key points

Cytomegalovirus is a double-stranded DNA virus which can cause severe disease or fatality in immunosuppressed or immunocompromised patients.

5.6 Bacterial tests for products stored at room temperature

Mandatory transfusion microbiology screening of donated blood has reduced the risk of transmission by transfusion of these viral contaminants to miniscule proportions (see Table 5.5). Bacterial contamination of blood and blood components remains the main infectious cause of transfusion reactions resulting in sepsis and death.

Fatalities due to bacterially contaminated blood components are now extremely rare. The majority of these are due to Gram-negative bacteria such as *Serratia liquifaciens* and *Yersinia*

TABLE 5.5 Estimates of the risks of infectious donations issued for transfusion in the UK for 2007–2009 *(Safe supplies: Testing the Nation Annual review 2009).*

Risk (1 per × million) due to:	HBV	HCV	HIV
All donations	0.79	0.035	0.14
New donors	2.23	0.133	0.18

enterocolitica and also Gram-positive coagulase-negative staphylococci. These organisms can proliferate at 2–6°C, the storage temperature of red cell components. The patients usually develop high temperature and chills during or shortly after transfusion, and death can occur within 24 hours.

Surveillance studies have shown that 1 in 1000–2000 units of platelets are contaminated with bacteria. However, the risk of death from bacterially contaminated platelet transfusion is between 1 in 7500 and 1 in 100,000. Fatality due to whole blood derived platelets is higher than that of single donor apheresis platelets. Passive surveillance studies in the UK, USA, and France show that Gram-positive bacteria account for 71% of transfusion transmission but Gram-negative organisms were implicated in 82% of the fatalities.

Fresh frozen plasma (FFP) and cryoprecipitate are rarely associated with transfusion-transmitted bacterial contamination. There are reports of both of these components acquiring bacterial infections when they were thawed in a contaminated water bath.

BOX 5.1 *Bacteria implicated in transfusion transmission by red cell and platelets*

Red cells	Platelets
Gram-positive bacteria	**Gram-positive bacteria**
Bacillus cereus	*Bacillus cereus*
Coagulase-negative staphylococcus	Coagulase-negative staphylococcus
Enterococcus faecalis	*Enterococcus faecalis*
Group B streptococcus	Group B streptococcus
Staphylococcus epidermidis	*Proprionibacterium acnes*
Proprionibacterium acnes	*Staphylococcus epidermidis*
Streptococcus species	*Staphylococcus aureus*
	Streptococcus species
Gram-negative bacteria	**Gram-negative bacteria**
Acinetobacter species	*Acinetobacter* species
Enterobacter species	*Enterobacter* species
Escherichia species	*Escherichia* species
Klebsiella species	*Klebsiella* species
Morganella morganii	*Pseudomonas* species
Proteus species	*Proteus* species
Serratia species	*Serratia* species
Yersinia enterocolitica	*Yersinia enterocolitica*

The sources of blood component bacterial contamination are:

- Skin contamination—this is due to inadequate decontamination of the skin prior to phlebotomy. Enhanced donor arm cleansing prior to venipuncture reduces bacterial risk posed by external skin surface.

- On occasions, there may be subcutaneous bacterial infection which is unaffected by the skin cleansing. During blood collection, the skin core or plug may become detached by the collection needle and contaminate the blood pack. Diversion of the first 20-30 ml of the donation into a sample pouch (used for blood grouping and microbiology screening) will reduce the contamination of the main pack.

- Asymptomatic donors—the donors are transiently infected as shown by elevated IgM or IgG antibody titres to bacteria, notably *Yersinia enterocolitica*.

- Contaminated blood bag—*Serratia marcescens* found in the dust of the manufacturing plant is thought to contaminate the outside of the blood collection bag. These multiply in the presence of moisture and nutrient, and possibly gain entry into the inside of the bag.

- Contaminated water bath—*Pseudomonas cepacia* and *Pseudomonas aeruginosa* in water baths used for thawing FFP and cryoprecipitate have been cultured from these components.

- Contamination during processing—this is extremely rare with the use of sterile connecting devices and integrated blood and satellite packs.

Screening for bacterial contamination

The detection of the bacteria in blood components depends on:

- Timing of sampling—low level contamination may not be detectable on the day of collection. These bacteria may proliferate over the succeeding days to sufficiently high numbers to cause severe adverse reactions in recipients. A decision has to be made as to the optimal day of sampling post-collection. This considers where the majority of bacterial contamination will be detected while still retaining a reasonable component shelf-life. This is usually a day or two after collection.

- Storage temperature of the blood component—most bacteria proliferate more rapidly at 20-24°C (for platelets) than at 2-6°C (for red cells).

- Sensitivity of the test system.

- Volume of the test sample—a larger volume is required to detect low level bacterial contamination.

Test systems

1. BacT/ALERT (BioMérieux, France)—this is an automated liquid culture system. It uses a broth bottle into which the sample is injected. The bottle has a colourimetric sensor which changes from blue to yellow with increasing CO_2 concentration as a result of bacterial proliferation. There are separate bottles for aerobic and anaerobic bacterial detection. Because the majority of fatalities are due to aerobic bacterial contamination and because of cost considerations, there is a preference for testing for aerobic bacteria only in some services.

2. Pall enhanced Bacterial Detection System (eBDS)—this is a closed culture system which relies on the consumption of oxygen as a result of bacteria proliferation.

Key points

Transfusions of blood components, predominantly platelets, contaminated with bacteria have been responsible for several fatalities. Some blood establishments have introduced automated blood culture systems to detect bacterial contamination of platelet components.

SELF-CHECK 5.4

Which blood component is more likely to transmit bacterial infections and why?

5.7 Emerging issues for blood safety

'Emerging infectious diseases' are defined by the Centre of Diseases and Communication as 'infections that have newly appeared in a population or have existed but are rapidly increasing in incidence or geographic range.'

International travel is one factor attributed to a microbial agent being carried from one country to another either by an infected human carrying the infectious agent or by introducing the host vector, e.g. insect. Donor deferral based on recent travel history is part of the strategy to guard against transfusion transmission of an emerging infection. This strategy is combined with surveillance programs to define at risk countries or regions.

In contrast to the viral pathogens discussed so far, for many of these agents there may be no long-term carrier or latent asymptomatic state. In further contrast, these agents may involve an insect to human or an animal to human life cycle, or be transmitted via the oral route (e.g. from 'contaminated' supplies). This latter is exemplified by the hepatitis virus agents, A (HAV) and E (HEV). Some agents may pose more risk to certain patient groups such as immunocompromised patients. It is noted in response to emerging issues that the English Blood Service will be providing HEV-negative components for solid organ and allogeneic stem cell recipients. Please refer to the Reference list: Howell D & Barbara JAJ *All Blood Counts* for a further overview.

The following section describes selected protozoan parasites, insect borne viruses, and prions which are among TTI agents.

BOX 5.2 *Potential transmission routes for agents transmitted by blood*

Malaria can be transmitted through:

- Female *Anopheles* mosquito transmitting from person to person
- Blood transfusion
- Sharing of needles to inject intravenous drugs, and
- From an infected mother to baby.

T. cruzi can be transmitted through:

- Insect vector bites human: after biting the victim, the insect ingests the human blood then defecates. *T. cruzi* is excreted in the faeces of the reduviid bug and is unknowingly rubbed into the bite wound, eyes, and mouth of the unsuspecting host.

- Congenital transmission—from mother to baby
- Organ transplant
- Blood transfusion in southern Mexico and South and Central America
- Accidental laboratory exposure, and
- Consumption of uncooked food which is contaminated with faeces from infected reduviid bugs.The class of viruses transmitted to humans by arthropods such as mosquitoes and ticks is referred to as Arboviruses. Arbovirus transmission by transfusion has been reported for Dengue fever virus, West Nile virus, Ross River virus, and Zika virus.

5.8 Insect/animal–borne pathogens

Malaria

Several parasitic diseases are potentially transmissible by transfusion: malaria is of most concern.

Malaria is a blood-borne infection which is transmitted from one person to another by female *Anopheles* mosquitoes. The infection is caused by a protozoan *Plasmodium* parasite of which the four common species are:

- *P. falciparum*
- *P. vivax*
- *P. malariae*
- *P. ovale.*

A fifth species, *Plasmodium knowlesi*, which has been known for a long time in primates has been identified in humans.

Human malaria is found predominantly in the tropical and subtropical regions of the world. There are 300–500 million cases of malaria resulting in between 1.5 to 2.7 million deaths annually. *Plasmodium falciparum* and *P. vivax* are the dominant species worldwide and are responsible for the more severe and lethal infections. The existence of the *Plasmodium* species in different parts of the world depends on the vector (mosquito) and biological and environmental factors such as humidity and temperature. For example, *P. vivax* stops developing below 15.5°C, whereas the temperature for *P. falciparum* is higher.

The parasite spends part of its life cycle in mosquitoes which transmit the infection to a human host while feeding on blood. The second part of the life cycle is in humans, where the parasite first invades the liver cells and multiplies. It may remain dormant in the liver for months. It is then released into the blood stream and infects the red blood cells, which cause the cells to burst. The symptoms of malarial infection, which occur 10–16 days after the mosquito bite, are chills, fever, and sweating. Sufferers may also experience headaches, nausea, and vomiting. Patients may suffer recurrent attacks, that is, every two days for *P. vivax* and *P. ovale* and every three days for *P. malariae*, which coincides with the infection and bursting of many red blood cells at the same time.

Apart from mosquitoes, malaria can also be transmitted through:

- Blood transfusion
- Sharing of needles to inject intravenous drugs, and
- From an infected mother to baby.

Tests for malaria include:

- Stained thick and thin smears of blood on a microscope slide to screen and identify the *Plasmodium* species. This is regarded as the 'gold standard' and is useful for current infection and to aid appropriate treatment.

- 'Dipstick' tests which detect products of plasmodial metabolism (such as lactate dehydrogenase) and plasmodial antigens (such as histidine rich protein 2). These tests are easy and quick to perform and require little technical skill.

- ELISA and immunofluorescence tests are used to detect immunity to *Plasmodium* species. ELISA tests are used in the UK blood transfusion services to screen donors for malaria antibodies between 6 and 12 months after return from a malarial endemic area.

- PCR techniques which can detect less than ten parasites in 10 µl of blood. This requires specialized equipment, trained staff, and takes longer to perform.

Key points

Malaria is caused by four species of the *Plasmodium* parasite—*P. falciparum*, *P. vivax*, *P. malariae*, and *P. ovale*. The disease is spread through the bite of the female *Anopheles* mosquitoes and is transmissible through blood transfusion.

SELF-CHECK 5.5

During what time period is the test required for malaria?

Trypanosoma cruzi (Chagas disease)

Chagas disease was discovered by Carlos Chagas in 1909 and is caused by the protozoan parasite *Trypanosoma cruzi* (*T. cruzi*). The disease is endemic in southern Mexico and South and Central America, where about 8–11 million people are infected. The parasite is transmitted to people and animals by insects of the *Triatoma* genus and the family Reduviidae, often referred to as reduviid or 'kissing bugs'. The reduviid bugs live in the cracks in walls and roofs of houses made of mud, straw, adobe, and palm thatch in the rural areas of the endemic countries. They emerge at night to feed on the faces of people while they are asleep. After biting the victim, they ingest their blood then defecate. *Trypanosoma cruzi* is excreted in the faeces of the reduviid bug and is unknowingly rubbed into the bite wound, eyes, and mouth of the unsuspecting host.

The acute phase of infection is usually asymptomatic, or the patient may exhibit mild symptoms such as fever, body ache, fatigue, headache, rash, loss of appetite, diarrhoea, and vomiting. If untreated, the infection is likely to resolve within a few weeks or months. However, the infection can cause death in children and immunocompromised people as a result of inflammation of the heart muscle and brain. There is a chronic phase during which the infection remains dormant for decades or life. About 10–30% of patients develop cardiac and/or intestinal complications which can be fatal.

Trypanosoma cruzi can be transmitted through:

- Insect bites with the vector in the faeces
- Congenital transmission—from mother to baby
- Organ transplant
- Blood transfusion in southern Mexico and South and Central America. Migrants from these areas may pose a transfusion risk in non-endemic areas

- Accidental laboratory exposure, and
- Consumption of uncooked food which is contaminated with faeces from infected reduviid bugs.

Testing

In the acute phase of infection when there are circulating parasites, diagnosis of Chagas disease can be made by examination of Giemsa-stained blood films. Diagnosis in the chronic phase is made by testing with two serological assays to detect antibodies to the *T. cruzi* parasite. Antibody tests used are indirect fluorescent antibody (IFA) and enzyme immunoassay (EIA).

In the UK, blood from donors who have lived or work in rural areas of Chagas endemic countries (for four weeks or more) must be negative for antibodies to *T. cruzi* at least six months after their return using an EIA. This includes donors whose mothers were born in southern Mexico, and South and Central America. In the absence of a test, the donor is deferred indefinitely.

Key points

Trypanosoma cruzi is transmitted through the faeces of the reduviid bug which lives in mud huts in South and Central America. The infection can cause the death of children and immunocompromised people.

SELF-CHECK 5.6

Why are tests for antibodies to malaria and Chagas performed on selected donors?

5.9 Arthropod (insect)-borne viruses, i.e. ARBO viruses

ARBO viruses (derived from ARthropod-BOrne) include Flaviviruses such as yellow fever, dengue fever, West Nile, Japanese encephalitis, and Zika virus. They also include Alphaviruses such as Chikungunya and Ross River virus. Four viruses are discussed here. The risk for transfusion transmission of these insect borne viruses emerged this century with reports for transmission of West Nile virus in the USA, dengue fever virus in Hong Kong and Singapore, and Ross River fever virus in Australia.

West Nile virus (WNV)

Since its isolation in 1937, WNV has been recognized as being responsible for epidemics in southern Europe, Africa, the Middle East, Russia, western and south Asia, and more recently in America. It is transmitted by a wide range of female mosquito species of which the *Culex* is the most predominant vector. It is a member of the Flaviviridae family and genus *Flavivirus*. West Nile virus is a small, spherical, lipid-enveloped virus which contains a single-stranded, positive-sense RNA virus.

An estimated 20–30% of infected individuals display symptoms such as fever, headache, rash, nausea, vomiting, eye pain, myalgia, flaccid paralysis, and lymphadenopathy. A small proportion will progress to a more severe disease, culminating in encephalitis and meningoencephalitis.

The virus can be transmitted by transfusion of red cells, platelets, and FFP. It is unlikely to be transmitted by fractionated plasma products because of the heat and solvent detergent treatment used. West Nile virus has also been transmitted by solid organ transplant and breastfeeding. The transfusion transmission of WNV has prompted blood centres in the USA to defer donors for 28 days if they display symptoms of WNV infection. On 1 July 2003, mini-pool NAT for WNV was introduced in the USA and Canada. Low–titre viraemia donations may not be detected by the mini-pool NAT.

The only known risk of WNV entering the blood supply in countries such as the UK is either from returning travellers who may be incubating the virus or from FFP imported from the USA. The following are in place to reduce the risk:

- Asymptomatic donors are deferred for 28 days after leaving an endemic area with ongoing WNV transmission in humans. Alternatively, a validated WNV NAT on the donation must be negative. The UK Blood Services have introduced mini-pool (pools of six samples) NAT for WNV from May 2012 for donors who are returning from affected areas.
- Donors with a history of WNV and/or a positive WNV NAT test should be temporarily deferred for clinical microbiology investigations. These donors may donate after six months without the requirement for a WNV NAT test.
- A negative WNV NAT test is required for all FFP imported from the USA. They are also subjected to methylene blue treatment which has been shown to reduce the WNV viral load by at least 6.5 $\log_{10}$.

Key points

Transfusion transmitted West Nile virus has been implicated in the deaths of patients in North America. This virus is not currently a risk to the UK blood supply.

Dengue fever virus

Dengue fever virus life cycle includes a mosquito to human to mosquito cycle. The mosquito host for the virus is limited but includes *Aedes aegypti* and *Aedes aldopicta*. The virus is endemic in these vectors in many tropical and subtropical countries. In other regions, such as Australia, mosquito species are present in some subtropical regions; however, the virus has not established in these species (non-endemic).

The growth of international travel has resulted in an increase of spasmodic outbreaks in non-endemic areas over the last 25 years. Strategies to contain these outbreaks include prompt notification of each suspected dengue case to health authorities; community education and effective water management systems to minimize breeding grounds for mosquitoes; and controlled mosquito eradication programs.

The dengue transmission cycle starts with the mosquito, *Aedes aegypti*, biting an infected person. The mosquito becomes infected ten days later. The infected mosquito bites a human who becomes infective four to thirteen days post–infection. Clinical manifestations range across the full spectrum from asymptomatic to febrile illness that lasts five to seven days. There can be sudden onset, extreme malaise, muscle, back and limb pain (called breakbone fever) with nausea, vomiting and headache, and ocular pain. At the extreme end there can be development of dengue hemorrhagic fever and death. There is no long–term carrier state. There are four types of dengue viral types and infection by one type does not confer immunity to the other viral types. In contrast a secondary infection with a different type can result in 'enhanced immune mediated' cell response in which clinical symptoms and sequelae are more severe. There are no licensed blood donor screening assays to detect dengue viral infections. However, very sensitive and specific diagnostic assays are available commercially.

At least two transfusion transmissible cases of dengue have been documented following transfusion from infected donors. As dengue fever virus is endemic in countries where the malaria parasite is prevalent, the deferral of donors based on past travel history will also result in deferral of donors potentially at risk.

In the event of local isolated outbreaks in non-endemic areas, temporary procedures for additional geographical restrictions on donor selection may be applied as an added precautionary measure.

Chikungunya virus

Chikungunya virus (also known as CHIKV) was first isolated in Tanzania in 1952 and has since been found in several African countries, India, South-East Asia, Saudi Arabia, and Mediterranean countries. Since 2004 there have been outbreaks in Indian Ocean islands and north-eastern Italy.

Chikungunya virus is an alphavirus which is transmitted to humans by several species of mosquitoes, usually *Aedes aegypti* and *A. albopictus*. Infections may be asymptomatic or patients may present with symptoms such as fever, headache, vomiting, rash, thrombocytopenia, muscle and joint pain, and weakness. In rare cases other complications such as encephalitis, fulminant liver failure, and death have been reported.

It is possible that CHIKV may be transmitted by blood transfusion or tissue or organ transplantation. Visitors to most Chikungunya endemic areas will be excluded from donating for six months under the current malaria guidelines. In most Chikungunya endemic areas where malaria is not a problem, visitors must not donate:

- For six months after their return to the UK if they have been or may have been infected with the virus, or
- For four weeks if they have not presented with symptoms of infection.

Zika virus

Recently, Zika (another mosquito-borne virus) appears to have been transmitted by transfusion and appropriate donor exclusion policies are being put in place. The reader is referred to the Reference list (Jimenez A, Shaz BH & Bloch EM *Zika Virus and the Blood Supply: What do we know?*).

5.10 Transmissible spongiform encephalitis, prions, and variant Creutzfeldt–Jakob disease

The first case of a variant CJD (vCJD) was described in 1996. Accumulated clinical, neurological, epidemiological, and scientific evidence points to an abnormal prion protein being the causative agent and is of the same strain as bovine spongiform encephalitis (BSE).

Prion protein normally exists as PrP^c (cellular form) predominantly in nerve cells where it may help to maintain neuronal function. It can also be found in varying concentrations in plasma, platelets, white cells, and erythrocytes. Abnormal prions (or PrP^{sc} after scrapie) are the infectious protein particles lacking in nucleic acid which can invariably cause fatal neuro-degenerative diseases. Prion diseases have been found in sheep, cats, cattle, mink, mule deer, elk, greater kudu, nyala, oryx, and also in humans, and are associated with an accumulation of abnormal prion protein in the brain.

Human prion disease can be classified into the following categories:

1. *Sporadic CJD:* this is the most common form of CJD, with an annual incidence of one in a million worldwide. The cause of sporadic CJD is unknown, but a popular theory is that it may arise from spontaneous conversion of normal prion protein in the brain to the abnormal form. The average age of onset of the disease is 65, with progressive dementia and death within about six months.

2. *Acquired CJD:* this includes accidental exposure to abnormal prion through medical and surgical procedure (iatrogenic CJD) such as human growth hormones and gonadotropin, inadequately sterilized electrodes, corneal transplants, and 'dura mater' grafts. It is also transmitted through cannibalistic funeral rites of the Fore tribe of Papua New Guinea, resulting in a disease called kuru. This practice has since stopped, which resulted in a reduction in the number of kuru cases.

3. *Inherited CJD:* this accounts for about 15% of human prion disease and is caused by an inherited abnormal gene. At least 20 different mutations in the human prion protein gene (PRNP) have been found.

4. *Variant CJD (vCJD):* as of 11 June 2012, there have been 176 deaths due to definite or probable cases of vCJD in the UK. Forty-nine fatal cases have been identified in other parts of the world, including 25 in France.

The possibility of transmission of vCJD by blood transfusion was raised following the first reported case of the disease. The UK Spongiform Encephalopathy Advisory Committee (SEAC) advised the use of universal leucoreduction as a precautionary measure to reduce the theoretical risk of transfusion transmitted vCJD infection. Experiments have previously shown prion infectivity in buffy coat. Subsequently there have been no reports of cases, suggesting that leucodepletion is an effective intervention. Although leucodepletion in an animal model only removed about half the prion, the concentration of prion in blood is relatively low compared with levels of viraemia in viruses such as HVB or HCV.

Also, donors who have two or more members in the family with familial CJD or were transfused since 1 January 1980 cannot donate. The UK also started importing plasma for fractionation predominantly from the USA and from other countries from October 1999.

To date there have been five cases of transmissions of vCJD by blood transfusions. All cases were prior to leucodepletion. Two cases have been associated with two donations from the same donor. The fifth case has been reported in a haemophilia patient. Box 5.3 sets out microorganisms/agents implicated in transmission by blood transfusion. A screening test for abnormal prion is not yet available, and there is a CE marked RBC prion reduction filter under evaluation.

Key points

Variant CJD is caused by an abnormal prion protein which was transmitted through contaminated meat products and has resulted in over 200 deaths worldwide, mostly in the UK. The abnormal prion is also transmitted through blood transfusion.

BOX 5.3 *Summary of microorganisms/agents implicated in transmission by blood transfusion:*

Bacteria:	Endogenous (not fungi)
	Exogenous
Parasitic protozoa:	Malaria
	Chagas disease
	Toxoplasmosis
	Babesiosis
Prions: (an agent)	? CJD
Viruses:	Dengue fever virus
	Hepatitis viruses A, B C, E
	Herpes (EBV, CMV, HHV8)
	Retroviruses: HIV1, HIV2; HTLV 1, HTVL II
	Parvovirus B19
	Ross River virus
	West Nile virus
	Zika virus

SELF-CHECK 5.7

What is the causative agent of vCJD and how is it transmitted from one individual to another?

5.11 **Quality control and blood safety**

The overwhelming majority of donor samples will be non-reactive for the mandatory microbiology markers. For blood safety the quality for each sample test result is assured by the blood service applying an effective quality management system which covers all the activities. These elements commence with donor education and selection. For example a donor with a recent infection and feeling unwell is contributing to blood safety by self-deferring. Self-deferral/exclusion by 'at-risk' donors avoided a significant number of HIV transmissions prior to the introduction of specific tests. A similar situation is extant for other TTIs and donor education and self-deferral remains an important step in maintaining a safe blood supply. Selection is also based on medical and (as just discussed) travel history.

Other elements include test kit evaluation, use of automated systems, quality control samples, validation and assessment of results, and staff knowledge and skills. Aspects of lot release of the reagent test kit and use of quality control samples, combined with external quality assurance schemes (EQAS) are discussed here.

To increase confidence that rare weakly reactive samples are detected, microbiology test kits should meet nationally agreed minimum criteria for specificity and sensitivity. The National Blood Service Microbiology Kit Evaluation Group with representatives from the UK Blood Transfusion Service (BTS) and the Health Protection Agency (HPA) evaluate microbiology kits and integrated test systems for their suitability for donation testing.

Each batch of tests must include the manufacturer's positive and negative controls for which the correct results must be obtained for the sample test results to be valid. In addition, a British Working Standard (BWS) is included in each batch of tests to demonstrate that an acceptable level of sensitivity is achieved. The BWS is produced by the National Institute of Biological Standards and Controls (NIBSC) but controls available from the HPA or an in-house control can be used. The BWS, HPA, or in-house controls, if used, should be reactive for the test results to be valid.

Statistical process control is used to monitor the performance of the microbiology assays by plotting the sample optical density to cut-off ratio (S/CO) of the working standard on a Shewhart chart. Commercial software is available to automate this process and display the points on a chart with 'warning' and 'out of control' limits set at two and three standard deviations. Plotting the S/CO of the working standards daily will give an early warning when the assay performance is deviating from normal. Thus, the operator can investigate the cause of the deviation and correct it before the assay fails.

The S/CO of the BWS and reagent batch number are reported to NIBSC and are used to compare the performance of each test equipment/assay of the transfusion centre with each other. A report of the analysis is sent to the transfusion centre so that they are aware of how the equipment/assay performance compares with others and take appropriate actions, if necessary.

SELF-CHECK 5.8

Why are internal and external controls used?

Batch pre-acceptance testing (BPAT)

Before each batch of microbiology or other assay kits are used, routinely **batch pre-acceptance testing** (BPAT) is performed to ensure that:

- It meets the minimum standard of sensitivity and specificity
- It has not deteriorated during transportation, and
- It provides information on batch to batch variation.

In the National Health Blood and Transplant Service (NHSBT), lot release testing is centrally performed at the National Transfusion Microbiology Reference Laboratory (NTMRL) before delivery of the kits to the transfusion centres. If the kits have passed the lot release test, the BTS will perform a delivery acceptance test before the kits are used for donation (or patient) testing. The delivery acceptance test is required to show that the kits have not deteriorated during transportation and that the specificity is within the contracted level.

Assay kits which fail lot release or delivery acceptance test should not be used for routine testing but returned to the supplier.

> **Batch pre-acceptance testing**
> Tests performed to show batch of test kits/reagents received meets pre-defined criteria such as sensitivity and specificity and has not deteriorated during transportation.

SELF-CHECK 5.9

Why is 'pre-acceptance' testing performed?

Infection surveillance

All blood transfusion centres in the UK report the number of initial and repeat reactive, new and known donors, and confirmed positives each month to the NHSBT/HPA Infection Surveillance Unit. The manufacturers of the kits and batch numbers are also collected. This information is used to prepare a monthly report which allows the users to compare equipment performance for each batch of kits, batch to batch variation, and is also used to estimate the risk of an infected donation being transfused (see Table 5.5).

Sample archive

Blood transfusion centres in the UK maintain sample archives either in the form of deep well microplate (for 96 samples with up to 1 ml of plasma/serum per sample) format or in blood collection tubes, containing gel spacers that permit freezing directly after centrifuging. The spacer separates the red cells from the plasma, permitting recovery of plasma on thawing the sample. The sample archives are kept below –20°C either at in-house or commercial storage for a minimum of three years. The main reason for retaining an archive sample is to allow retesting if a recipient develops a transfusion transmissible infection following transfusion.

5.12 Strategies for the future and conclusion

Blood donation testing for mandated TTIs has reduced the residual risk of a transfusion transmission such that the risks cannot be measured by prospective follow-up studies but are instead calculated using mathematical modelling. However, there will always be a risk associated with blood transfusion. The risk associated with transfusion infection is only a small part of overall transfusion risks which have not been considered in this chapter.

New infectious agents are continually emerging and some of these have potential to pose a threat to transfusion safety. Surveillance and reporting of post-transfusion infections will be an important step to safeguard and prepare for emergence of new threats. Internationally, 'haemovigilance' schemes are extant in all developed countries having been initiated in France. In the UK the 'SHOT' scheme (Serious Hazards of Transfusion) ensures reporting of adverse events following transfusion. This provides a crucial measure of clinically apparent complications, including TTIs.

In parallel new technologies are emerging which have the potential to assist in meeting these emerging threats. Emerging technologies include pathogen reduction, proteomic and nano technologies, and massively parallel sequencing (MPS). These technologies have potential to augment microbial and blood group testing to redefine donation testing in the future.

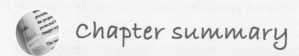

Chapter summary

- The mandatory infectious disease tests required for the release of blood and blood components are HBsAg, anti-HIV, anti-HCV, anti-syphilis, anti-HTLV, and NAT for HCV RNA, HIV RNA, and, for some countries, HBV DNA.

- Discretionary tests are performed for anti-CMV, anti-malaria, anti-Chagas (T. cruzi), and anti-HBc.

- All tests are performed on individual donations. In some countries testing by NAT and for anti-HTLV may be conducted on pools of 24 samples (or less) particularly where the prevalence of the viral agent is low.

■ The tests are performed on automated systems using ISBT 128 barcoded samples and the results are uploaded to the host computer online to reduce transcription errors.

■ Tests for syphilis are either performed on a Beckman Coulter blood testing analyser by TPHA or TPPA, or by ELISA.

■ All other serological tests are performed on automated systems using ELISA or chemiluminescent methods.

■ In the UK, NAT is performed on the Roche cobas s201 using a multiplex assay for HBV DNA and HCV, and HIV RNA.

■ All reagents used are subjected to batch pre-acceptance testing to ensure that they meet minimum standards of quality.

■ External or in-house controls should be included in each batch of tests.

■ Any donation which is serologically reactive (initial reactive) is retested in duplicate on the same system and same manufacturer assay. If both duplicate tests are negative, the donation and all components can be released for transfusion. Otherwise, all components from that donation must be discarded and a sample referred to a reference centre for confirmatory testing.

■ Donors who are confirmed by the reference centre as microbiology positive for any marker must be removed from the donor panel. Donors must be notified as a preventative health measure.

■ The commonest microbiological risk to the blood supply is bacterial contamination. Some blood transfusion centres test platelet components for these using automated culture systems.

■ Testing for West Nile virus is not a requirement for blood collected in the UK, but plasma products imported from the USA must be negative WNV NAT.

■ Variant CJD is a threat to the UK blood supply and leucodepletion has been introduced as a precaution to reduce transfusion transmission. Also, donors who have two or more members in the family with familial CJD or were transfused since 1 January 1980 cannot donate. A test is not currently available and CE-marked prion reduction filters for RBCs are under evaluation.

 ## Further reading

● Barbara JAJ, Regan FAM & Contreras MC (eds) 'Chapter 17 Quality in the screening of donations for transfusion transmissible infections', in *Transfusion Microbiology*. Cambridge University Press, Cambridge (2008), 217–26.

The specific elements associated with blood screening for TTIs that help to ensure the overall safety of the blood supply are explained in Chapter 17. These elements commence with donor selection through to national haemovigilance feed-back systems.

● British Blood Transfusion Society. *An Introduction to Transfusion Science Practice.* 5th edition. British Blood Transfusion Society, Manchester (2009). www.bbts.org.uk.

● Hewitt PE, Ijaz S, Brailsford SR, et al. Hepatitis E virus in blood components: a prevalence and transmission study in southeast England. *Lancet* 384 (2014), 1766–73.

● Hewitt PE, Llewelyn CA, Mackenzie J & Will RG. Creutzfeldt-Jakob disease and blood transfusion: results of the UK Transfusion Medicine Epidemiological Review study. *Vox Sang* 91 (2006), 221–30.

- Hoad VC, Speers DJ & Keller AJ, et al. First reported case of transfusion-transmitted Ross River virus infection. *Med J Aust* 202 (2015), 267–70.

- Howell D & Barbara JAJ. 'Chapter 2 Transfusion transmitted infections', in Thomas D, Ridler B, Thompson J (eds) *All Blood Counts—A manual for blood conservation and patient blood management*.TFM Publishing Limited, Shrewsbury (2014).

  This chapter provides an account of current risks of infectious complications following transfusion. It is noted that these TTI risks are minimal compared to the risks associated with the overall transfusion process.

- Jimenez A, Shaz BH & Bloch EM. Zika virus and the blood supply: what do we know? *Transfus Med Rev* 31 (2017), 1–10.

- Medicines Control Agency. *Rules and Guidance for Pharmaceutical Manufacturers and Distributors 2002*, 6th edition. The Stationery Office (Norwich), 2002.

- Petersen LR & Busch MP. Transfusion-transmitted arboviruses. *Vox Sang* 98 (2009), 495–503.

  This review paper considers arboviruses producing high incidence of clinically significant human disease, transfusion risk models, the lessons learnt from the West Nile virus, and future prospects.

- Soldan K, Barbara JAJ, Ramsey ME & Hall AJ. Estimation of the risk for hepatitis B virus, hepatitis C virus and human immunodeficiency virus infectious donations entering the blood supply in England 1993–2001. *Vox Sang* 84 (2003), 274–86.

- Stramer SL. Current perspectives in transfusion-transmitted infectious diseases: emerging and re-emerging infections. *ISBT Sci Ser* 9 (2014), 30–36.

- Stramer SL & Dodd RY. AABB Transfusion-transmitted diseases emerging infectious diseases subgroup. Transfusion-transmitted emerging infectious diseases: 30 years of challenges and progress. *Transfusion* 53 (2013), 2375–83.

- Tambyah PA, Koay ESC & Poon MLM, et al. Dengue hemorrhagic fever transmitted by blood transfusion. *N Engl J Med* 359 (2008), 1526–1527.

  This letter to the editor is of value to the student because it shows how prompt recognition through a donor call back system led to a favourable clinical outcome. It exemplifies the important contribution of donor education to ensure a safe blood supply. This case also illustrates the difficulties encountered when attempting to ensure a safe blood supply in the face of emerging flavivirus threats worldwide.

- UK Blood Transfusion and Tissue Transplantation Services. *Guidelines for the Blood Transfusion Services in the United Kingdom*, 8th edition. The Stationery Office, Norwich (2013).

- www.tsoshop.co.uk or at www.transfusionguidelines.org.uk. See also

- www.transfusionguidelines.org.uk/red-book/chapter-9-microbiology-tests-for-donors-and-donations-general-specifications-for-laboratory-test-procedures/9-2-microbiology-screening

Answers to the questions in this chapter are provided on the book's accompanying website:

Go to www.oup.com/uk/avent2e

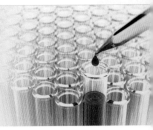

6

Human Platelet Antigens (HPA) and Human Neutrophil Antigens (HNA) and Their Clinical Significance

Geoff Lucas

Learning objectives

By the end of this chapter you should be able to:

- Describe the nomenclature of human platelet antigens (HPA) and human neutrophil antigens (HNA).

- List the most important HPA and HNA.

- Understand the principles, techniques, and problems in detecting HPA and HNA and the associated antibodies.

- Detail the most important clinical conditions in which platelet and granulocyte antibodies occur.

- Have a detailed understanding of the clinical management and problems associated with the management of neonatal alloimmune thrombocytopenia (NAIT) cases.

- Understand the role of platelet transfusion in other platelet immune disorders.

- Understand the processes of immune destruction affecting platelets.

- Describe the other types of clinical interventions that are used to manage the range of clinical conditions associated with HPA and HNA antibodies.

Introduction

In Chapter 2 you learned the range of different antigens that are found on red cells, the techniques used to identify them, and the antibodies against these antigens that occur following transfusion, pregnancy or as the result of autoimmune disease. Subsequent chapters (3–5) explored the different facets of blood transfusion and the clinical disorders.

This chapter examines similar principles again but in the context of platelets and granulocytes as the cells of interest. There are many common principles involved in the immunohaematology of red cells and the immunohaematology of platelets and granulocytes. Equally, there are some key differences which have resulted in different strategies both for typing and for antibody detection and identification. Some differences arise from the nature of the cells, for example both cell types are physiologically active and prone to aggregation *in vivo*; other differences occur because human platelet antigens (HPA) and human neutrophil antigens (HNA) occur on cells also expressing other common immunological target antigens, for example HLA class I, which are widely distributed antigens (see Chapter 9). The antigens uniquely expressed on platelets or neutrophils are implicated in immune-mediated thrombocytopenias and neutropenias respectively. Alloantibodies against HPA or against HNA formed during pregnancy, following transfusion or bone marrow transplantation may cause alloimmune thrombocytopenia or neutropenia respectively. Platelet and granulocyte antibodies can also arise as part of an autoimmune process, as the result of an immune response following drug administration, or as an isoimmune response, when a patient with a congenital absence of a membrane protein makes an immune response following exposure to that protein as the result of pregnancy or transfusion. Allo- and autoimmune thrombocytopenias can also occur in recipients following organ transplantation where immunocompetent cells from the donor are transferred within the transplanted organ. The detection and determination of the specificity and nature of such antibodies in these different scenarios is therefore important in determining the appropriate clinical treatment for the patient.

Autoantibodies

Antibodies that react with 'self' antigens.

Alloantibodies

Antibodies that react with an inherited antigenic characteristic that is lacking in the recipient.

Isoantibodies

Antibodies that react with an antigen that is normally found in all individuals but which is lacking in the patient.

Drug-dependent antibodies

Antibodies that react with a drug directly or with an antigenic structure created when the drug binds to a naturally occurring structure (known as haptenization).

6.1 Overview of platelet and granulocyte antigens

Antigens on human platelets and granulocytes can be categorized according to their biochemical nature into:

1. Carbohydrate antigens on glycolipids and glycoproteins:

    (a) A, B, and O

    (b) P and Le on platelets; I on granulocytes

2. Protein antigens:

    (a) human leucocyte antigen (HLA) class I (A, B, and C)

    (b) glycoprotein (GP) IIb/IIIa, GPIa/IIa, GPIb/IX/V, etc. on platelets

    (c) FcγRIIIb (CD16), CD177, etc. on granulocytes

3. Hapten-induced antigens, for example those associated with the following drugs:

    (a) quinine, quinidine

    (b) penicillins and cephalosporins

    (c) heparin

These antigens can be targeted by some or all of the following types of antibodies:

- **Autoantibodies**
- **Alloantibodies**
- **Isoantibodies**
- **Drug-dependent antibodies**

Many antigens on platelets and granulocytes are also found on other cells, for example ABO and HLA class I (Table 6.1); other antigens, however, are largely, but not exclusively, restricted to platelets and granulocytes and these are known as **human platelet antigens (HPA)** and **human neutrophil antigens (HNA)**. The genetic basis of all HPAs and most HNAs has been resolved, allowing DNA-based typing of patient, donor, and fetus. Techniques for high–through-put DNA-based typing of blood donors have dramatically improved the availability to HPA selected blood products in England and has made clinical support with these products a reality.

> **Human platelet antigen (HPA)**
> The term given to allelic forms of platelet membrane glycoproteins that give rise to an alloimmune response.
>
> **Human neutrophil antigen (HNA)**
> The term given to allelic forms of granulocyte membrane glycoproteins that give rise to an alloimmune response.

TABLE 6.1   The distribution of major platelet and granulocyte glycoproteins amongst peripheral blood cells.

Antigens	Erythrocytes	Platelets	Neutrophils	B lymphocytes	T lymphocytes	Monocytes
A, B, H	+++	(+)/++	−	−	−	−
I	+++	++	++	−	−	−
Rh*	+++	−	−	−	−	−
K	+++	−	−	−	−	−
HLA class I	−/(+)	+++	++	+++	+++	+++
HLA class II	−	−	−/+++ [§]	+++	−/+++ [§]	+++
GPIIb/IIIa	−	+++	(+)[‡]	−	−	−
GPIa/IIa	−	+++	−	−	++	−
GPIb/IX/V	−	+++	−	−	−	−
CD109	−	(+)/++ [§]	−	−	−/++ [§]	(+)
FcγRIIIb (CD16b)	−	−	+++	−	−	−
CD177	−	−	+++ [a]	−	−	−
CTL2	−	+ (personal observations)	+++	++ (B and T lymphocytes not separated)		?
CD11b/18	−	−	++	−	−	++[b]
CD11a/18	−	−	++	++	++	++

+++, ++, + Indicates level of antigen expression in decreasing order (+) indicates weak expression.

? Indicates not known.

* Non-glycosylated.

[§] On activated cells.

[‡] GPIIIa(β_3) in association with an alternative α chain α_v.

[a] Expressed on a sub-population of neutrophils.

[b] Also expressed on natural killer cells.

Key points

Allo-, auto-, iso-, and drug-induced antigens may be found on platelets and neutrophils and are implicated in a range of different immune cytopenias.

SELF-CHECK 6.1

What is the distinction between the following terms: white blood cells, granulocytes, and neutrophils?

Biallelic

A gene with two alternative alleles.

Allele

One of two or more alternative forms of a gene that arise by mutation and are found at the same place on a chromosome.

Codominant

Relating to two alleles of a gene that are both fully expressed in a heterozygote.

Immunoprecipitation

The isolation of immune complexes (usually with monoclonal antibodies) to identify membrane or intracellular components.

Monoclonal antibody immobilization of platelet antigens (MAIPA) assay

An ELISA assay which uses monoclonal antibodies against platelet antigens as the basis of detection and identification of platelet–specific antibodies.

Polymerase chain reaction (PCR)

An enzyme reaction utilizing Taq polymerase to amplify the copy number of a given DNA sequence and hence enable detection of a genetic characteristic.

Neonatal alloimmune thrombocytopenia (NAIT)

Thrombocytopenia in a neonate (or fetus) caused by the maternal–fetal transfer of platelet–specific antibodies recognizing either HPAs or platelet glycoproteins inherited by the fetus from the father but absent in the mother.

6.2 Human platelet antigens (HPA)

Inheritance and nomenclature

All the HPAs reported to date (with the exception of HPA-14) have been shown to be **biallelic**, with each **allele** being **codominant**. Historically, platelet-specific antigens were named by the authors first reporting the antigen, usually using an abbreviation of the name of the propositus in whom the alloantibody was first detected. Some systems were published simultaneously by different investigators and several names were assigned to the same antigen, for example Zw and PlA, and Zav, Br, and Hc, were later found to be the same polymorphism, that is, HPA-1 and HPA-5 respectively. In 1990, the working party for platelet immunology within the International Society of Blood Transfusion (ISBT) agreed the HPA nomenclature for platelet-specific alloantigens and subsequently the international Platelet Nomenclature Committee published guidelines for the naming of newly discovered platelet-specific alloantigens. In this nomenclature, each system is numbered consecutively (HPA-1, -2, -3, and so on) (Table 6.2) according to its date of discovery, with the major allele in each system being designated 'a' and the minor allele 'b'. Antigens are only included in a system if antibodies against the alloantigen encoded by both the major and minor alleles have been reported; if an antibody against only one allele has been reported, a 'w' (for workshop) is added after the antigen name, for example HPA-10bw (Metcalfe et al., 2003). Use of techniques such as **immunoprecipitation** of radioactive labelled platelet membrane proteins, the **monoclonal antibody-specific immobilization of platelet antigens (MAIPA) assay** and the **polymerase chain reaction (PCR)** have enabled the genetic and molecular basis of all HPAs to be elucidated (Figure 6.1 and Table 6.2). For all but one of the 29 HPA systems, the difference between the two alleles is a **single nucleotide polymorphism (SNP)** which changes the amino acid in the corresponding protein (Table 6.2). Twelve of the HPAs are grouped into six HPA systems (HPA-1 to 5 and HPA-15) and for all of these, except HPA-3 and HPA-15, the minor allele frequency is ≤0.2 and consequently homozygosity for the minor allele is relatively rare. There are also some very rare c alleles that have been documented for HPA-1, -5 and -7, where there is different amino acid substitution.

Most of the 29 HPA polymorphisms were first discovered during the investigation of cases of **neonatal alloimmune thrombocytopenia (NAIT)**. The majority of the antigens are located on the IIIa sub-unit of the platelet glycoprotein GPIIb/IIIa (CD41/CD61), which is a high abundance (~1%) and physiologically important component of the platelet membrane as it is the main platelet receptor for fibrinogen and critical to the final phase of platelet aggregation. The other HPAs are located on the IIb sub-unit of GPIIb/IIIa, on GPIa/IIa (CD49b), on GPIb/IX/V (CD42a,b,c,d), and CD109. Three of these receptor complexes are critical for haemostasis

TABLE 6.2 The human platelet antigen (HPA) systems.

HPA system	Antigen	Alternative names	Phenotype frequency* (%)	Glycoprotein	SNP	SNP rs number	Amino acid change
1	1a	Zw^a, Pl^{A1}	97.9	GPIIIa	T^{196}	rs5918	L^{33}
	1b	Zw^b, Pl^{A2}	28.8		C^{196}		P^{33}
2	2a	Ko^b	>99.9	GPIbα	C^{524}	rs6065	T^{145}
	2b	Ko^a, Sib^a	13.2		T^{524}		M^{145}
3	3a	Bak^a, Lek^a	80.95	GPIIb	T^{2622}	rs5911	I^{843}
	3b	Bak^b	69.8		G^{2622}		S^{843}
4	4a	Yuk^b, Pen^a	>99.9	GPIIIa	G^{526}	rs5917	R^{143}
	4b	Yuk^a, Pen^b	<0.1		A^{526}		Q^{143}
5	5a	Br^b, Zav^b	99.0	GPIa	G^{1648}	rs10471371	E^{505}
	5b	Br^a, Zav^a, Hc^a	19.7		A^{1648}		K^{505}
6	6bw	Ca^a, Tu^a	0.7	GPIIIa	G^{1564}	rs13306487	R^{489}
					A^{1564}		Q^{489}
7	7bw	Mo^a	0.2	GPIIIa	C^{1267}		P^{407}
					G^{1267}		A^{407}
8	8bw	Sr^a	<0.01	GPIIIa	T^{2004}		R^{636}
					C^{2004}		C^{636}
9	9bw	Max^a	0.6	GPIIb	G^{2603}		V^{837}
					A^{2603}		M^{837}
10	10bw	La^a	<1.6	GPIIIa	G^{281}		R^{62}
					A^{281}		Q^{62}
11	11bw	Gro^a	<0.25	GPIIIa	G^{1996}		R^{633}
					A^{1996}		H^{633}
12	12bw	Iy^a	0.4	GPIbβ	G^{141}		G^{15}
					A^{141}		E^{15}
13	13bw	Sit^a	0.25	GPIa	C^{2531}		T^{799}
					T^{2531}		M^{799}
14	14bw	Oe^a	<0.17	GPIIIa	Δ AAG$^{1929-1931}$		Δ K^{611}
15	15a	Gov^b	74	CD109	C^{2108}	rs10455097	S^{703}
	15b	Gov^a	81		A^{2108}		Y^{703}
16	16bw	Duv^a	<1	GPIIIa	C^{517}		T^{140}
					T^{517}		I^{140}
17	17bw	Va^a	<0.4	GPIIIa	C^{622}		T^{195}
					T^{622}		M^{195}
18	18bw	Cab^a	<1	GPIa	G^{2235}		Q^{716}
					T^{2235}		H^{716}

(Continued)

TABLE 6.2 Continued

HPA system	Antigen	Alternative names	Phenotype frequency* (%)	Glycoprotein	SNP	SNP rs number	Amino acid change
19	19bw	Sta	<1	GPIIIa	A^{487} C^{487}	ss120032848	K^{137} Q^{137}
20	20bw	Kno	<1	GPIIb	C^{1949} T^{1949}	ss120032852	T^{619} M^{619}
21	21bw	Nos	<1	GPIIa	G^{1960} A^{1960}	ss120032849	E^{628} K^{628}
22	22bw	Sey	<1	GPIIb	A^{584} C^{584}	rs142811900	K^{164} T^{164}
23	23bw	Hug	<1	GPIIIa	C^{1942} T^{1942}	rs139166528	R^{622} W^{622}
24	24bw	Cab^{2+}	<1	GPIIb	G^{1508} A^{1508}		S^{472} N^{472}
25	25bw	Swi^{a}	<1	GPIa	C^{3347} T^{3347}		T^{1087} M^{1087}
26	26bw	Sec^{a}	<1	GPIIIa	G^{1818} T^{1818}		K^{580} N^{580}
27	27bw	Cab^{3a+}	<1	GPIIb	C^{2614} A^{2614}	rs149468422	L^{841} M^{841}
28	28bw	War	<1	GPIIb	G^{2311} T^{2311}	ss550827881	V^{740} L^{740}
29	29bw	Kha^{b}	<1	GPIIIa	C^{98} T^{98}	ss1221285311	T^{7} M^{7}

* Frequencies based on studies in Caucasians.

SNP: single nucleotide polymorphism; rs: the reference SNP number in the international dbSNP database; ss: the submitted SNP reference number in the international dbSNP database.

and are responsible for the stepwise process of platelet attachment to the damaged vessel wall. GPIb/IX/V is the major receptor for von Willebrand factor (vWF) and is implicated in the initial binding of platelets to damaged endothelium. The GPIbα-bound vWF interacts with collagen, facilitating the interaction of collagen with its signalling (GPVI) and attachment receptors (GPIa/IIa). GPVI–related signalling leads to a change in the platelet integrins GPIIb/IIIa and GPIa/IIa, exposing high-affinity binding sites for fibrinogen and collagen respectively. The function of platelet CD109 has not been elucidated. These proteins are represented pictorially in Figure 6.1.

Glanzmann's thrombasthenia and Bernard–Soulier syndrome are two rare and severe, usually autosomal recessive, platelet bleeding disorders caused by mutations in the genes encoding GPIIb and GPIIIa, and GPIbα, GPIbβ, and GPIX respectively. These mutations result in either an absence, a numerical reduction, or altered function of these proteins, which typically results in either a loss of function but, occasionally, a gain of function.

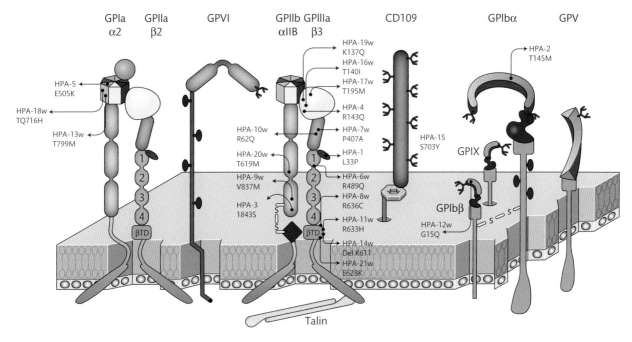

FIGURE 6.1

Representation of the platelet membrane and the glycoproteins (GP) on which the human platelet antigens (HPA) are localized. The major functional protein complexes (GPIa/IIa, GPVI, GPIIb/IIIa, CD109, and GPIbβ/X/bα/V) are depicted from left to right. The diagram also illustrates the transmembrane nature of these proteins and the interaction with the platelet cytoskeleton (represented by the protein talin), which is responsible for platelet shape change that occurs in response to external stimuli such as von Willebrand factor and fibrinogen. The positions of the HPA systems are indicated by black dots, with the amino acid change indicated by single letter code, and by residue number in the expressed protein. (Adapted from Practical Transfusion Medicine Fourth Edition, 2013, Wiley-Blackwell.)

The glycoprotein IIb/IIIa complex

The GPIIb/IIIa complex is a member of the integrin family of proteins and is composed of two polypeptide chains. GPIIIa (CD61) is a 90 kDa glycoprotein consisting of three major domains: a large extracellular N-terminal region containing 28 disulphide bonds, a transmembrane domain, and a short cytoplasmic segment. GPIIb (CD41) is also a transmembrane protein consisting of an extracellular 116 kDa heavy chain associated by a single disulphide bond with a 22 kDa light chain. There are approximately 50–80,000 copies of GPIIb/IIIa per platelet. This complex requires Ca^{2+} ions for its function and upon platelet activation undergoes a conformational change that enables it to bind fibrinogen and fibronectin, vitronectin, and vWF. X-ray crystallography studies of GPIIb/IIIa have revealed that this glycoprotein has distinct structural and functional regions.

The glycoprotein Ib/IX/V complex

The GPIb/IX/V complex (CD42) is involved in the initial stages of platelet adhesion via vWF to damaged subendothelium of the vessel wall under conditions of high shear stress. The vWF receptor is composed of four transmembrane components. GPIbα (CD42b) and GPIbβ (CD42c) are linked by a single disulphide bond and are associated with GPIX (CD42a) and GPV

(CD42d). There are approximately 25,000 copies of GPIb/IX and 12,000 copies of GPV per platelet. The primary vWF binding site has been localized within GPIbα, but there is evidence that the other three components also contribute to receptor function.

The glycoprotein Ia/IIa complex

The GPIa/IIa (CD49/CD29) complex is another dimeric, transmembrane protein and member of the integrin family that is structurally similar to GPIIb/IIIa. It is also found on activated T lymphocytes and several other cell types as well as platelets. The principal ligand of this heterodimer is collagen in exposed sub-endothelium. There are approximately 800–2800 copies of GPIa/IIa per platelet.

The CD109 protein

CD109 is a single chain, transmembrane 170kDa protein with variable expression on platelets. There are approximately 500–2000 copies of CD109 per platelet but variations of up to a 100-fold between donors has been reported. CD109 is also found on activated T cells and endothelial cells. On platelets, CD109 has a glycophosphotidylinositol (GPI) anchor (defined in Section 6.3) and is readily cleaved from the platelet membrane by proteases. The function of platelet CD109 is incompletely understood but, on endothelial cells, has a negative regulatory feedback for transforming growth factor-beta and is associated with improved collagen architecture during wound healing.

Incidence of platelet alloantigens in different populations

There have been few comprehensive large-scale studies to assess the frequency of platelet alloantigens in different populations, but small–scale studies show significant differences in the prevalence of some antigens, e.g. the HPA-1b is present in Caucasians but largely absent in Far Eastern populations, while the converse applies to the HPA-4b. Consequently, it is important to take ethnicity into account when investigating clinical cases of suspected HPA alloimmunization.

Key points

Alloantigens on platelets are known as human platelet antigens (HPAs).

HPA typing

Until the early 1990s, HPA typing was performed by serology (phenotyping) using monospecific human antisera. These antisera were relatively uncommon as the majority of immunized individuals produced HLA class I antibodies in addition to the HPA antibodies. The development of more advanced assays such as the MAIPA assay (Figure 6.2) that were able to elucidate complex mixtures of antibodies against different glycoproteins permitted more extensive phenotyping, but antisera against many HPA specificities remained scarce and were unavailable for most laboratories.

DNA-based typing techniques have largely replaced HPA phenotyping in most laboratories. **polymerase chain reaction with sequence-specific primers (PCR-SSP)** (Cavanagh et al., 1997) is a reliable technique for small-scale patient testing but has begun to be replaced by commercially available kits, and other types of technique such as polymerase chain reaction with sequence based typing, which avoid the use of agarose gels containing ethidium bromide. High-throughput donor HPA typing techniques with automated readout, such as Taqman assays, have been used routinely and have reduced the cost of large-scale typing. **Microarray techniques** for the simultaneous detection of numerous SNPs have been developed (Bugert et al., 2005) while **next generation sequencing** is likely to emerge as a cost-effective alternative for transfusion services requiring mass donor typing capability for multiple alleles.

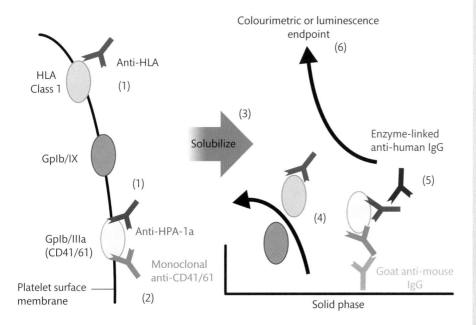

FIGURE 6.2

Monoclonal antibody-specific immobilization of platelet antigens (MAIPA) assay. This diagram demonstrates the detection of HPA-1a antibodies in the presence of HLA class I antibodies, a laboratory scenario that may not readily lead to the determination of HPA antibody specificity using a whole-cell assay such as the platelet immunofluorescence test. The sequence of the assay is as follows: 1) Target (HPA-typed) platelets are incubated with the test serum. The HPA-1a antibodies in this example will bind to HPA-1a (+) platelets but not to HPA-1a (–) platelets. 2) After washing, platelets are incubated with a platelet glycoprotein-specific monoclonal antibody (anti-GPIIb/IIIa is used in this example because this is the carrier molecule for the HPA-1 polymorphism—Table 6.2). 3) After washing, the platelets are solubilized. 4) After centrifugation, the resultant supernatant is added to a microtitre plate previously coated with goat anti-mouse IgG antibodies. 5) The solubilized complex of platelet glycoprotein, murine antibody, and human antibody of interest is captured by the immobilized goat anti-mouse antibodies on the microplate. 6) After washing, the presence of human antibodies is detected by the addition of enzyme-linked anti-human antibodies.

Polymerase chain reaction with sequence specific primers (PCR-SSP)

The polymerase chain reaction using primers that recognize a DNA sequence encoding a unique heritable genetic characteristic—typically an SNP.

Microarray techniques

An assay system using labelled probes to simultaneously identify a range of different characteristics.

Next generation sequencing

High-throughput DNA sequencing techniques which produce thousands or millions of sequences from DNA fragments from different individuals simultaneously. There a number of different strategies, e.g. sequencing the entire genome (exosome) of a single individual, sequencing a 'focused' exosome which looks at a range of genes of known clinical importance for a small number of individuals or sequencing a limited range of clinically important polymorphisms simultaneously from a large number of individuals. Where DNA from many individuals is analysed the DNA fragments from individuals are 'indexed' with a marker (incorporated by PCR) to ensure that an individual's DNA can be identified. The amplified fragments are analysed by computer to provide a continuous sequence for each individual and compared with the known sequence. The process should ensure that multiple overlapping fragments are obtained at each site (somewhere between 20 and 50 copies—this is referred to as coverage) so that the results, especially for heterozygous individuals, can by interpreted with confidence. This technique is still advancing and currently there remain problems with differentiating different forms of homologous genes. More details on NGS are described in Chapter 2.

Genotyping of fetal DNA from amniocytes or from chorionic villus biopsy samples is of clinical value in cases of HPA alloimmunization in pregnancies where there is a history of severe NAIT and the father is heterozygous for the implicated HPA. Non-invasive HPA genotyping assays based on the presence of trace amounts of fetal DNA in maternal plasma, as developed for red cell antigens and the prevention of haemolytic disease of the newborn (see Chapter 3), reduce the risk to the fetus from invasive sampling procedures and have been introduced for determining HPA-1 alleles by some reference centres.

SELF-CHECK 6.2

What are the risks associated with amniocentesis or fetal blood sampling?

SELF-CHECK 6.3

Why have laboratories concentrated on HPA-1a for free fetal maternal DNA typing?

Platelet isoantigens, autoantigens, and hapten-induced antigens

In addition to the HPAs there are other antigens that can lead to the production of antibodies against platelets. GPIV is absent from the platelet membrane in 4% of Black Africans and 3–10% of Japanese. If these individuals are exposed to normal, GPIV-positive platelets as a consequence of pregnancy or transfusion they may produce GPIV isoantibodies. These antibodies may cause NAIT or platelet refractoriness, and may be responsible for non-haemolytic febrile transfusion reactions in multi-transfused recipients. Similarly, formation of isoantibodies against GPIIb/IIIa and GPIb/IX/V can complicate the pregnancies and transfusion support of patients with Glanzmann's thrombasthenia and Bernard–Soulier syndrome respectively. The non–HPA Mou^a antigen is a polymorphism which has currently not been localized to a glycoprotein and the genetic basis is unknown. Anti-Mou^a has been implicated in three cases including both NAIT and platelet transfusion refractoriness.

GPIIb/IIIa and GPIb/IX/V, which carry the HPAs, are often the target of autoantibodies in autoimmune thrombocytopenia. Such autoantibodies bind to the platelets of all individuals regardless of their HPA type. Platelet autoimmunity can be associated with haematopoietic malignancies and following haemopoietic stem cell transplantation during immune cell re-engraftment. The presence of platelet autoantibodies may also contribute to platelet transfusion refractoriness. Solid organ transplantation, mostly associated with liver transplant, has been associated with the horizontal transmission of autoantibodies if the organ donor was a patient with immune thrombocytopenia.

SELF-CHECK 6.4

How would you distinguish between platelet-specific allo- and autoantibodies in a transfused patient?

SELF-CHECK 6.5

What interventions might be used to reduce the impact of platelet autoantibodies in patients with platelet transfusion refractoriness?

SELF-CHECK 6.6

Why are liver transplants from patients with autoimmune thrombocytopenia more likely than other organs to be associated with the horizontal transfer of ITP?

Some drugs too small to elicit an immune response in their own right may bind to platelet GPs *in vivo* and act as a **hapten**. In some patients, the haptenized platelet GP can trigger the formation of antibodies that only bind to the GP in the presence of hapten. A classic example is quinine and its stereo-isomer, quinidine. Typically, quinine-dependent antibodies bind to either GPIIb/IIIa and/or GPIb/IX/V, although other GPs are sometimes the target. Many other drugs, particularly heparin and several antibiotics, have been associated with hapten-mediated thrombocytopenia. In haemato-oncology patients, who often receive a spectrum of drugs, unravelling the causes of persistent thrombocytopenia or poor responses to platelet transfusions can be complex because of the many possible causes of thrombocytopenia. If the thrombocytopenia is drug (hapten) mediated, withdrawal of the drug will result in rapid recovery of the platelet count.

> **Hapten**
> A substance that is unable to elicit an immune response by itself (usually because it is too small) but which can do so when combined with a larger molecule.

SELF-CHECK 6.7

What is a stereo-isomer?

6.3 **Human neutrophil antigens (HNA)**

There are fewer recognized antigens on the membrane of human **neutrophils** compared to platelets but, as with platelets, these can also be divided into different categories. There are common antigens which have a wider distribution on other blood cells and tissues, for example I, Le^x, and sialyl-Le^x (CD15) blood group systems and HLA class I. There are 'shared' antigens which have a limited distribution amongst other cell types, for example the HNA-4 and HNA-5 polymorphisms associated with CD11/18. There are also a small number of truly neutrophil-specific antigens, for example the HNA-1 polymorphisms on FcγRIIIb (CD16). The current nomenclature for the HNA systems includes polymorphisms that are both cell-specific and 'shared' (Table 6.3).

> **Neutrophils**
> Together with eosinophils and basophils these circulating white cells are collectively known as granulocytes or polymorphonuclear cells. In normal healthy adults, neutrophils account for >90% of all granulocytes. Most granulocyte immunology laboratories do not attempt to separate these three cell types prior to antibody testing so any antibodies detected are more correctly called granulocyte-specific. Nonetheless, HNA-1 and -2 have been shown to be truly neutrophil-specific in that they are expressed on neutrophils but not eosinophils or basophils.

Nomenclature

The current human neutrophil antigen (HNA) systems are described by Flesch et al (2016) and includes both neutrophil-specific and more widely distributed antigens that are present on other circulating white cells and tissues. This HNA nomenclature is an allele and **epitope**-based rather than antigen-based system in order to accommodate more recent findings. Different alleles can encode more than one epitope and more than one allele can encode the same epitope. Other antigens that have not been incorporated into the HNA system, because of insufficient scientific information, continue to be referred to by the original acronym assigned at the time of discovery.

FcγRIIIb (CD16) and the HNA-1 system

The human FcγRIII (CD16) molecule is a member of the immunoglobulin superfamily which is distinct from other human Fc receptors for IgG (FcγR). FcγRIII exists in two non-allelic forms: FcγRIIIa and FcγRIIIb, encoded by separate genes but which nonetheless share a high degree of homology at both the DNA and protein level, which can cause particular problems when genotyping. FcγRIIIb is linked to the neutrophil plasma membrane via a **glycosylphosphatidylinositol (GPI) anchor**, and has low affinity for IgG (Figure 6.3).

> **Glycophosphotidylinositol (GPI) anchor**
> A chemical linkage between some glycoproteins and the cell membrane which can be readily cleaved under certain conditions thereby releasing the glycoprotein from the cell surface.

TABLE 6.3 The human neutrophil antigen (HNA) alleles and epitopes.

Allele	Nucleotide positions of the corresponding alleles	Amino acid positions of the corresponding glycoproteins	Epitopes	Glycoprotein/ CD classification	Phenotype frequency %*
FCGR3B*01	108G 114C 194A 233C 244G 316G	36R 38L 65N 78A 82D 106V	HNA-1a	FcγRIIIb/CD16	46
FCGR3B*02	108C 114T 194G 233C 244A 316A	36S 38L 65S 78A 82N 106I	HNA-1b HNA-1d**	FcγRIIIb/CD16	88
FCGR3B*03	108C 114T 194G 233A 244A 316A	36S 38L 65S 78D 82N 106I	HNA-1b HNA-1c	FcγRIIIb/CD16	5
FCGR3B*04	108C 114C 194G 233C 244G 316A	36S 38L 65N 78A 82D 106I	HNA-1a	FcγRIIIb/CD16	
FCGR3B*05	108C 114T 194G 233C 244G 316A	36S 38L 65S 78A 82D 106I	HNA-1bv	FcγRIIIb/CD16	
FCGR3B*null	Gene deletion—no allele	No glycoprotein			
CD177	Allelic variation in this gene does not code for different serological phenotypes		HNA-2§	CD177	97
SLC44A2*01	451C 455G	151L 152R	HNA-3a	CTL2	94.5
SLC44A2*02	451C 455A	151L 152Q	HNA-3b	CTL2	35.9
SLC44A2*03	451T 455G	151F 152R	HNA-3av¶	CTL2	
ITGAM*01	230G	61R	HNA-4a	CD11b	99.1
ITGAM*01	230A	61H	HNA-4b	CD11b	
ITGAL*01	2372G	766R	HNA-5a	CD11a	>99
ITGAL*02	2372C	766T	HNA-5bwΨ	CD11a	

* Frequencies based on studies in Caucasians.

** This can be considered as the **antithetical** antigen to HNA-1c.

¶ Variation in reactivity with human antisera can be observed.

Ψ HNA-5bw is not included in the current HNA nomenclature because no antibodies with this specificity have currently be described. However, for practical purposes, it is useful to be able describe the gene product.

§ HNA-2 null phenotype is due to incorrect splicing resulting in mRNA strands containing introns with stop codons.

Note that a number of nucleotide positions are different from those described in the first edition of this book. These have arisen because different transcript variants have subsequently been recognized.

Antithetical

One of two or more alternative antigens.

In immunoprecipitation and SDS-polyacrylamide gel electrophoresis studies, FcγRIIIb migrates as a broad band with a molecular weight between 50 kDa and 80 kDa. This variation in apparent molecular weight is the result of variations in glycosylation between FcγRIIIb^{HNA-1a} and FcγRIIIb^{HNA-1b} forms. At the DNA level, there are five nucleotide differences between the FcγRIIIB^{HNA-1a} and FcγRIIIB^{HNA-1b} genes, but only four of these substitutions give rise to the changes in amino acids arginine/serine, asparagine/serine, aspartic acid/asparagine, and valine/isoleucine substitutions at positions 36, 65, 82, and 106, respectively, that define the difference between HNA-1a and -1b (Figure 6.3).

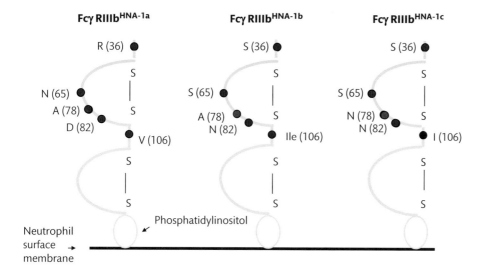

FIGURE 6.3

Representation of the amino acid substitutions that result in the HNA-1a, -1b, -1c, and 1d epitopes found on FcγRIIIb. The positions of the amino acid substitutions arising from the allelic variation of the *FCGR3B* gene are depicted by black dots. Amino acid changes are identified as one-letter symbols. The single amino acid substitution which accounts for the difference between HNA-1b and HNA-1c epitopes are represented by a red dot. The HNA-1d epitope is formed by two amino acids 78Alanine and 82Asparagine and can be considered as the antithetical epitope to HNA-1c. The intra-chain disulphide bonds create two domains which are closely related to the C-terminal heavy chain domains of IgG. Adapted from the illustration published by Salmon et al. (1996). The positions of the amino acids are noted according to the numbering system of Ravetch & Perussia (1989).

A single amino acid substitution alanine/asparagine at position 78 defines the HNA-1c polymorphism (see Figure 6.3). The recently described HNA-1d epitope is also expressed by individuals that express HNA-1b. The two cases in which antibodies to the HNA-1d epitope have been detected have been found in individuals that are HNA-1a(+), 1b(-), and HNA-1c(+) whose immune systems 'see' the HNA-1d epitope as foreign. Despite considerable homology between the different forms of FcγRIIIb, the immune system is able to recognize the epitope created by the unique combination of the two amino acids at positions 78 (alanine) and 82 (asparagine) (see Figure 6.3). The specificity of antisera to HNA-1d and the subtle differences in the HNA-1 system can be further understood by studying the granulocyte test reaction patterns presented in Figures 6.9a and 6.9b.

HNA-1a is the most immunogenic of the polymorphisms on neutrophil FcγRIIIb (CD16). Gene duplication appears to have led to the creation of HNA-1c, and consequently HNA-1c(+) individuals often have three rather than two *FCGR3B* genes (Koene et al., 1998). Normally there are between 100,000 and 200,000 copies of FcγRIIIb per neutrophil, but HNA-1c(+) individuals frequently have increased expression of FcγRIIIb because of the additional gene. Large-scale studies of the incidence of the HNAs in different ethnic groups have not been performed, but the available data indicate that the frequency of the HNA-1a antigen is more common in Japanese, Chinese, and Korean populations than in Caucasians.

The FcγRIIIb 'null' phenotype (~1:2000 Caucasians) arises from an absence of the *FCGR3B* genes. A maternal deficiency of FcγRIIIb on neutrophils can cause immune neutropenia in the newborn due to maternal transfer of FcγRIIIb isoantibodies formed in response to paternally inherited FcγRIIIb (de Haas et al., 1995).

SELF-CHECK 6.8

What is meant by the term 'degeneracy of the genetic code'?

HNA-2 alloantigen

HNA-2 is localized on a 58–64 kDa glycoprotein (CD177) expressed as a glycosylphosphatidylinositol-anchored membrane GP found both on the neutrophil surface membrane and on secondary granules from 97% of the population. The percentage of neutrophils expressing HNA-2 varies between individuals, and HNA-2 alloantibodies typically give a bimodal fluorescence profile with granulocytes from HNA-2 positive donors (Figure 6.4). The HNA-2 status can be determined by phenotyping with human polyclonal or murine monoclonal antibodies. Recently, preliminary studies have suggested that a point mutation in the splicing region of this gene can be used to genetically determine HNA-2 status, but further work is required. There is no antithetical antigen to HNA-2.

HNA-3 system

HNA-3a (previously known as 5[b]) was originally described using antisera obtained from women immunized during pregnancy and was reported as being widely distributed on granulocytes, platelets, lymphocytes, kidney, spleen, and lymph node tissue. Biochemical techniques localized the HNA-3a antigen to a granulocyte glycoprotein with a molecular weight of 70–95 kDa. This polymorphism has been subsequently localized to choline transporter like protein 2 (CTL2) and a single point mutation at amino acid 154 (HNA-3a encoded by arginine and HNA-3b encoded by glutamine) (Greinacher et al., 2010).

The genes encoding the HNA-3a and HNA-3b polymorphisms are referred to as SLC44A2*01 and *SLC44A2*02* and have associated frequencies of 0.792 and 0.207, respectively, in the German population, with 64.1% of individuals as homozygous HNA-3a, 5.5% homozygous HNA-3b, and 30.4% heterozygous. Antibodies to HNA-3a have been associated with transfusion

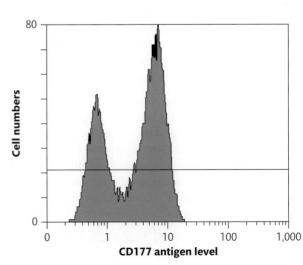

FIGURE 6.4

Characteristic bi-modal binding pattern of HNA-2 antibodies to granulocytes. There is a population of cells expressing low levels of HNA-2 (on the left) and a population of cells expressing high levels of HNA-2 (on the right). The ratio between these two peaks varies between individuals as does their relative positions, i.e the amount of HNA-2 on the neutrophils varies.

related acute lung injury (TRALI) and in neonatal alloimmune neutropenia (NAIN). Antisera to HNA-3b (previously known as 5[a]) have been described but the clinical significance of these antibodies is unknown. A further mutation, *SLC44A2*03*, causes a change in an adjacent amino acid which can affect the binding of some HNA-3a specific antisera.

HNA-4 and HNA-5

HNA-4a and HNA-5a are polymorphisms encoded by the genes for CD11b and CD11a respectively. CD11b and CD11a exist non-covalently with CD18 as heterodimeric proteins and belong to the integrin family of proteins. Alloantibody formation against the HNA-4a and 5a polymorphisms has been observed in transfusion recipients, and recently cases of neonatal alloimmune neutropenia due to HNA-4a, HNA-4b, and HNA-5a alloantibodies have also been described. HNA-4a has a calculated gene frequency of 0.906 and is expressed on granulocytes, monocytes, and a sub-population of T lymphocytes. The HNA-5a antigen is expressed on granulocytes, monocytes, T, and B lymphocytes in 91.8% of a Dutch population.

Other antigens

There are a number of other incompletely described antigens reported to be located on granulocytes, for example LAN, SR, SL, 9a, ND, and NE.

> **Key points**
>
> Alloantigens on neutrophils and granulocytes are known as human neutrophil antigens (HNAs).

6.4 **Antibody detection**

Techniques for the detection of HPA and HNA antibodies have evolved from non-specific and insensitive tests, for example the platelet agglutination test, to non-specific and sensitive tests, for example the **platelet immunofluorescence test (PIFT)** and the **granulocyte immunofluorescence test (GIFT)**, and onwards to specific and sensitive assays that use purified or captured GPs, for example the MAIPA assay or **monoclonal antibody immobilization of granulocyte antigen (MAIGA) assay** and other solid-phase ELISA assays. **Fluorescent bead based assays** are now becoming available that will potentially simplify the detection of HPA and HNA antibodies. These assays utilize beads coupled either to recombinant antigens bearing the major HPA/HNA or beads coupled to purified membrane GPs carrying these antigens. Some of these assays are now commercially available and will help streamline laboratory investigations and offer an additional tool to detect and identify antibody specificities. These techniques offer significant advantages to non-specialist laboratories, and mass screening, but the cost/test for the commercial kits is currently high. An understanding of the technical limitations of these assays is just beginning and so, currently, it is important that more traditional techniques are also maintained. An alternative development has seen the application of surface-plasmon resonance (Socher et al., 2009) to enable detection of low-affinity HPA antibodies which can be removed by the multiple wash steps used in other types of assay.

Platelet immunofluorescence test (PIFT)
A whole-cell immunofluorescence assay capable of detecting platelet reactive antibodies.

Granulocyte immunofluorescence test (GIFT)
A whole-cell immunofluorescence assay capable of detecting granulocyte reactive antibodies.

Monoclonal antibody immobilization of granulocyte antigens (MAIGA) assay
An ELISA assay which uses monoclonal antibodies against granulocyte antigens as the basis of detection and identification of granulocyte specific antibodies.

Fluorescent bead based assays
These assays utilize fluorescently dyed beads which have been coupled with either recombinant or isolated human glycoproteins from platelet or granulocyte membranes.

SELF-CHECK 6.9

What is the difference between antibody avidity and affinity?

Detection of HPA antibodies

Numerous techniques have been described for the detection of platelet antibodies. This text will describe in detail the two previously mentioned techniques, that is, PIFT and MAIPA, which have gained widespread use and have proven track records in quality assessment schemes. However, there are also alternative antigen capture and solid phase red cell adherence assays which are used by many laboratories.

It is generally accepted that reliance on a single technique is a sub-optimal investigation strategy for the detection of platelet specific antibodies and a combination of a whole–cell assay with an antigen capture assay offers significant diagnostic advantages. Despite an inability to distinguish between platelet-specific and HLA antibodies, the PIFT with a flow cytometric endpoint remains a simple, sensitive and widely used assay. The principles of the PIFT are described below.

Typical results obtained by microscopy and by flow cytometry are shown in Figures 6.5 and 6.6 respectively.

METHOD Basics steps of the platelet immunofluorescence test (PIFT)

The steps in the assay procedure include:

- Initial incubation of washed platelets with the serum sample being investigated
- Subsequent washing
- Addition of fluorescent labelled anti-human immunoglobulin
- Further washing

The endpoint of the assay can be determined manually using a fluorescence microscope or more usually a flow cytometer.

METHOD Results of the platelet immunofluorescence test (PIFT)

A histogram plot of forward scatter (FS) and side scatter (SS) is used to define the population of platelets for analysis (histogram 1) and this should be confirmed using a fluorescently labelled platelet glycoprotein-specific monoclonal antibody. The results of fluorescence binding for a negative control sample are shown in histogram 2.1; a weak positive HPA-1a antiserum from a NAIT case in histogram 2.2; and a strong positive HPA-1a antiserum from a case of PTP in histogram 2.3. The results of the assay can be represented in different ways, either as the percentage of cells occurring above a certain threshold (typically >95% of a normal population) in region B or as the mean channel fluorescence values obtained for region C.

(a) 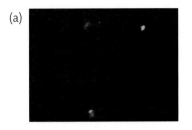   (b)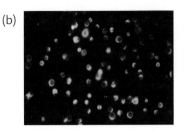

FIGURE 6.5

The results of microscopic analysis of the PIFT showing typical fluorescent staining with (a) negative control serum and (b) a strongly reactive HPA-1a antiserum.

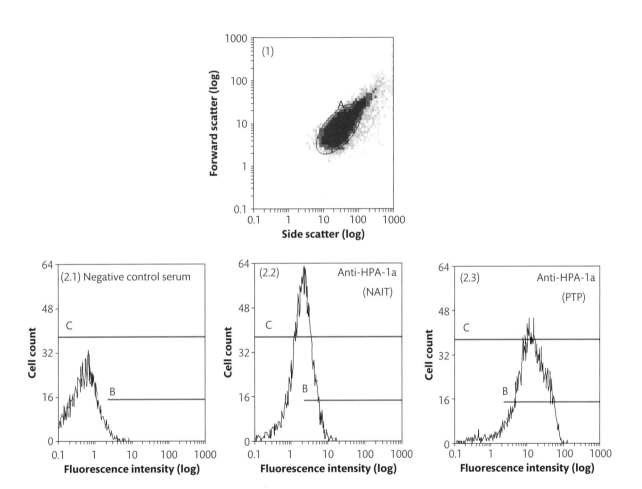

FIGURE 6.6

Typical results of flow cytometric analysis of the platelet immunofluorescence test (PIFT). A histogram plot of forward scatter (FS) and side scatter (SS) utilizes the ability of cells to scatter laser light on the basis of cell size and granularity. This type of plot can be used to define the population of cells (in this case platelets) for analysis (histogram 1). The identity of the cell population should be confirmed using a fluorescently labelled platelet glycoprotein-specific monoclonal antibody. The results of fluorescence binding for a negative control sample (histogram 2.1), a weak positive HPA-1a antiserum from a NAIT case (histogram 2.2), and a strong positive HPA-1a antiserum from a case of post-transfusion purpura (PTP) (histogram 2.3). The results of the assay can be represented in different ways, either as the percentage of cells occurring above a certain threshold (typically >95% of a normal population) in region B or as the mean channel fluorescence values (from the X axis) obtained for region C.

METHOD *The procedure of the monoclonal antibody immo-bilization of platelet antigens (MAIPA) assay*

- Target platelets and the human serum sample to be investigated are incubated together (1).

- After washing to remove unbound antibodies, a murine monoclonal antibody directed against the glycoprotein being investigated, that is, GPIIb/IIIa is added. This step creates a trimolecular complex consisting of murine antibody, GPIIb/IIIa, and the HPA-1a antibody (2).

- After washing to remove unbound murine monoclonal antibody, the platelets are solubilized using a non-ionic detergent and the lysate is centrifuged to remove any particulate material (3).

- The resultant supernatant is added to a microtitre well which has been previously coated with goat anti-mouse IgG antibodies (4).

- After further incubation, the trimolecular complex created in step (2) is captured to the solid phase by the goat anti-mouse antibody binding to the murine GPIIb/IIIa antibody.

- The other unbound platelet glycoproteins (e.g. GPIb/IX) and other bound antibodies, for example HLA class I antibodies bound to the appropriate antigen are removed from the microtitre well by washing.

- An enzyme-linked goat anti-human IgG antibody is added to the microtitre well. After appropriate incubation and washing, an enzyme substrate is added and positive reactions are determined using a colorimetric or chemiluminescence endpoint (5).

The careful selection of reagents is critical to the performance of this assay, for example there must be no cross reactivity between the goat anti-mouse IgG antibody and human IgG antibodies or between the enzyme-conjugated anti-human IgG antibody and either murine anti-GPIIb/IIIa antibodies or the goat anti-mouse IgG used to coat the solid phase. Equally, the selection of the glycoprotein-specific antibodies in step (2) is critical as it must have an epitope binding site that does not compete with the binding site of the human antibodies to be detected.

The use of platelets expressing different HPA and different murine monoclonal antibodies, for example anti-GPIb/IX or GPIa/IIa instead of anti-GPIIb/IIIa, makes it possible to routinely investigate and elucidate the presence of complex mixtures of platelet reactive antibodies in a way that is not possible with whole–cell assays such as the PIFT.

However, assays based on the use of purified/captured GPs are now the cornerstone for the detection and identification of HPA antibodies. The MAIPA assay (Kiefel et al., 1987) captures specific GPs using monoclonal antibodies and can be used to analyse complex mixtures of platelet–reactive antibodies in patient sera. The principle of this assay is shown in Figure 6.2.

The MAIPA assay requires considerable technical expertise in order to ensure maximum sensitivity and specificity, and selection of appropriate screening cells is critical, since the use of platelets heterozygous for the relevant antigen or from donors who have a low expression of particular antigens, for example HPA-15, may result in the failure to detect clinically significant alloantibodies. The combination of PIFT and MAIPA assay together with a panel of HPA typed platelets currently remains the most reliable, cost-effective strategy for detecting and identifying platelet reactive antibodies.

Fluorescent bead based assays for platelet antibodies offer significant potential advantages to the PIFT and MAIPA assays, but further work is required to fully understand their limitations. The beads are labelled with differing amounts of two fluorescent dyes to create an array of beads with different emission characteristics when activated by laser. Typically, a 100 different beads are prepared each with its own unique combination of dyes, which can be visualized at unique position by its fluorescent emission characteristics (Figure 6.7) using an instrument similar to a flow cytometer. Each bead is coupled to an isolated protein, e.g. GPIIb/IIIa from a HPA genotyped donor or a recombinant protein expressing a HPA. Different beads are coupled to

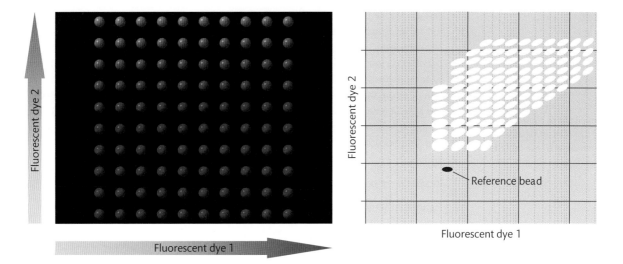

FIGURE 6.7

A hundred different microbeads, each defined by differing amounts of two fluorescent dyes, are prepared (Figure 6.7, left) and have different emissions characteristics when analysed by laser (Figure 6.7, right). A reference bead is included to help calibrate the instrumentation. Each bead is coupled with a different platelet antigen (or other protein of interest from a granulocyte, red cell, lymphocyte, or other tissue). Different beads are mixed together and then incubated with control or test serum sample. The beads are then washed prior to incubation with an anti-globulin reagent coupled to a third fluorescent dye. Antibody binding is assessed by laser and the position of the beads identify to which protein the antibodies have bound. This technology has the potential to transform immunohaematology investigations with red cell, HLA platelet, and granulocyte antibodies being detected and identified simultaneously by the same methodology and instrumentation.

different proteins and these are then mixed together. The bead mixture is then mixed with test serum and, after washing, any antibodies binding to a bead/protein are detected using an anti-human IgG or IgM reagent conjugated to a third fluorescent label. Beads that have elevated levels of anti-human IgG can then be identified as having antibodies against the protein on a given microbead. Similar technology has already been in routine use for a number of years for detecting antibodies against HLA class I and class II antigens.

Detection of HNA antibodies

The reliable detection and identification of neutrophil antibodies is technically and, often, logistically difficult. The main problems are the abundant expression (typically 100–300 K per cell) of low–affinity FcγR receptors for the constant domain of human IgG, which increases the binding of immunoglobulins to the cell surface and the requirement for fresh, typed donor neutrophils as panel cells, since neutrophils cannot be stored. Considerable technical expertise is required to investigate suspected cases of antibody-mediated neutropenia and only a few laboratories worldwide undertake these investigations to a high standard.

Many techniques for neutrophil/granulocyte antibody detection have been evaluated over the years. Early assays such as the granulocyte cytotoxicity and granulocyte agglutination tests had low specificity, although the latter test appears to have particular advantages in detecting some HNA-3a-specific antibodies. The granulocyte immunofluorescence and granulocyte chemi-luminescence tests have the advantage of good sensitivity but are not specific, that is, they cannot readily distinguish between granulocyte-specific and HLA class I antibodies without further investigations. A combination of two techniques, usually the granulocyte immunofluorescence test (GIFT) and **granulocyte agglutination test (GAT)**, together with an HNA typed panel, is currently recommended as the optimal approach for antibody detection. For HNA systems expressed on CD16, CD177, and C11/18, MAIGA assays can be applied to investigation of serum samples that also contain HLA class I antibodies. The principles of the GIFT and the MAIGA assay are analogous to the equivalent platelet tests (PIFT and MAIPA) described earlier. An example of the forward scatter/side scatter histogram obtained with granulocytes and lymphocytes is shown in Figure 6.8.

The GAT brings together fresh, viable granulocytes with test samples and after a prolonged incubation of between 2 and 6 hours, agglutination is assessed using microscopy.

Figure 6.9a shows the GAT results obtained after incubation with a HNA-1b antiserum.

i.   Granulocytes from a donor typed as *FCGR3*01*. Negative reaction indicated by a monolayer of individual granulocytes.

ii.   Granulocytes from a donor typed as *FCGR3*02*. Positive reaction indicated by agglutinated granulocytes.

iii. Granulocytes from a donor typed as *FCGR3*01; FCGR3B*02*. Positive reaction indicated by agglutinated granulocytes.

iv.   Granulocytes from a donor typed as *FCGR3*01; FCGR3B*03*. Positive reaction indicated by agglutinated granulocytes. Note the weaker reaction with these cells.

Granulocyte agglutination test (GAT)

A simple test that brings together small volumes of isolated granulocytes and human test or control where the agglutination endpoint is measured by eye using a microscope.

METHOD *The granulocyte agglutination test (GAT)*

- Isolated, viable granulocytes (1 μl) are incubated with test or negative and positive control serum (3 μl) in a microplate under mineral oil (to prevent evaporation) at 30°C for between 2 and 6 hours.

- In the presence of granulocyte reactive antibodies, the granulocytes slowly coalesce around each other to form agglutinates around the edge of the test well due to electrostatic interactions.

- The amount of granulocyte agglutination is assessed by eye using a microscope.

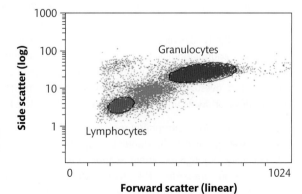

FIGURE 6.8

Results of flow cytometric analysis of granulocytes and lymphocytes identified by forward scatter (FS) and side scatter (SS) characteristics as described previously for platelets (see legend of Figure 6.6). The cell population between the lymphocytes and granulocytes represents co-isolated monocytes.

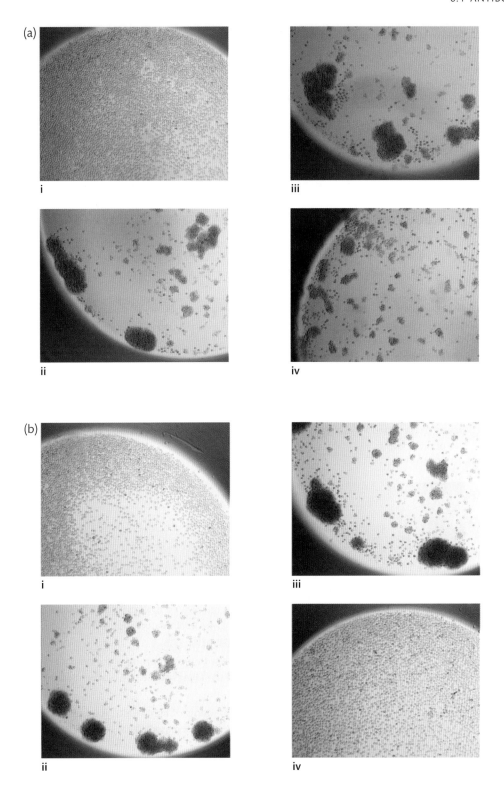

FIGURES 6.9a AND 6.9b
The results obtained with two HNA specific antibodies using the GAT (images kindly provided by Dr Angelika Reil, German Red Cross Blood Service West, Hagen, Germany).

SELF-CHECK 6.10

Why is there reactivity of the HNA-1b antiserum with granulocytes from the donor typed as *FCGR3*01; FCGR3B*03* in Figure 6.9a iv? And why is the agglutination less than that observed with the *FCGR3*02* donor in Figure 6.9a ii?

Figure 6.9b shows the GAT results obtained after incubation with a HNA-1d antiserum.

i.   Granulocytes from a donor typed as *FCGR3*01*. Negative reaction indicated by a monolayer of individual granulocytes.

ii. Granulocytes from a donor typed as *FCGR3*02*. Positive reaction indicated by agglutinated granulocytes.

iii. Granulocytes from a donor typed as *FCGR3*01; FCGR3B*02*. Positive reaction indicated by agglutinated granulocytes.

iv. Granulocytes from a donor typed as *FCGR3*01; FCGR3B*03*. Negative reaction indicated by a monolayer of individual granulocytes. Note the weaker reaction with these cells.

SELF-CHECK 6.11

Why does the HNA-1d antiserum not react with the donor typed as *FCGR3*01; FCGR3B*03* in Figure 6.9b iv?

Granulocyte chemiluminescence test (GCLT)

A biological assay that utilizes human monocytes to detect granulocyte antibodies bound to the membrane surface.

In contrast to the immunochemical assays commonly used in immunohaematology, the **granulocyte chemiluminescence test (GCLT)** is a biological assay (Lucas, 1994). The assay measures the biochemical activity of human monocytes initiating the phagocytosis of opsonized (antibody coated) granulocytes (Figure 6.10a) and was developed with the objective of providing a better indicator of clinical significance.

METHOD The granulocyte chemiluminescence test (GCLT)

Figure 6.10a shows the principle of the GCLT:

• Opsonized granulocytes (i.e. granulocytes coated with antibodies after incubation with test serum containing granulocyte reactive antibodies) are introduced to washed human monocytes. (The granulocytes are heat treated prior to opsonization to inactivate the phagocytic potential of these cells.)

• The FcR receptors on the monocytes interact with the Fc portion of the bound antibodies and via a process of trans-membrane signalling activate the biochemical processes in the monocyte to initiate phagocytosis.

• The biochemical pathways generate small amounts of light, which is amplified by an acceptor molecule (luminol) and the resultant increased signal is measured in a luminometer.

Figure 6.10b shows the kinetics of the interaction between opsonized granulocytes and human monocytes over 30–40 minutes. The three lines represent the light generated by inert serum (red line), HNA-1a antibodies (blue line), and an HLA antiserum (green line):

- There is an initial lag phase as the monocytes initiate phagocytosis of opsonized granulocytes.
- The release of light peaks at 8–15 minutes depending on antibody class, antibody concentration, and antigen density.
- The reaction begins to subside as the biochemical reserves of the monocytes become exhausted.

(a) **Mechanism**

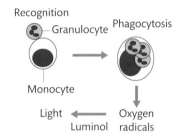

(b) **Kinetics**

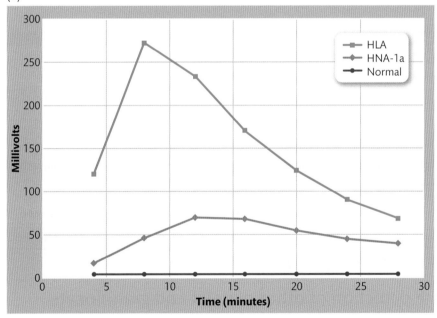

FIGURE 6.10

The granulocyte chemiluminescence test. Granulocytes incubated with antibody containing sera are washed and then introduced to isolated human monocytes. The monocytes recognize and are activated by the Fc portion of the bound antibodies to initiate phagocytosis. The monocytes produce small amounts of light which is amplified by the electron acceptor (luminol) and is measured in a luminometer (a type of spectrophotometer). The granulocytes are heat treated prior to incubation with the test sera to inactivate their own inherent phagocytic potential. (The enzymes which comprise the biochemical process of phagocytosis are temperature sensitive.)

The bead based assay technology described for detecting platelet antibodies has also been applied for the detection of HNA specific antibodies in a commercial kit for the detection of HLA class I, HLA class II, and HNA antibodies. The commercial impetus for this development was provided by the introduction of HLA and HNA antibody donor screening of blood donors by blood transfusion services as part of the strategy to reduce the incidence of TRALI. This kit provides a streamlined alternative for antibody screening compared to traditional techniques for granulocyte antibodies and overcomes the problems of obtaining fresh granulocytes from typed donors, which can be particularly difficult for low-frequency antigens such as HNA-1c and HNA-3b3b. These kits are relatively new and currently there is little experience of its sensitivity and specificity, although preliminary results suggest that sensitivity is reduced compared to traditional techniques, especially for HNA-3 reactive antibodies. In addition, a number of centres have described development of rHNA cell lines. These assays utilize a cell line into which the gene encoding the antigen of interest has been inserted. The resultant transfected cell line then expresses the antigen and can either be stored frozen or maintained in continuous culture. Selection of the host cell line is important to ensure that the cells can be readily grown and that any potentially confounding antigens, e.g. HLA class I, are absent.

Typing for HNAs traditionally utilized monospecific alloantisera or more recently HNA-specific monoclonal antibodies, for example HNA-1a, -1b, and -2. Increased understanding of the molecular nature of HNA has enabled PCR based typing for HNA-1a, -1b, -1c, -3a, -3b -4a, -4b, -5a, and -5bw and the development of recombinant HNAs, which may transform the serological investigation of granulocyte alloantibodies.

SELF-CHECK 6.12

What do you understand to be the major challenges in undertaking *in vitro* serological investigations with granulocytes using traditional techniques?

SELF-CHECK 6.13

What would be the consequences of performing a sub-optimal number of washes in the PIFT or GIFT following incubation with patient serum?

SELF-CHECK 6.14

What problems might be encountered in using fluorescent microbeads coupled to HPA and HNA proteins/peptides for detecting platelet and granulocyte antibodies?

Key points

Reliable detection and identification of HPA- and HNA-specific antibodies currently requires the use of both whole-cell-type assays such as the PIFT, GIFT, or GCLT and antigen-capture type assays such as the MAIPA and MAIGA assays, together with access to a HPA/HNA typed cell panel. Fluorescent bead based assays are currently being evaluated.

The detection of other platelet and granulocyte antibodies

The diagnostic value of detecting autoantibodies against platelets and neutrophils has been much debated because of the limited clinical benefit of these tests for many patients and, consequently, laboratory investigation is only indicated in certain clinical conditions. In the autoimmune thrombocytopenias, the antibodies typically recognize epitopes on platelet glycoproteins GPIIb/IIIa or GPIb/IX/V, although antibody specificity is not routinely investigated. Autoantibodies against the HPAs have not been described. There is emerging evidence that antibody specificities in the immune thrombocytopenias may indicate response to treatment

(Zeng et al., 2012). Detection of isoantibodies is of clinical importance in thrombasthenia patients and individuals with GPIV deficiency, whilst the identification of drug dependent antibodies can also have a profound effect on patient management.

SELF-CHECK 6.15

What are the main problems in the detection and identification of platelet and granulocyte antibodies?

6.5 Clinical significance of HPA alloantibodies

HPA alloantibodies are implicated in the following clinical conditions:

- Neonatal alloimmune thrombocytopenia
- Post-transfusion purpura
- Platelet transfusion refractoriness
- Persistent post-bone marrow transplant thrombocytopenia.

Unlike red cell and granulocyte immunohaematology, platelet antibodies with HPA allospecificity have not been implicated in autoimmune thrombocytopenias.

SELF-CHECK 6.16

Give some examples of red cell antigens that are targets for autoantibodies.

Neonatal alloimmune thrombocytopenia (NAIT)

Neonatal alloimmune thrombocytopenia (NAIT) is by far the most important of the clinical conditions discussed in this chapter in terms of the number of suspected cases referred for laboratory investigation, the potential impact upon health and social care services, and the impact upon blood transfusion service resources for HPA selected blood products. Accordingly, more emphasis is given to this condition.

Neonatal alloimmune thrombocytopenia is the platelet equivalent of **haemolytic disease of the fetus and newborn (HDFN)** and the first case was described in 1959. Neonatal alloimmune thrombocytopenia had been long suspected on clinical grounds, but laboratory confirmation had proved difficult because platelet antibody detection was technically more demanding than for red cell antibodies. Today, NAIT is a distinct clinical, but probably underdiagnosed, entity with an estimated incidence of severe thrombocytopenia due to maternal HPA antibodies of between 1 in 1000 and 1200 live births. Unlike HDFN, about 30% of NAIT cases occur in the first pregnancy.

> **Haemolytic disease of the fetus and newborn (HDFN)**
>
> A disease associated with the fetomaternal transfer of red cell antibodies that cause haemolysis and red cell destruction in the infant (see Chapter 3).

Definition and pathophysiology

Neonatal alloimmune thrombocytopenia is usually due to maternal HPA alloimmunization caused by fetomaternal incompatibility for a fetal HPA inherited from the father but which is absent in the mother. Maternal IgG alloantibodies against the fetal HPA cross the placenta and bind to fetal platelets, thereby causing reduced platelet survival and thrombocytopenia.

Severe thrombocytopenia in the term neonate, accompanied by haemorrhage, is generally caused by HPA-1a antibodies if the mother is of Caucasian or African origin. Antibodies against HPA-4 antigens are generally implicated in cases of Far Eastern ethnicity. In the latter group and in patients of African origin, maternal GPIV deficiency should also be investigated. HPA-5b antibodies have been documented in all major ethnic groups but generally these cause mild thrombocytopenia, although intracranial cerebral haemorrhage (ICH) has been reported.

Neonatal alloimmune thrombocytopenia due to alloantibodies against the other HPAs is infrequent. HLA class I antibodies, present in 15–25% of multiparous women, are generally not thought to cause NAIT and although a number of individual case reports have been described, larger scale studies have not provided confirmatory evidence. Destruction of IgG-coated fetal platelets is assumed to take place in the spleen through interaction with mononuclear cells bearing Fcγ receptors for the constant domain of IgG. HPA-1a is known to be expressed on fetal platelets from 16 weeks' gestation, with placental transfer of IgG antibodies occurring from 14 weeks, so thrombocytopenia can occur early in pregnancy. ICH has been reported as early as 16 weeks' gestation. The duration of thrombocytopenia in an untreated infant following delivery is variable—typically in the order of about a week, but can be a long as four weeks. It is therefore important to ensure that the platelet count is carefully monitored during the first few weeks of life and after any transfusions. In some cases, the nadir platelet count occurs at about 3–5 days of life because splenic function takes a few days to efficiently remove antibody-coated platelets.

Incidence

Prospective screening of pregnant Caucasian women has shown that about 1 in 1200 neonates have severe thrombocytopenia (platelet count $<50 \times 10^9$/l) because of alloimmunization against HPA-1a (Williamson et al., 1998). The approximately 120 cases a year of serologically confirmed, clinically referred NAIT cases in England is below the anticipated ~450 cases predicted from population studies and suggests that NAIT remains under-diagnosed. HPA-5b antibodies are frequently found in pregnant women, but they are generally of less clinical significance than HPA-1a antibodies, possibly due to the lower copy number of the GPIa/IIa complex on platelets (1–2000 compared to 50–80,000 for GPIIb/IIIa).

Clinical features and differential diagnosis

There are many causes of neonatal thrombocytopenia, including bacterial or viral infections, premature delivery, intrauterine growth retardation, diabetes, inadequate megakaryopoiesis, asphyxia at birth, inherited chromosomal abnormalities (particularly trisomy 21), and maternal autoimmune thrombocytopenia. In addition, platelet type von Willebrand's disease, in which there is a tendency for *in vitro* platelet aggregation, and a variety of technical problems, for example platelet clumping in EDTA, can also lead to falsely low platelet counts.

Typically, a full-term infant with NAIT presents with skin bleeding (purpura, petechiae, and/or ecchymoses), or more serious haemorrhage such as ICH, and an isolated thrombocytopenia, but is otherwise healthy with a normal coagulation screen. Less commonly, ventriculomegaly, cerebral cysts, and hydrocephalus may be discovered **in utero** by routine ultrasound. Hydrops fetalis has also been reported in association with NAIT and this diagnosis should be considered if there are no other obvious reasons for the hydrops.

in utero
Literally within the uterus.

The precise incidence of ICH due to NAIT is unknown, but conservative estimates suggest that it is as low as 1 in 20,000 live births, which equates to approximately 35 cases per annum in the UK. Nearly 50% of severe ICHs occur *in utero*, usually between 30 and 35 weeks' gestation, but sometimes before 20 weeks. Severe NAIT (platelet count $<30 \times 10^9$/l) is a serious condition and appropriate management (see later in this section) is essential to prevent ICH and the possibility of lifelong disability. Conversely, at the other end of the clinical spectrum, NAIT can be discovered incidentally when a blood count is performed for other reasons.

Laboratory investigations

The cause of severe thrombocytopenia in an otherwise healthy neonate should be determined with urgency and investigation for maternal HPA antibodies must be carried out by techniques with appropriate sensitivity and specificity. The use of the indirect PIFT and the MAIPA assay, together with a panel of HPA typed platelets is the current preferred option for many reference laboratories, but bead based assays are also now available. In England, HPA antibodies are detected in approximately 15% of referrals of suspected NAIT. The most frequently detected specificities are anti-HPA-1a and anti-HPA-5b which are implicated in about 85% and 10% of confirmed cases of NAIT respectively. The ability of an HPA-1a-negative mother to form anti-HPA-1a is partly controlled by the *HLA DRB3*01:01* allele. HPA-1a-negative women who are *HLA DRB3*01:01* positive have a one in three chance of making HPA-1a compared to a frequency of 1 in 300 for DRB3*01:01 negative women. This highly significant association between an HLA class II type and the formation of HPA-1a alloantibodies has not been observed for any of the other antigens on platelets, red cells, or leucocytes.

Molecular typing of the parents and neonate for HPA-1, -2, -3, -4, -5, -6, -9, and HPA-15 should be performed and the results reviewed in conjunction with the results of the antibody investigations. Particularly, in patients of Far Eastern origin, HPA-4 immunization should be considered if there is a discrepancy between the parental genotypes. Anti-GPIV antibodies and GPIV expression on platelets should also be investigated if HPA antibodies are not detected but the clinical presentation is convincing.

Alloimmunization against low-frequency HPAs, for example HPA-9bw, can cause NAIT and should be considered in referrals that have a negative antibody screen for the common HPA antibody specificities but a strong clinical history. Screening all suspected NAIT referrals for antibodies against low-frequency HPAs is not cost-effective and a recent study of more than 1000 paternal DNA samples from NAIT referrals showed the presence of HPA-bw alleles in fewer than ten paternal samples. Investigations for alloimmunization against rare HPA-bw alleles should therefore be reserved for clinically severe cases of NAIT where there is a strong index of suspicion of NAIT and no alternative clinical diagnosis (Ghevaert et al., 2007). Genotyping of the paternal DNA sample for low-frequency HPA is a pragmatic approach in this clinical setting. The use of fluorescent beads coupled to GPIIb/IIIa mutated to carry a large number of low-frequency HPAs also has considerable potential in cases where DNA typing has identified a low frequency feto/maternal mismatch.

At present, there is no predictive test linking a characteristic of HPA-1a specific antibodies detected in NAIT with clinical outcome of a pregnancy. Attempts have been made to associate antibody titre with the degree of thrombocytopenia as has been done for anti-D and the severity of HDFN but results have been inconsistent. Similarly, there have been attempts to associate clinical outcome with IgG subclass or glycosylation of HPA-1a IgG antibodies. A recent proposal has suggested that the presence of antibodies against vitronectin integrin (α_v/β_3), which is expressed on endothelial cells and shares 74% amino acid homology with GPIIb/IIIa (αIIb/β_3) on platelets, may be a critical factor that predisposes to bleeding and ICH.

Key points

Neonatal alloimmune thrombocytopenia is a common disorder and HPA-1a or HPA-5b antibodies are responsible for approximately 95% of Caucasian cases.

The immunogenicity of HPA-1a

There are a number of factors that may influence the immunogenicity of HPA-1a in NAIT compared to other HPAs including:

1. The relatively distal position of this polymorphism from the cell membrane provides easier interaction and recognition by cells of the immune system.

2. The greater distance from the cell surface also reduces electrostatic repulsion between cells, again facilitating cell:cell interactions.

3. The introduction of a proline for a leucine at amino acid position 33 introduces a major change in the secondary structure of the protein. Proline is frequently associated with tight turns in protein structures or kinks in alpha helices because it is connected to the protein backbone twice. The proline and leucine forms of this protein have distinct secondary structures which change the electron cloud of surrounding amino acids and make the other form more 'visible' to the immune system.

Neonatal management

A neonatal platelet count of $<100 \times 10^9/l$ should be confirmed and a blood film examined. The neonate should be carefully examined for skin or mucosal bleeding if a low platelet count is confirmed. If the platelet count is $<30 \times 10^9/l$ or if there are signs of bleeding, it is strongly recommended that the neonate is transfused with HPA-1a(-) and 5b(-) platelets, as these will be compatible with the maternal HPA alloantibody in over 95% of NAIT cases. The transfusion of HPA-1a(-) and 5b(-) platelets in NAIT caused by HPA-1a or HPA-5b antibodies results in a higher increment and more prolonged platelet survival than transfusion of random donor (HPA-1a-positive) platelets (Allen et al., 2007). However, if HPA-1a(-) and 5b(-) platelets are not immediately available and there is an urgent clinical need for transfusion then random ABO and RhD compatible donor platelets suitable for neonatal use should be used in the first instance. Figure 6.11 illustrates the clinical advantage frequently observed as a result of using HPA-1a(-)5b(-) platelets to support infants with NAIT due to HPA-1a antibodies. A follow-up platelet count should be performed approximately one hour after the transfusion is completed, and at least daily thereafter until the platelet count has normalized. In a typical case, the platelet count should recover to normal within a week, although a more protracted recovery can occur. Intravenous immunoglobulin (GIVIgG) is not recommended as first-line treatment as there is a delay of 24–48 hours before a satisfactory count is achieved, in contrast to the immediate effect of transfusing HPA-compatible donor platelets. A cerebral ultrasound scan of the baby should be considered if the platelet count is $<50 \times 10^9/l$, and is recommended when the platelet count is $<30 \times 10^9/l$.

Key points

Optimal post-natal treatment of NAIT is the transfusion of HPA-1a(-) and 5b(-) donor platelets.

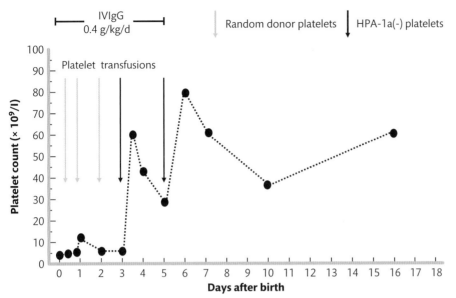

FIGURE 6.11
Neonatal platelet counts for an infant with NAIT due to HPA-1a antibodies. Initial treatment with random platelets and IvIgG did not produce a satisfactory platelet increment and only the use of HPA-1a(-) platelets resulted in the desired correction to the infant's platelet count.

Antenatal management

In a subsequent pregnancy of a mother with a previous pregnancy affected by NAIT, the pregnancy should be managed by an appropriately experienced fetal medicine team. The treatment strategy is based on the clinical history and outcome in previous pregnancies.

There are two main antenatal treatment options: high-dose IVIgG to the mother, or *in utero* platelet transfusion of the fetus, with the former being generally recognized as the safest, most effective current intervention to reduce the risk of ICH in the fetus. Maternal IVIgG (1 g or 0.5 g/kg body weight) is given at weekly intervals, usually commencing between 12 and 20 weeks of gestation, depending on the history of previous pregnancies. Early commencement of treatment is indicated in those cases where there is a history of antenatal ICH. A beneficial effect of IVIgG on the fetal platelet count occurs in approximately 70% of cases. Some treatment centres subsequently perform a fetal blood sampling (FBS) to ascertain the platelet count, usually after eight weeks' of treatment with IVIgG, but the recent trend is to minimize invasive treatment wherever possible. If a safe fetal platelet count has not been achieved at the time of sampling, the pregnancy may be managed by increasing the dose of IVIgG and/or adding corticosteroids (prednisolone, 0.5 mg/kg body weight) or augmenting treatment with fetal platelet transfusions as required to maintain the platelet count. *In utero* transfusions of irradiated platelets, carried out with FBS, carry a significant risk of fetal morbidity and mortality. This treatment should not be chosen as first-line treatment but as a rescue regime or in the management of pregnancies with a history of treatment failure on IVIgG. The intrauterine transfusion of platelets has more complications compared to red cell transfusions for HDFN, for example bradycardia and post-needle withdrawal cord bleeds, and the risk increases since this technically demanding procedure may need to be repeated on a weekly basis (see Figure 6.12) because of the short half-life of platelets.

SELF-CHECK 6.17

Why are irradiated platelets used for intrauterine transfusions?

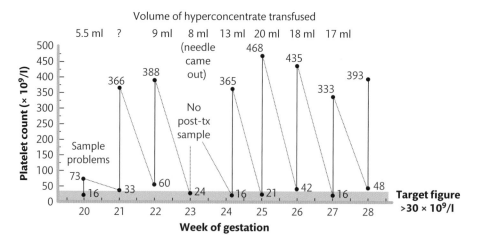

FIGURE 6.12

Third pregnancy of a mother with a history of NAIT due to HPA-1a antibodies. The first pregnancy was associated with intrauterine death. The second pregnancy resulted in an infant with moderate thrombocytopenia. The fetal platelet counts during the third pregnancy are shown with IUT commencing at week 20 and continuing on a weekly basis until delivery by Caesarean section. The objective of treatment was to maintain the platelet count of the fetus above 30×10^9/l and the target platelet count after transfusion was $>300 \times 10^9$/l.

Counselling

Couples with an index case of NAIT should be counselled about the risks of severe fetal/neo-natal thrombocytopenia in a subsequent pregnancy. Advice should be based on the severity of disease in the infant(s) and the outcome of immunological investigations as follows:

- Thrombocytopenia in subsequent cases can be as severe or more severe.
- The best predictors of severe fetal thrombocytopenia in a future pregnancy are the occurrence of antenatal ICH and severe thrombocytopenia (platelet count $<30 \times 10^9$/l) in a previous pregnancy.
- Antibody specificity, titre, or the bioactivity of HPA-1a antibodies do not reliably correlate with the severity of NAIT, and are probably of little value in informing clinical management (Ghevaert et al., 2007b).
- The HPA zygosity of the partner.

SELF-CHECK 6.18

What is meant by the term zygosity?

Key points

Optimal antenatal treatment in women known to be HPA alloimmunized has yet to be determined, but maternal IVIgG administration is generally preferred to intrauterine transfusion of platelets.

HPA typed platelet donor panels

Establishing donor panels for fetal and neonatal platelet transfusion requires a major commitment from blood services and the availability of high-throughput DNA typing techniques. Although the frequency of HPA-1a-negative individuals amongst Caucasians is 2.5%, potential donors for fetal/neonatal transfusions must also be negative for the mandatory microbiological tests including hepatitis E virus and cytomegalovirus (CMV), negative for antibodies against red cells, platelets and leucocytes, and low titre anti-A and anti-B. Thus, in order to recruit one HPA-1a negative donor who is able to meet all of the above criteria approximately 1500–2000 donors will have to be typed for HPA-1a. A further 20% of donors will be ineligible for the HPA-1a(-)5b(-) panel because they will be HPA-5b(+).

Therapeutic platelets for fetal transfusion should also be RhD compatible, as small amounts of red cells present in platelet concentrates may immunize RhD-negative recipients, and ideally also be ABO compatible. In order to recruit a single RhD-negative, HPA-1a-negative donor whose platelets will be suitable for a first fetal platelet transfusion, where the fetal/neonatal blood group is unknown, approximately 15,000–20,000 donors need to be typed. In England, neonatal HPA-1a(-), 5b(-) platelets are routinely available to order on demand at five sites across the country.

Post-transfusion purpura (PTP)

Post-transfusion purpura is an acute episode of thrombocytopenia occurring 5–12 days after whole blood, red cell concentrate, or platelet transfusion. In 95% of cases, PTP affects middle-aged or elderly women who have been alloimmunized against HPA-1a during an earlier pregnancy. The transfusion causes a secondary immune response which boosts HPA-1a antibody levels; although the mechanism of destruction of the patient's own HPA-1a(-) platelets remains unproven there is evidence to support the simultaneous production of platelet autoantibodies during the strong secondary immune response. Post-transfusion purpura can occasionally affect men immunized by previous transfusion. An unusual case of PTP in a male patient, in whom three different HPA antibody specificities were detected in addition to HLA antibodies (Lucas et al., 1997), provides a useful example of the ability of the MAIPA assay (see Section 6.4) to elucidate complex mixtures of antibodies. Rarely, 'passive PTP' can occur immediately following infusion of plasma from a donor who has made HPA-1a antibodies following pregnancy.

> **Post-transfusion purpura (PTP)**
> An unexpected thrombocytopenia occurring 5–12 days after a blood transfusion that is associated with the presence of HPA-specific antibodies, usually in the recipient.

SELF-CHECK 6.19

How might platelet autoantibodies be generated following blood transfusion in PTP?

Cases of PTP should be reported to the **Serious Hazards Of Transfusion (SHOT)** scheme and historical data indicate that the incidence of PTP in the UK prior to universal leucodepletion was in the order of 1 in 0.5 million transfusions. The incidence has further reduced since leucodepletion by a factor of approximately 4 (Williamson et al., 2007).

SELF-CHECK 6.20

What is leucodepletion?

SELF-CHECK 6.21

How could leucodepletion have reduced the incidence of PTP?

The onset of thrombocytopenia in PTP is usually rapid, with the platelet count falling from normal to below 10×10^9/l within 24 hours or less of transfusion (Figure 6.13a). Haemorrhage is common, with widespread purpura (Figure 6.13b), bruising (Figure 6.13c), mucous membrane, gastrointestinal, and urinary tract bleeding. Post-transfusion purpura may be preceded by febrile non-haemolytic transfusion reactions. The natural history of PTP lasts between 7 and 28 days but early management is essential to reduce the risk of intracranial haemorrhage. High dose IVIgG over 2–5 days is the current treatment of choice, but platelet transfusions are not usually indicated unless the bleeding is severe. As the incidence of PTP is very rare, a diagnosis of heparin induced thrombocytopenia should be considered if the patient has received this drug.

Recurrence of PTP following further transfusions has been reported but is unpredictable. In order to minimize the risk of recurrence, patients requiring further transfusions should receive HPA compatible red cells or platelets, but if these are not available, leucocyte-depleted blood components are considered acceptable alternatives.

Platelet transfusion refractoriness and platelet selection

Platelet transfusion refractoriness

A suboptimal increase in circulating platelet count following platelet transfusion.

Platelet transfusion refractoriness may be defined as a failure to achieve a sustained increase in platelet count following a platelet transfusion. The criteria for a successful platelet transfusion vary. Generally, transfusion of an adult dose of platelets should result in an increase of 30–50,000 in an average adult. In a clinical setting, an increase of $\geq 20 \times 10^9$/l at 24 hours is considered a successful outcome, while an increase of $<10 \times 10^9$/l is not. Determination of the corrected count increment:

$$(CCI) = \frac{\text{Platelet cnt}_{(\text{post-transfusion})} - \text{Platelet cnt}_{(\text{pre-transfusion})} \times \text{Body surface area} (m^2)}{\text{No. of platelets transfused} (\times 10^{11})}$$

provides a more objective guide to the success or otherwise of a platelet transfusion but is seldom performed routinely.

Platelet transfusions are not normally given to adult patients unless the platelet count is $\leq 10 \times 10^9$/l or there is a risk of haemorrhage or surgery is planned.

FIGURE 6.13

The main features of post-transfusion purpura (PTP). Figure 6.13a illustrates the typical crash in platelet count following blood transfusion and the prompt recovery following IVIgG administration (usually within seven days). In the absence of IVIgG treatment the recovery of the platelet count may take 1–2 months. Figures 6.13b and 6.13c illustrate typical manifestations of petechiae and ecchymoses associated with low platelet count.

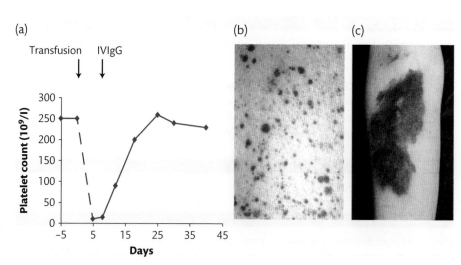

In the majority of cases, platelet refractoriness is due to 'non-immune' factors such as consumption due to coagulation problems, for example disseminated coagulation, or following surgery, concomitant bacterial infections, or increased sequestration of platelets as occurs in hypersplenism. When immunological destruction of platelets does occur, there is a hierarchy of potential agents. Platelet transfusion refractoriness to random platelets should be initially addressed by providing ABO compatible platelets to avoid the action of anti-A and anti-B. If this does not result in a satisfactory platelet increment on two occasions, the presence of HLA class I antibodies should be investigated. HLA-A and HLA-B antigens are expressed on platelets and, in England, provision of HLA selected platelets is based both on the HLA-A and HLA-B type of the recipient and the HLA antibody specificities detected in the patient's circulation. It is not necessary to try and match exactly for the genes encoding these proteins (there are currently over 2900 HLA-A alleles and more than 3600 HLA-B alleles), because these antigens express only a limited number of epitopes recognized by antibodies, which are clustered into cross-reacting antigens (CREGS). Platelets are selected from the CREGS which avoid the antibody specificities detected in the patient, although it is often not possible to provide optimally selected platelets and partial matches may need to be used. The grade of selection (or match) can be classified into: 'A' grade—no mismatch at HLA-A or HLA-B; 'B1' grade—one mismatch at the HLA-A or HLA-B loci; or 'B2' grade—two mismatches at the HLA-A or HLA-B loci, although there are other classifications. It is not usual to match for HLA-C antigens. In countries where platelets from HLA typed donors are not available, it is necessary to crossmatch patient serum with candidate platelet units to determine the units that give the least reaction.

In a small proportion of patients, HLA selected platelets may not result in a satisfactory increment because of the presence of HPA antibodies. The reported incidence of HPA antibodies in platelet transfusion refractory patients varies between 0–20% in different studies and the methodologies used to detect platelet antibodies. Typically, HPA antibodies occur together with HLA antibodies, although very occasionally (<1% of cases) only HPA antibodies are detected. The HPA specificities usually detected in this setting are HPA-1b, HPA-2b, and HPA-5b. Platelet autoantibodies, i.e. antibodies with platelet glycoprotein rather than HPA specificity, can also occur in this context since many patients have underlying immune dysregulation, e.g. myelodysplastic syndromes, aplastic anaemia, chronic lymphocytic leukaemia. It is not possible to provide compatible platelets for patients with platelet autoantibodies.

Despite their low incidence, HPA antibodies, are often highly clinically significant and in alloimmunized patients with both HLA and HPA antibodies, where platelet selection may be difficult because of low antigen frequencies, it may be necessary to choose HPA selected platelets in preference to optimally HLA selected platelets in order to achieve satisfactory increments and/or prevent/reduce haemorrhage.

HPA alloimmunization can also occur in the post-bone marrow transplant setting and these may have an adverse impact on megakaryocyte engraftment and/or transfusion management in the recovery period (Lucas et al., 2010). Liver transplantation has also been associated with passive, transient transfer of HPA immunization due to the presence of passenger lymphocytes/plasma cells in the transplanted organ with thrombocytopenia resulting in the recipient.

Immune destruction of platelets

The destruction of platelets following binding to platelet antibodies has been most extensively studied in the context of autoimmune thrombocytopenia (AITP) but is likely to be similar for other immune thrombocytopenias. The primary sites of destruction are the reticuloendothelial system in the spleen and liver, which is analogous to the immune destruction of red cells. The removal of the spleen was for many years the primary treatment for AITP. The success of this treatment was because splenectomy:

- removed a major site of platelet destruction
- removed a major site of antibody production.

Marginating platelets were released into the circulation (~30% of all platelets in a normal invidual marginate in the spleen).

Intraveneous immunoglobulin G (IVIG) treatment

IVIgG treatment has found a role in NAIT, PTP, platelet tranfusion refractoriness, and autoimmune thrombocytopenias. The immuno-modulatory effects of IVIgG are multifactorial and may vary in importance from patient to patient but include as a minimum:

- IVIgG provides negative feedback to 'turn off' the IgG production in the recipient, therefore dampening down production of antibodies binding to platelets.
- Blockade of the Fc receptors of the cells in the reticuloendothelial system to prevent phagocytosis of opsonized platelets.
- Coating of platelets to prevent antibody binding/recognition by Fc receptors.
- Anti-idiotype interactions to improve regulation of the immune system.

6.6 Clinical significance of HNA antibodies

HNA alloantibodies are implicated in the following clinical conditions:

- Neonatal alloimmune neutropenia
- Non-haemolytic febrile transfusion reactions
- Transfusion-related acute lung injury
- Transfusion-related alloimmune neutropenia
- Autoimmune neutropenia
- Persistent post-bone marrow transplant neutropenia

Neonatal alloimmune neutropenia (NAIN)

Neonatal alloimmune neutropenia is the neutrophil equivalent of HDFN but like NAIT can occur in the first pregnancy. Maternal alloimmunization against neutrophil-specific alloantigens on fetal/neonatal neutrophils is rare, with an estimated incidence of 0.1–0.2% of live births. Clinical presentation primarily manifests after delivery, as bacterial infections associated with an isolated neutropenia, unless the mother has a systemic infection during pregnancy. Severe neutropenia in the newborn may require treatment with antibiotics and/or granulocyte colony stimulating factor (GCSF) to control bacterial infections and quickly achieve a normal

Neonatal alloimmune neutropenia (NAIN)

Neutropenia in a neonate (or fetus) caused by the maternal fetal transfer of granulocyte-specific antibodies recognizing either HNAs or granulocyte glycoproteins inherited by the fetus from the father but absent in the mother.

neutrophil count. In untreated NAIN cases, prior to the availability of GCSF, the neutropenia caused by HNA-1a, -1b, and -2 antibodies has been reported to extend up to 28 weeks (Figure 6.14). This extended period of neutropenia contrasts sharply with the comparatively short period of thrombocytopenia usually associated with NAIT. There a number of factors that may influence the duration of neutropenia including:

- The target antigens HNA-1 and HNA-2 are restricted to the neutrophil compartment and the antibodies cannot be adsorbed by other tissues.

- The HNA-1 and -2 antigens are expressed on marrow precursor cells (metamyelocytes and myelocytes respectively), so there may be an effect similar to that seen with anti-Kell, red cell production and HDFN.

- If the infant's immune system is slow to mature, the production of IgG can be delayed which reduces the catabolic rate of IgG causing any maternally transferred antibodies to persist longer.

Non-haemolytic febrile transfusion reactions (NHFTR), transfusion-related acute lung injury (TRALI), and transfusion-related alloimmune neutropenia (TRAIN)

These three conditions are distinct entities but have some overlapping clinical characteristics, which means they can be discussed together. **Non-haemolytic, febrile transfusion reactions (NHFTRs)** are usually caused by bacterially contaminated blood products, particularly platelet concentrates, but can occasionally be associated with the presence of HLA, HPA, and/or HNA alloantibodies in the recipient. In the UK, where there is universal leucocyte-depletion of blood products, investigations for bacterial contamination and IgA deficiency should initially be carried out. The clinical management of NHFTRs, if pre-medication with anti-histamines and corticosteroids is not effective, is to alter product specification by using red cells or platelets with reduced plasma content. Serological investigations for platelet, HLA, and granulocyte antibodies are of limited clinical value as the diagnostic specificity of these tests for NHFTRs is low. Nonetheless, testing for HNA (and HPA/HLA) antibodies may be required in the rare cases in which a severe NHFTR cannot be otherwise explained and plasma-reduced components have proved ineffective.

> **Non-haemolytic febrile transfusion reactions (NHFTRs)**
> An increase in temperature >1°C following a blood transfusion but which is not associated with red cell haemolysis.

Transfusion-related acute lung injury (TRALI) is a severe and sometimes life-threatening transfusion reaction that should by reported by the hospital to SHOT. There are two categories of TRALI recognized—immune TRALI, which involves donor derived antibodies and 'non-immune' TRALI, which is less severe and involves the transfusion of bioactive lipids arising from the storage of blood products. The majority of 'immune TRALI' cases are caused by donor leucocyte alloantibodies against alloantigens present on the patient's leucocytes, although patient alloantibodies have been involved in some cases. In most 'immune' TRALI cases, HLA class I and II specific antibodies are implicated, but HNA antibodies, particularly HNA-1a and HNA-3a, have also been implicated as causal agents. Transfusion-related acute lung injury (TRALI) investigations are logistically complex but should initially include a screen for both HLA and HNA alloantibodies in samples from donors and, in a small number of cases if non-leucodepleted blood has been transfused, the patient. In some cases, a crossmatch between the donor's sera and the patient's granulocytes and lymphocytes may be required.

> **Transfusion-related acute lung injury (TRALI)**
> Difficulty in breathing associated with *de novo* chest X-ray changes observed within six hours of transfusion that is not associated with transfusion overload or cardiac insufficiency.

The incidence of TRALI notified to SHOT has reduced in recent years (Chapman et al., 2009). It is important to distinguish between TRALI and transfusion associated circulatory overload (TACO) due to fluid from excessive transfusions leaking into the lungs.

Reducing the incidence of TRALI

The exact mechanism of 'immune' TRALI is incompletely understood, but there is a clear association between the incidence of TRALI and the use of plasma-rich blood products from female donors. Consequently, transfusion services have introduced a variety of strategies to reduce the incidence of TRALI. In England, there is a programme to screen all female platelet apheresis donors for HLA class I, HLA class II, and HNA-specific antibodies and only donors without these antibodies are able to donate apheresis platelets. In addition, pooled platelets are resuspended using plasma from male donors. Other transfusion services have taken different approaches, including banning female blood donors form donating plasma or platelets. The use of platelet additive solutions to supplement human plasma in the resuspension of platelets from buffy coats has further reduced the exposure of patients to plasma and the risk of TRALI.

SELF-CHECK 6.22

What samples and which laboratory techniques would you use to investigate a suspected case of TRALI?

Transfusion-related alloimmune neutropenia (TRAIN)

A transient neutropenia following infusion of a blood product due to the action of neutrophil-specific antibodies but which does not develop the symptoms of TRALI.

The first documented case of **transfusion-related alloimmune neutropenia (TRAIN)** occurred following the infusion of 80 ml of plasma-reduced blood after surgery on a four-week-old infant (Wallis et al., 2002). The plasma from the female blood donor was found to contain HNA-1b alloantibodies, and resulted in an absolute neutropenia in the infant, who typed as HNA-1a(+), 1b(+). The neutropenia was resolved after seven days by treating the infant with GCSF. The phenomena has also now been described in other patients. The condition is of interest since it demonstrates that, in some circumstances, infused passive HNA antibodies can trigger neutropenia rather than TRALI.

Autoimmune neutropenia

An autoimmune disease in which the antibodies form target granulocytes. These antibodies can recognize HNAs, especially in children.

Autoimmune neutropenia

Autoimmune neutropenia is a rare condition which can occur as a transient, self-limiting autoimmunity in young children (typically presenting from 18 months to four years of age)

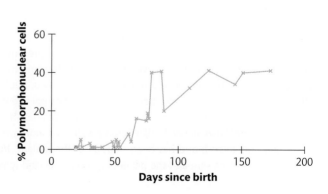

FIGURE 6.14

Sustained neutropenia in an infant affected by neonatal alloimmune neutropenia due to HNA-1b antibodies. There was a degree of compensation in the proportion of other white cells; the white cell count ranged between $9.8–13.0 \times 10^9/l$ during this period.

(Bux et al., 1998) or in a chronic form in adults (Shastri & Logue, 1993). The condition may be primary, that is, the sole presenting feature, or secondary to other conditions, for example rheumatoid arthritis, or systemic lupus erythematosus. The autoantibodies tend to target the FcγRIIIb (CD16), CD177, or CD11/18 molecules, but can also be HNA specific, typically HNA-1a, especially in children. The most sensitive method for the detection of autoantibodies is to test the patient's neutrophils using the direct immunofluorescence test. However, a combination of severe neutropenia, difficulties of cell isolation, and the requirement for a fresh sample limit the applicability of this test in adults and make it virtually impossible in children. Screening of a patient's serum sample with a panel of typed neutrophils in the indirect granulocyte immunofluorescence and granulocyte chemiluminescence or granulocyte agglutination tests provides a suitable alternative investigative strategy, and in some studies this approach has been found to be only slightly less sensitive than using direct test. The value in identifying these antibodies in children is that the condition is usually readily managed by use of antibiotics or GCSF and confirmation of antibodies avoids the need for expensive investigations, including a bone marrow biopsy for leukaemia where neutropenia can be a prodromal symptom.

Persistent neutropenia after bone marrow transplantation

Antibody-mediated neutropenia may be a serious complication of bone marrow transplantation. In this context, the neutrophil antibodies may be autoimmune and/or alloimmune in nature and laboratory investigation requires serological and typing studies to elucidate the nature of the antibodies involved. Granulocyte-specific antibodies in the post-bone marrow context can cause lineage specific delay in engraftment, which requires specific clinical management.

Granulocyte transfusions

Granulocyte transfusions are implicated for only a small number of profoundly neutropenic patients who are refractory to antibiotic treatment. Granulocyte transfusions are usually restricted to children because of the problem of obtaining sufficient granulocytes for treating adults. In England, buffy coat concentrates are prepared from 20 ABO identical donors and must be used within 24 hours. Often, a clinical effect of the transfusion may be observed without an increase in the circulating neutrophil count. An alternative approach has been to collect GCSF mobilized granulocytes from volunteer donors, usually relatives, but concerns about possible side effects of GCSF on healthy donors has tended to restrict this practice.

Other clinical consequences of HPA and HNA polymorphisms

Until recently, the importance of platelet and granulocyte polymorphisms was restricted to their ability to induce the formation of alloantibodies and thereby clinical conditions discussed earlier in this chapter. However, there is also evidence that certain platelet and granulocyte polymorphisms may affect cellular function and may be associated with increased risk of disease. On platelets, HPA-13bw (+) platelets have reduced response to collagen, as revealed by aggregation studies, and reduced ability to spread on a collagen surface. On granulocytes, the HNA-1a and -1b antigens can influence the function of the immunoglobulin FcγRIIIb receptor; granulocytes from HNA-1a individuals exhibit greater levels of phagocytosis than granulocytes from HNA-1b individuals, while prelimary evidence suggests that the HNA-1c form of FcγRIIIb binds more effectively to IgG.

 Chapter summary

- Platelets and granulocytes have unique antigens (HPA and HNA respectively) on their surface.

- The advent of biochemical and molecular analysis of glycoproteins on platelets and granulocytes has enabled the elucidation of the HPA and HNA systems and provided investigative procedures for antigen typing and antibody detection.

- Many of the techniques developed differ from those used in red cell immunohaematology laboratories because of the different biologic and antigenic characteristics of platelets and granulocytes.

- HPA and HNA give rise to immunological responses which typically result in either thrombocytopenias or neutropenias respectively, although, in some cases, more systemic pathology can also be initiated, for example TRALI.

- The clinical conditions caused by HPA and HNA antibodies are largely well-characterized but there remain areas of uncertainty, for example assessing the clinical significance of these antibodies, the optimal antenatal management of NAIT, and the precise mechanism and reasons for susceptibility to TRALI.

- Advances in technology have led to improved treatment options for many of the clinical problems caused by immune responses to HPA and HNA, for example the provision of HPA selected platelets and use of IVIgG in NAIT and the use of GCSF in the treatment of the more severe cases of NAIN and autoimmune neutropenia.

- The interplay between clinical observation, for example isolated cytopenias in a neonate or following transfusion, and development of technological advances in the laboratory have been crucial in improving the treatment of these conditions and increasing under-standing of the immunopathology of these disorders.

- The link between antigens, immune response, and biological function of target mol-ecules has had significance for the understanding of the basic biology of platelets and granulocytes.

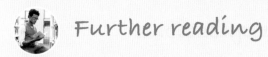 Further reading

• Coller BS & Shattil SJ. The GPIIb/IIIa (integrin αIIbß3) odyssey: a technology-driven saga of a receptor with twists, turns and even a bend. *Blood* 112 (2008), 3011–3024.

A 'tour de force' review of the biochemical, clinical, and physiological importance of the GPIIb/IIIa receptor.

• Fung YL, Minchinton RM & Fraser JF. Neutrophil antibody diagnostics and screening: review of the classical versus the emerging. *Vox Sang* 101 (2011), 282–290.

An overview of the techniques used in granulocyte immunology.

• Hod E & Schwartz J. Platelet transfusion refractoriness. *Br J Haematol* 142 (2008), 348–360.

A review of the factors impacting on patients with platelet transfusion refractoriness.

• Hayashi T & Hirayama F. Advances in alloimmune thrombocytopenia: perspectives on current concepts of human platelet antigens, antibody detection strategies, and genotyping. *Blood Transfusion* 13 (2015), 380–390.

A review of the current key issues and advances in alloimmune thrombocytopenia.

• Kjeldsen-Kragh J, Killie MK, Tomter G, et al. A screening and intervention program aimed to reduce mortality and serious morbidity associated with severe neonatal alloimmune thrombocytopenia. *Blood* 110 (2007), 833–839.

An alternative approach to antenatal management and prospective study of NAIT.

• Peterson JA, McFarland JG, Curtis BR & Aster RH. Neonatal alloimmune thrombocytopenia: pathogenesis, diagnosis and management. *Br J Haematol* 161 (2013), 3–14.

A recent review of NAIT.

• Poles A, Woźniak MJ, Walser P, Ridgwell K, Fitzgerald J, Green A, Gilmore R, Lucas G. A V740L mutation in glycoprotein IIb defines a novel epitope (War) associated with fetomaternal alloimmune thrombocytopenia. *Transfusion* 53 (2013), 1965–1973.

Description of the discovery of a novel human platelet antigen system—HPA-28bw.

• Porcelijn L, Huiskes E, Comijs-van Osslen I, Chhatta A, Rathore V, Meyers M & de Haas M. A new bead-based human platelet antigen antibodies detection assay versus the monoclonal antibody immobilization of platelet antigens assay. *Transfusion* 54 (2014), 1486–1492.

An evaluation of a beads based assay for HPA antibodies

• Vlaar APJ & Juffermans NP. Transfusion-related acute lung injury: a clinical review. *Lancet* 382 (2013), 984–994.

An extensive of overview of the incidence, presentation, and clinical management of TRALI and implications for blood transfusion services.

Discussion questions

6.1 There is an antenatal screening programme to identify women at risk of HDFN. What would be the key elements for a screening programme to identify women at risk of having an infant due to HPA antibodies? Identify the limitations of such a strategy including any ethical issues.

6.2 Explore the different strategies for reducing the incidence of TRALI.

6.3 Discuss the advantages and disadvantages of commercial companies supplying test kits for a niche area of blood transfusion such as platelet and granulocyte immunology.

Answers to the questions in this chapter are provided on the book's accompanying website:

 Go to www.oup.com/uk/avent2e

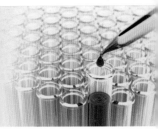

7

Compatibility Testing and Adverse Effects

Malcolm Needs

Learning objectives

After studying this chapter you should be able to:

- Describe the process of compatibility testing and how it applies to each type of blood component.
- Describe the various crossmatch methods used in laboratories to determine compatibility.
- Describe and explain when and why each crossmatch method either may or may not be used.
- Describe how blood is issued in an emergency.
- Outline the various national guidelines regarding pre-transfusion compatibility testing.
- Describe what constitutes an adverse reaction.
- Outline the role the laboratory has in the investigation of an adverse reaction.
- List the actions that might be taken by the laboratory in the event of an adverse reaction occurring.
- Distinguish between the UK Serious Hazards of Transfusion (SHOT) reporting scheme and the incident reporting requirements of the Medicines and Healthcare products Regulatory Agency (MHRA).

Introduction

This chapter builds on the knowledge gained from previous chapters, and shows how these procedures form a vital part of the process of providing as safe as possible blood for the patient. You will learn that compatibility testing is not just one test, but a multi-factorial process, starting when the patient has their sample collected, and completed when the blood and/or blood component is transfused.

Within the laboratory, the process starts with sample acceptance and finishes with the issue of the appropriate red cell, plasma, or cellular product.

The safety of the overall process relies on the combined input of many different staff groups.

Unfortunately, even when the compatibility testing process has been performed correctly, adverse reactions can occur, and these can vary in severity from mild to life-threatening. We can, however, learn by properly investigating these events, collating data on a national basis, and publishing a synopsis of the events in an anonymized report; this was the basis for setting up the UK haemovigilance system SHOT.

In this chapter we refer to a number of UK regulations, guidelines, and recommendations, but these will not necessarily apply in other countries where other regulations might be in place.

7.1 Compatibility testing (serological and non-serological)

Compatibility testing

Compatibility testing within the laboratory covers the processes by which donor red blood cells (RBCs), plasma, and/or cellular components are either tested or checked to ensure that incompatible RBCs or blood components are not issued or released from the laboratory for transfusion to patients.

Compatibility testing within the laboratory covers the processes by which donor red blood cells (RBCs), plasma, and/or cellular components are either tested or checked to ensure that incompatible RBCs or blood components are not issued or released from the laboratory for transfusion to patients.

Compatibility testing is performed using serological or non-serological methods.

The purpose of compatibility testing is to minimize the possibility that the component selected will harm the patient and that when the component is transfused, it will have an acceptable survival *in vivo* so as to deliver the desired clinical outcomes. The transfusion of an incompatible unit of RBCs may either decrease the survival of the RBCs, or, indeed, cause a reaction so severe that it can lead to the death of the patient (for more detail of how this may come about, see Chapter 8).

Blood transfusion laboratories may use a variety of methods to determine compatibility between RBCs (and/or blood components) and a potential recipient. The methods should be compliant with the British Society for Haematology (BSH) guidelines for pre-transfusion testing which have been used extensively as a source of recommendations throughout this chapter and validated for use within your laboratory (see Figure 7.1).

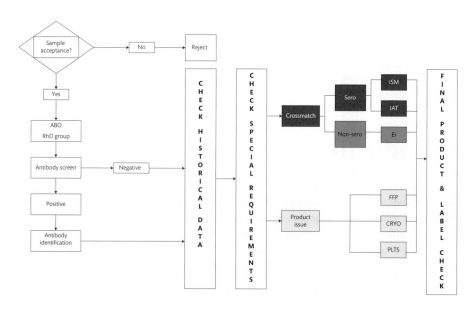

FIGURE 7.1

Blood and blood component compatibility process overview.

Sample acceptance

The integrity of the request and the sample is usually the responsibility of the clinical staff or the phlebotomy team. It is important that blood samples are taken and labelled according to BSH guidelines, and that a system of positive patient identification is used wherever possible. This may be facilitated by the use of electronic barcode readers that allow scanning of the patient details from the wrist band that are then printed out as a label at the bedside, and *immediately* attached to the sample tube.

The greatest areas of risk affecting the process of compatibility testing are clerical, documentation, or identification failures. In recognition of this fact, the UK National Patient Safety Agency (NPSA) specification 14 stated that all staff involved in the transfusion process should be subject to appropriate and regular competency assessment. This has now been superseded by a recommendation by the National Blood Transfusion Committee (NBTC) Recommendations for Training and Assessment in Blood Transfusion that states all staff involved in the transfusion process must receive training as a minimum every three years, and that knowledge and understanding assessments must be performed at least every three years.

All laboratories should have a sample acceptance policy that is known to the users of pathology services. Upon receipt into the laboratory, the sample information and request information are checked and compared to ensure that they both contain the following matching minimum data:

- Last (family) name
- First (given) name
- Date of birth
- NHS number/hospital number/accident and emergency (A&E) number/major incident number.

The sample must be identified by at least four independent data items to confirm from whom the sample has been taken. The list above shows the national minimum requirements. In areas such as Wales, however, where a large percentage of the population have the same family name, additional data items are also required, such as an address.

The person who performs the venepuncture should label the sample immediately at the bedside. It should also be dated and signed by that person. Samples that do not meet the laboratory's minimum standards should not be processed, but dealt with as stated in the individual laboratory's protocol. For patient safety reasons, there must be zero tolerance, however difficult this may be to introduce and maintain.

Obviously, in some situations, such as trauma calls from A&E, unconscious or confused patients, or during a major incident, the patient's identity may not be known, and the sample cannot be labelled with the patient's demographics, as described above. There must be at least one unique identifier, however, which may be the hospital number, A&E number, or the major incident number. In addition to this, the gender of the patient should be identified on the sample label. An indication of the patient's age is also helpful, as this may help with the decision making regarding red cell selection, e.g. K-negative RBCs for females of child-bearing potential (0–50 years). As above, the sample should be labelled immediately at the bedside by the person who performed the venepuncture, and also dated and signed by that person.

In pre-transfusion testing, the **importance of careful checking** is paramount and cannot be over-emphasized.

Age of sample

The sample used for grouping, antibody screening, and crossmatching of RBCs should represent, as closely as possible, the patient's current *in vivo* immunological status.

Once an individual has been exposed to foreign RBC antigens, they may be immunized to produce antibodies against these antigens. A RBC transfusion is a source of foreign antigens. It is not, however, only this that can cause such an exposure but any transfusion of a component that may contain RBCs such as platelets or granulocytes. Do not forget that platelets can stimulate the production of antibodies directed against human platelet antigens (HPA), and leucocytes can stimulate the production of antibodies directed against human leucocyte antigens (HLA) and human neutrophil antigens (HNA). Such exposures can change the patient's *in vivo* immunological status, thus invalidating any previous antibody screen results for subsequent RBC selection.

Appropriate timing of samples taken for grouping and antibody screening and crossmatching is therefore critical and a maximum of three days (when the sample is stored between 2 and 8°C) is recommended.

During pregnancy, fetal RBCs may be found in small numbers in the maternal circulation via a feto-maternal haemorrhage (FMH), which may be apparently 'silent' (i.e. may not be caused by an overt sensitizing event, such as abdominal trauma). The fetal RBCs will almost certainly differ antigenetically from the mother's RBCs as they are likely to express antigens of paternal origin that are not expressed on the maternal RBCs. These foreign antigens may stimulate an immune response in the mother.

This is why, after three days (again, when the sample has been stored between 2 and 8°C) the antibody screen on samples from pregnant women is not considered representative of the woman's current *in vivo* immune status.

The **'three-day rule'** applies if the patient has been transfused and/or has been pregnant within the previous three months. Each laboratory will have their own documented protocol based on the BSH guidelines on the subject.

A formal deviation from this recommendation is also included in these guidelines. Such a deviation must include a risk assessment for each individual patient. This risk assessment must be recorded in the laboratory information management system (LIMS) and in the patient's notes. These deviations may be considered for chronically transfused patients, following multiple, repeated transfusion episodes, with either annual review, or immediate review, if there is a change in serological status. These deviations allow samples to remain acceptable for up to seven days.

Similarly, this principle may be extended to pregnant women with no clinically significant antibodies who require blood standing by for potential obstetric emergencies, e.g. *placenta praevia*, but again, a formal risk assessment is required for each individual pregnant woman.

Confirmatory samples

As discussed earlier, the greatest area of risk with regard to receiving a blood transfusion is that the wrong patient has been bled. This could lead to a patient receiving RBCs or components that have been issued on the basis of a different patient's blood results which could lead to an ABO-incompatible unit being transfused. To minimize the risk of this type of error going undetected, it is recommended that before any routine transfusion the laboratory has tested

two blood samples from the patient, collected at different times and preferably by two different individuals.

Sadly, it is important to recognize that some individuals will try to get around this by taking two samples at the same time but sending them to the laboratory for testing at different times, an extremely dangerous practice. Some laboratories have tried to mitigate against this happening by handing a second, empty sample tube with a different-coloured top to the person delivering the initial sample and not accepting a second sample unless it is in this second tube. Even then, however, it will not stop a determined miscreant from emptying the contents of the second sample, taken at the same time as the initial sample, into this second tube. It is extremely important, therefore, to educate any person authorized to take blood samples as to why a second sample should be taken from the patient at a different time.

Key points

It is very important that any sample for compatibility testing is taken from the correct patient and correctly labelled immediately at the bedside. When the sample and request form are received in the laboratory they are checked to ensure that they meet stringent requirements to ensure errors have not been made.

SELF-CHECK 7.1

Why are pregnant women considered as a special group with regard to the timing of sample collection prior to transfusion?

ABO and D grouping and antibody screening

RBCs of the pre-transfusion samples are grouped, as a minimum, for the ABO and D antigens and the plasma screened for the presence of RBC alloantibodies using two or three examples of antibody-screening RBCs by the indirect antiglobulin technique (IAT). Patients who have been tested previously within the laboratory have the results of their ABO and D groups compared against previous testing results as a further safeguard against sample/patient identification errors. This checking is usually carried out automatically by the LIMS, and staff are alerted to any discrepancies.

The RBCs selected for antibody screening have probable homozygous expression for all the major clinically significant RBC antigens except the K antigen. The K antigen is usually represented by a RBC having heterozygous expression of the antigen so that even weak alloantibodies are likely to be detected. If the antibody screening test is positive, further tests are required to identify the specificity and probable clinical significance of the antibody or antibodies present.

It is important to note that different areas of the world may require different antigens to be expressed on the screening and antibody identification RBCs to reflect the antigens commonly expressed within their own populations, e.g. Mur and Di^a in the Chinese populations, and C^x, Ul^a, and LW^b in the Finnish population.

Unless there is an emergency requirement for RBCs (e.g. the patient is exsanguinating) the results of the group, the antibody screen, and antibody identification must be obtained before blood can be issued. For antibodies that are considered to be clinically significant, for example anti-E, anti-S, anti-K, anti-Fy^a, and anti-Jk^a, RBC units that have been tested and found to be negative for the cognate antigen are selected and crossmatched by IAT. For clinically insignificant antibodies, such as anti-Lu^a, random ABO and D compatible units, which have not been specifically antigen typed, can be transfused, if crossmatched by IAT and found to be compatible.

ABO and D group selection of RBCs

Whatever crossmatch technique is used, the same rules apply regarding ABO blood group selection. It is best to use the same ABO group as the patient; however, this is not always possible (e.g. when another ABO compatible unit is the only unit available that lacks a high prevalence antigen, such as In^b). Table 7.1 shows the ABO groups that should be selected in order of preference.

When supplies of D-negative units are limited, D-positive units may be selected for D-negative recipients. D-positive RBCs should not, however, be issued to D-negative females of childbearing potential (unless they are exsanguinating, and only then under a physician's orders), or patients who have, or are known historically to have anti-D.

Although group O RBCs can be given to those of other ABO groups (except O$_h$ individuals), this practice is avoided if possible, as there are limited supplies of group O RBCs. If group O RBCs are used, provided they are in additive solution, they do not need to be negative for high titre (HT) haemagglutinins (see later for a full description), as the volume of residual plasma is too small to cause significant haemolysis. Indeed, the risk is considered so small that only units of RBCs destined for paediatric use, paediatric exchange transfusions, and intrauterine transfusions are now so labelled by NHSBT.

Special requirements

An increasing number of patients have special requirements for the components they need. The following section is not a list of all the possible special requirements, and you should always refer to a local standard operating procedure (SOP), recommendations from the Advisory Committee on the Safety of Blood, Tissues and Organs (SaBTO), or the current BSH guidelines regarding indications for special requirements.

There are some special requirements that are indicated by the patient demographic. For example, the UK Department of Health requires that children born after 1996 who require FFP should receive pathogen-reduced FFP of non-UK origin such as methylene blue-treated FFP. Other special requirements, however, can only be known if the requesting clinician provides such relevant clinical information to the laboratory. Special requirements, such as those of irradiated or cytomegalovirus (CMV)- negative components, should be indicated on the request form.

TABLE 7.1 Selection of red cells according to donor and recipient ABO blood group.

Recipient's RBC group	O	A	B	AB
First choice	O	A	B	AB
Second choice	-	O	O	A or B
Third choice	-	-	-	O

Once these special requirements have been notified to the laboratory and recorded on the LIMS, it should automatically bring these, and any demographically mandated requirements, to the attention of the laboratory staff. Ideally, rules should prevent allocation of components that do not meet these special requirements. Where the LIMS has a rule-based prevention, however, there should be a facility for exceptional issue to override a rule by the use of controlled log-in, passwords, or some other security method, and this facility should be available to all lone workers such as on-call staff.

Other non-mandatory but advisable requirements, for example K-negative RBCs for females of child-bearing potential, may be highlighted by the LIMS rules system.

Key points

Pre-transfusion testing includes ABO and D grouping, antibody screening, and possible antibody identification. On the basis of these tests, blood is selected for cross-matching, but also taking into account other special requirements the patient may have.

Crossmatching

The term 'crossmatch' is used in this chapter in relation to the selection and issue of RBCs. The crossmatch initially referred to the serological testing, usually by a tube technique, of RBCs from the donor unit against the recipient's plasma and testing the donor plasma against the recipient's RBCs. The IAT is now the method of choice used to detect any serologically incompatibility of possible clinical significance between the donor RBCs and the recipient's plasma. The IAT crossmatch complements the IAT antibody screening process, it does not replace it.

The reason for this is twofold.

First, it is because, as stated above in the section 'ABO and D grouping and antibody screening', the RBCs used for antibody screening are selected to have probable homozygous expression for all the major clinically significant RBC antigens such as Jk(a+b-), whereas the donor unit(s) may have heterozygous expression of the antigen such as Jk(a+b+). If the patient's antibody is weak, therefore, a weak expression of the antigen, such as heterozygous expression (so-called dosage) may lead to a false negative crossmatch that, if the blood was transfused, could cause a transfusion reaction.

Second, the reagent RBCs used for antibody screening are kept in a preservative that is designed to optimize antigenic expression, whilst it is not designed to optimize oxygen carrying capacity. RBCs in a unit of blood, on the other hand, are in a preservative designed to optimize their oxygen carrying capacity, but this preservative is not designed to optimize antigenic expression. Once again, therefore, antigen expression on donor RBCs could be compromised which could lead to a false negative crossmatch, possibly leading to an adverse event, in the form of a transfusion reaction.

The crossmatch has evolved significantly over the years. In the recent past, all hospitals used, at the very minimum, the IAT to crossmatch RBCs, but now other serological or non-serological techniques are used to determine compatibility. Whatever technique is used, it is best practice for one person to carry out the crossmatching procedure from beginning to end. Where this is not possible, there should be an audit trail to show what each individual involved did at each stage of the procedure.

There are three key methods for checking compatibility but not all laboratories may use all of these methods. These are:

- IAT crossmatch

- Immediate spin crossmatch (ISXM)

- Electronic issue (please note that the correct terminology is electronic issue, and not electronic crossmatch, as no physical crossmatch is involved in this method).

SELF-CHECK 7.2

Why does the crossmatch not replace the antibody screen?

IAT crossmatch

This is a serological method for crossmatching, as the recipient's plasma is directly tested against the donor RBCs. An IAT crossmatch is sometimes called a 'full crossmatch'. This method should detect incompatibilities between donor RBCs and recipient's plasma due to ABO and IgG antibodies. This technique must be used if the recipient's plasma is known currently or historically to contain RBC alloantibodies in certain other situations, such as when the recipient has received a stem cell transplant.

The IAT has been greatly adapted over the years from the original tube technique to techniques that can be used in column agglutination technologies (CAT) or microplate technologies. The technique, and indeed the technologies, have evolved due to a need for automation which provides decreased turnaround time (TRT) and increased reproducibility and security.

Advantages

- Incompatibilities between donor RBCs and recipient plasma due to ABO and/or IgG antibodies can be detected by this method.

- Antibodies present in the recipient's plasma might be missed if the antigens are not expressed on the antibody screening RBCs used, for example, a low prevalence antigen such as Wr^a.

- Antibodies present in the recipient's plasma may be missed if the screening RBCs have only a single dose (heterozygous expression) or weak expression of the corresponding antigen if the screening RBCs do not fulfil the BSH guideline requirements.

- Antibodies present in the recipient's plasma may be missed due to a technical error in performing or reading the antibody screen. Therefore by performing an IAT crossmatch incompatible units should then be identified.

Disadvantages

- The length of time to issue RBCs for transfusion is usually about 35 minutes, but this is dependent upon the technology used.

- It is more expensive than the abbreviated methods due to reagent and staff costs.

Immediate spin crossmatch (ISXM)

This is a serological method for crossmatching. This technique involves the testing of the recipient's plasma directly against a 2–3% saline suspension of donor RBCs with a 2–5 minute incubation period at room temperature. This technique is used to detect ABO incompatibilities between donor RBCs and recipient's serum/plasma, but should not be used for patients where the ABO grouping reveals very weak anti-A and/or anti-B.

As incompatibility between donor RBCs and the recipient's plasma due to IgG antibodies is not detectable by an ISXM, this cannot be used if the patient has clinically significant RBC alloantibodies detected in either the current or in an historical sample. The current antibody screen, therefore, must be negative. The technique can, however, detect non-clinically significant cold-reacting IgM antibodies (such as the vast majority of examples of anti-A_1), which may delay the provision of blood whilst the cause of the incompatibility is investigated.

Advantages

- It will detect most ABO incompatibilities.
- The technique is simple.
- Improved TRT for issue of RBCs in comparison to the IAT crossmatch.

Disadvantages

- Any errors in the antibody screening that would lead to an incompatibility between donor and recipient will not be detected.
- It will detect incompatibilities due to cold-reacting, non-clinically significant antibodies.
- It is not a standardized technique.
- There are no controls performed with the test.
- Non-specific reactions can be detected.

Electronic issue (EI)

EI is a non-serological method for selecting compatible blood. There is no serological testing performed between the donor RBCs and the patient's serum/plasma. EI is the term given to the issue of RBCs by the LIMS comparison of the patient's current ABO and D grouping and antibody screening results with both the patient's historical results and the ABO and D group of the donor RBC units.

As the name suggests, this method can only be applied where the process of initial testing is automated and coupled with the electronic transfer of non-manually manipulated results from the analyser to the LIMS. This technique cannot be used if the patient has clinically significant RBC alloantibodies detected in either the current sample or in an historical sample. This method relies on the principle that any clinically significant RBC alloantibodies will be detected by the antibody screen and by checking the historical data in the LIMS system.

The UK National External Quality Assurance Scheme (NEQAS) found the use of routine EI in blood transfusion laboratories has increased from 10% in 2002 to 59% in 2015. Undoubtedly, the use of EI is on the increase as more laboratories meet the BSH guideline requirements and the MHRA requirements for EI.

There are a number of patient categories where the process of EI is not recommended and a full IAT serological crossmatch should be performed. These patient categories are summarized below:

- Patients who have a positive antibody screen.
- Patients with clinically significant alloantibodies, whether or not these antibodies are demonstrable in the current sample.

- Patients who have a group manually entered into the LIMS, for any reason.
- Patients where any of the results have been manually manipulated, for any reason.
- If the patient has received an ABO incompatible bone marrow or haemopoietic stem cell transplant.
- If the patient has received an ABO incompatible solid organ transplant in the previous three months due to the possible presence of passenger lymphocytes. Any IgG anti-A/B produced by the passenger lymphocytes will not be detected in the antibody screen.
- For neonates or fetuses where the mother has a clinically significant IgG alloantibody present in her plasma.

Advantages

- It is a simple technique.
- Improved TRT for issue of RBCs in comparison with either the IAT crossmatch or if the units of blood are held remotely from the blood transfusion laboratory, the ISXM.
- Decreased reagent and staff costs.

Disadvantages

- As this is a non-serological technique, any errors in either the ABO and D grouping or the antibody screening would lead to an incompatibility between donor and recipient.
- There is a requirement for automation.
- There is a requirement for an interface between the automation and the LIMS.

SELF-CHECK 7.3

What is the potential problem with performing the ABO and D testing on the same sample twice, and then issuing blood where there is no historical grouping record for the patient?

Fetal and neonatal K-negative crossmatch

Fetal or intrauterine transfusions (IUT) are only carried out in specialized hospitals where there are very specific procedures for determining compatibility. Neonatal transfusions occur in many more hospitals. The neonatal period is generally defined for transfusion purposes as from birth to four months as infants rarely produce antibodies until after four months. Antibodies present in the fetus or neonate originate from the mother, and it is these antibodies that can affect the compatibility of the fetal or neonatal transfusion. It is therefore appropriate to undertake pre-transfusion testing on samples from both the mother and the neonate but occasionally this is not possible.

The mother's sample should be tested for:

- ABO and D group.
- Alloantibodies.
- Alloantibody specification should the antibody screen be positive.

The neonate's sample should be tested for:

- ABO and D group.

- Direct antiglobulin test (DAT): if positive, use monospecific antiglobulin reagents.
- The presence of atypical RBC antibodies, if no maternal sample is available.

The blood for transfusion should be selected by reviewing the results of the above maternal and neonatal investigations, and should be compatible with, but not necessarily identical to, the neonate's own ABO and D group. It must also be compatible with any ABO or alloantibodies present in the maternal plasma, or in the neonate's plasma, if the maternal plasma is not available. Generally, most hospitals use only group O blood for neonatal transfusions. If the DAT on the neonate is positive, or the mother has a positive antibody screen, blood should be crossmatched by IAT.

If the neonate requires further small-volume transfusions then no further serological testing is required until the neonate is four or more months old. After four months of age the infant is capable of producing RBC alloantibodies; pre-transfusion testing is the same as for adults.

Emergency issue (including use of emergency group O, D-negative RBCs)

There are life-threatening occasions where RBCs are required prior to the completion of all the pre-transfusion and compatibility tests. These occasions are determined by the medical team in charge of the patient, not by the laboratory staff.

Each transfusion laboratory should have a SOP for this situation, based on the BSH guidelines. In the case of such an emergency, group O, K-negative RBCs may be issued before a blood sample is obtained or tested. If the patient is a female under 50 years of age (or estimated to so be, if they are unidentified) then the RBCs issued should also be D negative.

If RBCs are to be issued for transfusion prior to completion of all the pre-transfusion tests, then the patient's sample should be ABO and D grouped. A reverse group and a repeat cell group (using a different aliquot of the same sample) or an ISXM must be performed before the issue of ABO-matched RBCs. The antibody screen should be performed as soon as possible, and if it is negative, then it is not necessary to perform a retrospective crossmatch. If time allows, keep aliquots of the donor units so that, should the patient's plasma be found to contain an alloantibody, the RBCs can be tested for the cognate antigens against which the antibody or antibodies are directed.

In an emergency situation, it is vital that efficient and effective communication is established between the laboratory and the patient's medical team.

Key points

Before blood can be issued for transfusion to a patient, it must be crossmatched. The technique used depends on the results of the pre-transfusion testing. If the patient has been grouped twice, and there are no alloantibodies detected either in the current or historic sample, EI can be used, but otherwise a full serological crossmatch, using an IAT, is performed.

7.2 Selection of plasma products

HT negative status

In the UK, all plasma donations of all groups (apart from AB) are tested for high-titre anti-A and anti-B, and units found to be negative are labelled as 'HT negative'. There is no guarantee, however, that these components will not have the ability to cause ABO-related haemolysis; they are just less likely to so do.

Plasma from a non-HT negative donor is capable of causing acute haemolysis if transfused to an ABO-incompatible recipient. This is particularly important in large-volume transfusions to neonates and children, particularly if they are of small stature, and the same applies to transfusions of plasma-rich components, such as platelets.

Fresh frozen plasma (FFP) and cryoprecipitate (cryo)

FFP and cryo are plasma products. Compatibility is determined on the basis of the donor and recipient's ABO group and not by a crossmatch technique. The D status of the recipient is irrelevant as there are only small amounts of RBC stroma present in the component. RBC stroma are less immunogenic than intact RBCs, therefore even in D-negative females of child-bearing potential, D-positive FFP and cryo can be issued safely.

It is best to use the same ABO group of FFP as the patient. This, however, is not always possible. In an emergency situation, where the patient's group is not yet known, AB FFP can be issued, but this should just be used in an emergency as group AB FFP is in reasonably short supply. Table 7.2 shows the ABO groups that should be selected in order of preference.

When transfusing neonates or children it must be remembered that they have a small blood volume, so even when a small volume is to be transfused in absolute terms, this may constitute a large-volume transfusion to the recipient in relative terms. Transfusion of plasma that contains antibodies to their RBCs may cause passive immune haemolysis. For infants and neonates plasma should be free of clinically significant irregular RBC antibodies.

SELF-CHECK 7.4

Why is it preferable to use group A FFP for group B recipients and vice versa where ABO-identical FFP is not available?

TABLE 7.2 Selection of FFP according to donor and recipient ABO blood group.

Recipient's group	O	A	B	AB
First choice	O	A	B	AB
Second choice	A	AB	AB	A* HT negative
Third choice	B	B* HT negative	A* HT negative	B* HT negative
Fourth choice	AB	-	-	-

Group O FFP must only be given to group O recipients.
* HT negative—components that test negative for 'high titre' anti-A/B should be selected. Only suitable for emergency use in adults.Methylene blue-treated FFP (MBFFP) is used instead of standard FFP for patients born after 1 January 1996.

7.3 **Selection of cellular components**

Platelets

Platelets are a cellular component usually suspended in plasma, although some are issued washed and resuspended in platelet suspension medium (PSM). PSM is usually used when the recipient has anti-IgA to rid the component of IgA, but as a by-product, ABO antibodies will also be removed.

Compatibility of normal platelet units is determined on the basis of the donor and the recipient's ABO and D group, and not by a crossmatch technique. It is best practice to use the same ABO and D group of platelets as the recipient. This is not always possible and in an emergency situation ABO non-identical units may be given. ABO antigens are expressed on platelets (type 1 by passive adsorption from the plasma, and type 2 as an integral part of the membrane), so the recipient's ABO antibodies may react with ABO incompatible platelets which may then have a reduced survival *in vivo*. For example, a group A recipient transfused with group B platelets would result in the recipient's anti-B reacting with the B antigen on the platelets.

Using group O platelets for non-group O recipients should, however, be avoided as much as possible because the donor's anti-A,B will react with the recipient's A and/or B antigens, causing varying degrees of haemolysis. Should this scenario arise, the degree of haemolysis should be mitigated by the use of group O HT-negative platelets. Table 7.3 shows the ABO groups that should be selected in order of preference.

Only units labelled as HT-negative anti-A and/or anti-B should be transfused into ABO-non-identical, but ABO compatible recipients, for example O into A, B or AB, A into AB, or B into AB. Measurement of HT antibodies is, however, a guide only, and caution should be observed if high volumes of group O platelets are transfused into non-group O recipients (particularly infants and children) as clinically significant haemolysis may ensue. The use of group O platelets for non-O recipients should be avoided as much as possible for this reason.

HLA-matched platelets may by necessity be a different ABO group to the patient, and only units labelled as HT-negative for anti-A and/or anti-B should be transfused to ABO non-identical recipients.

Platelet concentrates contain small numbers of RBCs (pooled platelet units more than units of platelets collected by apheresis). D-negative platelet concentrates should therefore be given to D-negative females of child-bearing potential. If in an emergency, D-positive platelets are transfused to a D-negative female of child-bearing potential, anti-D immunoglobulin prophylaxis should be considered. The anti-D immunoglobulin will not compromise the *in vivo* survival of the platelets, as platelets do not express the D antigen.

TABLE 7.3 Selection of platelets according to donor and recipient ABO blood group.

Recipient's group	O	A	B	AB
First choice	O	A	B	AB (only by prior notice)
Second choice	B	B HT negative	A HT negative	A HT negative or B HT negative
Third choice	A	O HT negative	O HT negative	O HT negative

CASE STUDY 7.1 *Group O platelets to a group A patient*

- Three-year-old female with acute lymphoblastic leukaemia (ALL).
- Given one adult therapeutic dose (ATD) of group O apheresis platelets, as no group A available.
- Became unwell.
- Bilirubin rose from 40 µmol/l^{-1} to 102 µmol/l^{-1}.
- Haemoglobin (Hb) fell from 102 g/l^{-1} to 82 g/l^{-1}.
- Fully recovered.
- Donation tested positive for HT anti-A.

Buffy coats/granulocytes

Buffy coats and granulocytes are only transfused in specialized hospitals and usually only to patients with overwhelming infections. They are a cellular component containing RBCs. Compatibility is determined on the basis of the donor and the recipient's ABO and D group, and crossmatching. It is best practice to use the same ABO and D group of buffy coat/granulocytes as the patient. As viable T lymphocytes will almost certainly also be present in these components, they should be irradiated prior to transfusion.

7.4 **Visual inspection and labelling of the units**

The final stage of the compatibility process is the visual examination and labelling of the pack(s). Before any unit is issued it should be checked for the following:

- Leaks at the ports or the seams.
- Haemolysis in the plasma, if a RBC unit.
- Discolouration, if a RBC unit.
- Large clots, if a RBC unit.
- Turbidity or clumping of the contents if FFP, cryo, or platelets.
- It is vitally important to examine all platelet packs carefully as any abnormal appearance may indicate bacterial contamination.

If any of the above defects are detected, the units should not be issued but returned to the blood service for investigation. After all of the previous checks have been completed, the unit(s) are ready to be labelled. The label should be securely attached to the pack, and any previous labels should be removed. A compatibility report may additionally be issued by the transfusion laboratory. Any group substitutions or special requirements should be highlighted on this report. The labelled unit(s) and compatibility form, if used, should then be placed in the appropriate storage facility pending collection or return to stock, if not required.

7.5 **Traceability of blood components**

The Blood Safety and Quality Regulations (BSQR) of 2005 require a record to be kept of storage conditions and movements of any blood component, from the time of the original donation, from processing in the supplying blood centre, testing in the hospital laboratory, to the component being transfused or discarded, for whatever reason (so-called 'vein to vein'). Under the terms of BSQR, hospital transfusion laboratories are required to maintain an accurate record of the final fate of any component that they have issued to patients, transferred to another location, or discarded. Many hospitals are now investing in electronic systems that will track units from the time of receipt in the transfusion laboratory, right through to administration at the patient's bedside. Records should also be kept in the patient's notes of the transfusion process and any untoward outcomes, such as a transfusion reaction.

Key points

For components other than RBCs and buffy coats/granulocytes, a crossmatch is not needed. FFP and cryo are issued on the basis of the ABO group of the donor and the recipient, but they are issued on the basis of the ABO group alone for FFP and cryo; for platelets and buffy coats/granulocytes, the D group should also be considered.

7.6 **Adverse effects of transfusion**

As with any medical intervention, blood component transfusion has the potential for both benefit and risk to the patient, and the decision to transfuse in the first place must balance the benefits against the potential risks.

Transmission of viral and other infections through transfusion may make the headlines, but the actual risk estimates for the UK in 2010, as reported by the Health Protection Agency, are very small (and these have not changed):

- Hepatitis B   1 in 670, 000

- Human immunodeficiency virus (HIV)   1 in 5 million

- Hepatitis C   1 in 72 million

- Human T cell lymphotropic virus 1 (HTLV-1)   1 in 17 million

Indeed, infection via blood is now so rare that these figures are mathematical models rather than actual figures.

Although the probability of getting variant Creutzfeldt-Jakob disease (vCJD) is probably very low with a single blood transfusion, the risk of any infection will increase with additional blood transfusions. Within the UK, there have been just a handful of cases where patients are known to have become infected with vCJD from a blood transfusion.

Since 1996, there have been 43 cases of transfusion-transmitted bacterial infection (TTI) reported to SHOT, of which 11 recipients died due to the TTI. The majority of these cases (36) relate to platelet units, which are particularly prone to bacterial contamination, due to the need to store them at 22°C (± 2°C).

Despite careful testing of the donation and the compatibility testing, blood components may initiate a reaction when transfused. Non-infectious reactions can be conveniently divided into immune and non-immune, or into immediate or delayed, as shown in Table 7.4.

Adverse reactions can occur due to human procedural error at any stage within the transfusion process, and complications may even be due to a necessary constituent of the blood component such as the citrate in the anticoagulant solution. Transfusion reactions can be classified as follows:

- **Febrile non-haemolytic transfusion reactions (FNHTR)** are relatively common in blood transfusion. They are defined as a 1°C or greater temperature rise with or without chills, and some hypotension. They are thought to be caused by HLA or lymphocytotoxic antibodies, or cytokines released from leucocytes on storage, and so are much less common now that all the blood components (except of course buffy coats/granulocytes) are leucodepleted before issue. Most symptoms are relatively mild and benign, and transfusion may usually continue if the patient's temperature resolves with antipyretics such as paracetamol.

- **Allergic (or urticarial) reactions** are as commonly reported as FNHTRs, and are caused by histamine, an organic nitrogenous compound released from mast cells when the patient's immune system recognizes an allergen in the donor plasma (or vice versa). This causes swelling and raised red welts that may be intensely itchy, and are treated with antihistamine. The majority of allergic reactions are mild and not life-threatening, but they may occasionally be severe, and may necessitate the provision of plasma-deficient blood components to minimize the risk of reaction.

TABLE 7.4 Immune and non-immune adverse transfusion reactions.

Immune-mediated adverse events	
Immediate	**Delayed**
Febrile non-haemolytic transfusion reaction (FNHTR)	Delayed haemolytic transfusion reaction (DHTR)
Acute haemolytic transfusion reaction (AHTR)	Alloimmunization
Allergic reaction	Post-transfusion purpura (PTP)
Anaphylactic reaction	Transfusion-associated graft versus host disease (TA-GvHD)
Transfusion-related acute lung injury (TRALI)	Immunosuppression
Non-immune-mediated adverse events	
Immediate	**Delayed**
Transfusion-associated circulatory overload (TACO)	Iron overload
Physical change to RBCs	Air embolism
Dilution of coagulation factors and platelets	

- **Acute haemolytic transfusion reactions (AHTR)** most commonly occur very soon after the transfusion of incompatible RBCs but can occur up to 24 hours after the transfusion. The RBCs are rapidly destroyed, releasing free haemoglobin (Hb) and RBC stroma into the circulation (for more detail, see Chapter 8). Signs and symptoms can occur within minutes of starting a transfusion, and ABO-incompatible transfusions may be life-threatening, causing shock, acute renal failure, and disseminated intravascular coagulation (DIC).

- **Delayed haemolytic transfusion reactions (DHTR)** occur more than 24 hours after the transfusion, and are most often the result of an anamnestic response in a patient who has been previously sensitized against a particular antigen by transfusion, pregnancy, or transplant, and in whom antibody is not detectable by routine serological techniques during pre-transfusion testing. Clinical signs and symptoms are relatively mild compared to AHTRs, and any unexplained post-transfusion decreases in Hb in the absence of bleeding should be investigated as a possible DHTR (but see also hyperhaemolysis in Chapter 8).

- **Transfusion-associated circulatory overload (TACO)** is most frequently caused by the transfusion of too much volume at too fast a rate, leading to congestive heart failure and pulmonary oedema. Patients at particular risk of TACO include young children, elderly patients, patients with cardiac disease, and patients with chronic normovolaemic anaemia.

- **Transfusion-associated acute lung injury (TRALI)** is characterized by chills, cough, fever, cyanosis, hypotension, and increasing respiratory distress during, or within, six hours of transfusion of volumes of blood unlikely to cause circulatory overload (as in TACO, above). The symptoms are similar to those seen in acute respiratory distress syndrome (ARDS) and, initially, the diagnosis of TRALI is one of exclusion. The most likely mechanism for TRALI is the presence of leucocyte antibodies in the plasma of the blood component, initiating complement-mediated cell damage in the pulmonary capillary network.

- **Iron overload** is a longer-term complication of RBC transfusions, also known as transfusion haemosiderosis, and patients who are chronically dependent on transfusion therapy are particularly at risk. Accumulated iron begins to affect the function of the heart, liver, and endocrine glands, leading to symptoms including muscle weakness, fatigue, weight loss, jaundice, anaemia, cardiac arrhythmias, and mild diabetes. Removal of accumulated tissue iron stores without lowering Hb levels is achieved by the use of various chelating agents, but another strategy could be to use the freshest possible blood for this type of patient, thus reducing the frequency of transfusion and the donor exposure over their lifetime.

- **Immunosuppression** is a non-specific effect that reduces the activity of the recipient's immune system soon after transfusion of blood components. This may actually be beneficial to the patient, in that transfusion prior to renal transplantation has been shown to result in better graft survival. Alternatively, other studies have shown an increase in post-operative infections in patients who have been transfused.

- **Post-transfusion purpura (PTP)** is an acute episode of thrombocytopenia typically occurring between 5 and 12 days following transfusion of RBCs or platelets, associated with the presence in the patient of alloantibodies directed against antigens within the human platelet antigen systems (HPA). The platelet count can drop from normal to below $10 \times 10^9/l$ within 24 hours or less, leading to haemorrhage. Platelet transfusion is not usually indicated unless bleeding is severe, and high-dose IVIgG is the treatment of choice.

- **Platelet refractoriness** is a failure to achieve a sustained increase in platelet count following a platelet transfusion. In many cases, refractoriness may be due to 'non-immune' factors such as platelet consumption due to coagulation defects, increased sequestration of platelets in the spleen following surgery, or where there is bacterial sepsis. Where there is immune destruction of platelets, it is usually due to the action of HLA class 1 antibodies and in such cases, satisfactory platelet increments may be achieved by the provision of HLA-selected donations. Less frequently, antibodies directed against HPA or ABO antigens may be involved and it may be necessary to provide HPA-compatible and/or ABO compatible platelet donations in order to achieve satisfactory increments.

- **Transfusion-associated graft versus host disease (TA-GvHD)** is a rare but often life-threatening complication of transfusion caused by engraftment and clonal expansion of viable donor T lymphocytes in a susceptible host. It is characterized by fever, rash, liver dysfunction, diarrhoea, pancytopenia, and bone marrow hypoplasia occurring less than 30 days after transfusion. Mortality has been estimated at greater than 80% and death is generally due to infection and/or haemorrhage as a result of the bone marrow aplasia. Patients at risk of TA-GvHD such as those receiving treatment with purine analogues or with congenital immunodeficiency, should be transfused with irradiated cellular components. In certain cases, the cause is a shared HLA haplotype between the donor and the recipient in which case the recipient's immune system does not 'recognize' the donor-derived viable T lymphocytes as 'foreign', thus allowing the engraftment and clonal expansion to occur. This is much more commonly seen in certain areas of Eastern Asia than in other parts of the world; however, any cellular blood component derived from either a first- or second-degree relative throughout the world should be irradiated, as there is a much higher risk of shared HLA haplotypes in these cases.

- **Anaphylactic reactions** are immediate, immune-mediated reactions in which there are systemic symptoms, including hypotension, loss of consciousness, shock, and, less commonly, death. Around 1 in 700 of the general population are IgA deficient, half of whom have produced an anti-IgA but despite this apparent large group, anaphylactic reactions occur relatively infrequently. They are, however, much more likely with plasma-rich products, such as FFP or platelets than with RBC transfusions.

Key points

There are a number of causes of adverse transfusion reactions that can be broadly classified as immune or non-immune, and immediate or delayed.

SELF-CHECK 7.5

What are the most common adverse transfusion reactions and how are they caused?

CASE STUDY 7.2 Severe anaphylaxis following FFP infusion

- 75-year-old required FFP for post-operative bleeding.
- Developed anaphylactic reaction with rash, dyspnoea, and hypotension.
- Required cardiopulmonary resuscitation (CPR).
- Condition improved after treatment over the next 2.5 hours.

7.7 **Monitoring the patient during transfusion**

The 2009 BSH guideline on the administration of blood components requires hospitals to have a policy for the care and monitoring of patients receiving transfusions. This policy should define the staff responsible for the monitoring of the patient during transfusion, the information to be given to the patient about possible adverse effects of transfusion, and the recording of specific observations during the transfusion:

- Patients should be readily observable by members of the clinical staff while being transfused.

- The start and finish times of the infusion of each unit should be clearly indicated on observation charts.

- Vital signs (temperature, pulse, blood pressure, and respiration rate) should be measured and recorded before the start of each unit of RBCs or blood component and at the end of each transfusion episode.

- Temperature and pulse should be measured 15 minutes after the start of each unit of RBCs or blood components.

Further observations during the transfusion are at the discretion of each clinical area, and need only be taken should the patient become unwell or show signs of a transfusion reaction. Unconscious and anaesthetized patients, and babies are more difficult to monitor for signs of transfusion reactions as patients in these groups are unable to draw attention to the fact that they are feeling unwell. These patients should have formal observations taken more often, again at the discretion of the clinical area.

Adverse reactions to transfusion of blood components range from brief episodes of fever, to life-threatening haemolysis. The challenge for clinicians lies in recognition of these reactions, especially since the early signs and symptoms, such as fever and chills, may indicate either relatively benign febrile reactions, or potentially fatal intravascular haemolysis due to ABO incompatibility.

Making an accurate assessment of an adverse event involves taking a clear history, and recording of temperature, pulse rate, blood pressure, respiratory rate, and oxygen saturation. Few signs and symptoms are entirely diagnostic of a particular type of reaction, but accurate recording will help build a picture of what may be going on, as exemplified by the following examples:

- Mild febrile or allergic reactions which result in a temperature rise of less than 1.5°C above the pre-transfusion baseline, rigors, or urticarial rash are relatively common and rarely need investigation as long as the patient is more regularly monitored during the transfusion to ensure their condition does not worsen. A higher rise in temperature may indicate a more serious reaction.

- An increase in pulse rate (tachycardia) could be an indication that more serious problems are developing.

- A sudden drop in blood pressure (hypotension) may be seen in bacterial sepsis, AHTRs, anaphylaxis, TRALI, or citrate toxicity.

- Shortness of breath, excessively rapid breathing, and hypoxia may occur as a result of circulatory overload, TRALI, bacterial contamination, anaphylaxis, and acute intravascular haemolysis.

CASE STUDY 7.3 *Inappropriate transfusion of FFP for warfarin reversal results in anaphylaxis*

- 75-year-old given three units of FFP to reverse warfarin prior to amputation.
- Developed severe anaphylactic reaction, with rash, dyspnoea, and angiodema.
- Admitted to the Intensive Care Unit (ICU).
- Improved over next two hours.

- Swelling (oedema) of the lips, tongue, and airways may be associated with anaphylaxis, whereas swelling of the lower limbs could indicate circulatory overload.
- Chest pain or tightness may occur in circulatory overload, TRALI, and anaphylaxis, while back pain and pain at the infusion site may indicate acute intravascular haemolysis.
- Cramps and muscle pains, along with tingling in the fingers or lips, may be associated with citrate toxicity.

7.8 Investigation of transfusion reactions

In the event of an acute transfusion reaction (ATR) being suspected, the transfusion should be immediately discontinued, and the intravenous (IV) line maintained for fluid resuscitation if necessary. The patient should be clinically evaluated, monitored, and given immediate supportive care as appropriate. The bedside check of the patient identification wristband and pack labelling should be repeated to ensure that an administration error has not occurred and the units, and the giving sets, should be returned to the transfusion laboratory for investigation. If the patient has received more than one unit of RBCs or other components then all the packs are suspect, as are the giving sets, not just the one that happened to be infusing at the time the patient's symptoms were noted.

It is important to inform the hospital transfusion team (consultant haematologist, transfusion laboratory manager, and transfusion practitioner) as soon as possible after a suspected reaction so that appropriate actions and investigations can be carried out. Good communication between the clinical area and the laboratory is essential to ensure effective investigation of suspected adverse reactions to transfusion.

If the acute reaction is suspected due to bacterial infection it is also necessary to inform the blood supplier immediately, so that any other components made from the same donations are put into quarantine until the reaction is proved to be from another cause.

For the laboratory investigation to proceed, it is important to obtain a post-transfusion sample for grouping and a direct antiglobulin test (DAT), as well as a sample for a repeat full blood count (FBC). In addition to the grouping sample, which is usually anticoagulated to facilitate testing by automated analysers, it is also useful to take a clotted sample. Complement-fixing antibodies, such as anti-Vel, are better detected in serum than in plasma, where the anticoagulant typically chelates Ca^{++}, Mg^{++}, and Mn^{++} necessary for complement function. It is also of value to examine the first urine passed by the patient following the suspected reaction, as the presence of a dark tinge (haemoglobinuria or bilirubinuria) may indicate a haemolytic process. This may be confirmed by dipstick testing on the ward. In addition, a clotting screen should be performed so that there is early warning of a possible DIC.

Laboratories should have an SOP based on current national guidelines for investigating a case of suspected transfusion reaction, but in general the transfusion laboratory should:

- Check for any clerical, collection, or administration errors that may have occurred.
- Check for signs of visible haemolysis in samples and component packs.
- Investigate any possible serological incompatibility as soon as possible after stopping the transfusion.

The transfusion laboratory must first exclude the possibility of an administrative error, including the possibility that a patient received a component intended for a different recipient. If the investigation implicates a patient identification, issuing, or collection error, then the possibility that other patients are also at risk due to a component mismatch or sample labelling error must be considered and addressed.

It may be decided to ask for fresh samples on all patients received in the laboratory at approximately the same time as, or from the same location as, the suspect sample, and to quarantine all blood components issued at approximately the same time, in order to ensure that blood grouping results are correct and that components have been correctly labelled.

- Visual inspection of the patient's plasma after transfusion and comparison with a pre-transfusion sample is a sensitive method to detect intravascular haemolysis, as destruction of as little as 5 ml of transfused RBCs will produce a reddish tinge, indicative of haemoglobinaemia.
- Care must be taken in gross examination, however, as poor sample collection technique, as well as myoglobinaemia, seen in severe trauma, burns, or muscle injury may also cause red-tinged plasma unrelated to intravascular haemolysis.
- Icteric (dark yellow/brown) plasma caused by hyperbilirubinaemia may indicate a haemolytic process that has been going on for some hours, or may be a sign of coincidental liver disease.
- The presence of clots, discolouration, or significant haemolysis in the component pack or giving set could be consistent with bacterial contamination.
- The DAT has been reported to be positive in 90% of AHTRs. Where it is negative, it may be that all of the incompatible RBCs have already been destroyed and cleared, with associated signs of haemoglobinaemia or haemoglobinuria.
- A DAT should be performed on both the pre-transfusion sample, if available, and the post-transfusion sample for comparison. Where the DAT of only the post-transfusion sample is positive, elution of antibody from post-transfusion RBCs may aid either identification, or confirm specificities of antibodies detected in plasma or serum.
- Where an AHTR is suspected, the patient's blood group and antibody screen should be retested with both the pre- and the post-transfusion samples to ensure that they are the same blood group, and that a weak antibody has not been missed during the pre-transfusion screening. If using a serum sample for antibody screening, it is important to use a polyspecific anti-human globulin (AHG) reagent containing anti-C3d, as many test systems designed for anticoagulated samples use monospecific anti-IgG reagent.
- A serological compatibility testing should be either repeated (if originally performed), or undertaken (if EI was originally used) using both the pre- and post-transfusion samples.

This is to ensure all results were correct, and that no alloantibodies directed against low prevalence antigens were present, particularly in the case of EI.

- Where a DHTR is suspected, it is extremely unlikely that the implicated blood packs will still be available, so a repeat/initial crossmatch with pre- and post-transfusion samples will not be possible. In these cases, it is important to test a post-transfusion sample for the presence of atypical antibodies and perform a DAT. Sometimes it may not be possible to determine the clinical significance of a RBC antibody, or there may be clinical evidence of a haemolytic reaction in the absence of conclusive serology. More specialized tests, such as RBC survival studies may be useful in these cases.

- Where an immune antibody has been implicated in a reaction to RBCs, it is useful to perform a RBC phenotype (or, if necessary and available, a genotype) on both the pre-transfusion sample and the implicated unit, if still available, to confirm absence of the corresponding antigen in the patient and its expression on the RBCs of the unit.

- A post-transfusion full blood count (FBC) may be useful to establish baseline parameters, and it may also be possible to identify agglutinated RBCs on a film.

- A coagulation screen is useful in monitoring the development of a coagulopathy in either acute haemolysis or infection.

- If bacterial contamination is suspected, either originating from the unit or the giving set, then cultures for bacteria and fungi should be performed on both the patient's sample and the implicated component pack(s)/giving set(s). The pack(s)/giving set(s) should be returned to the laboratory as soon as possible, and should be forwarded, without delay, to the blood service for further testing.

- Renal function tests and urinary output are useful measures of the onset of renal impairment and other metabolic disorders. Raised bilirubin, lactate dehydrogenase (LDH), and low haptoglobin (Hp) levels are useful markers of haemolysis, and a low level of ionized calcium is consistent with citrate toxicity.

- In cases of anaphylactic reactions, samples may need to be sent to reference laboratories to test for platelet and/or HLA antibodies, or for IgA deficiency and anti-IgA.

Careful records should be kept of all investigations performed, and also of those performed by a reference laboratory, as it may be necessary to report the results to SHOT and/or the MHRA, as detailed in the next section.

Key points

In the event of an ATR reaction being suspected, the transfusion should immediately be discontinued and an investigation initiated. Checks should be made to ensure the correct component is being given to the correct patient. Laboratory testing includes repeating the compatibility testing on a pre-transfusion sample, if available, and with a freshly collected post-transfusion sample.

SELF-CHECK 7.6

What are the initial laboratory tests to be carried out if a haemolytic transfusion reaction is suspected?

7.9 **Haemovigilance in the UK**

Haemovigilance is defined as the systematic surveillance of adverse reactions and adverse events related to transfusion, and is aimed at improving safety throughout the transfusion chain from donor to patient. Across the European Union (EU), there is a legal requirement to submit data on **serious adverse reactions** (SAR) and **serious adverse events** (SAE) to the EU Commission, under the terms of the EU Directives 2002/98/EC and 2005/61/EC.

These directives have been transposed into UK law as the Blood Safety and Quality Regulations (BSQR).

- A SAR is defined within the regulations as 'An unintended response in a donor or in a patient that is associated with the collection or transfusion of blood or blood components that is fatal, life-threatening, disabling or incapacitating, or which results in, or prolongs, hospitalisation or morbidity.'

- A SAE is defined as 'Any untoward occurrence associated with the collection, testing, processing, storage and distribution of blood or blood components that might lead to death or life-threatening, disabling or incapacitating conditions for patients, or which results in, or prolongs hospitalisation or morbidity.'

Within the UK, the MHRA has been appointed as the 'competent authority' to oversee the regulations on behalf of the Secretary of State. In its regulatory role, the MHRA emphasis is on the quality management systems (QMS) in place in blood establishments and hospital laboratories, and its legislative remit extends to the point where the laboratory responsibility ends. The MHRA has to provide total numbers of reactions and events on an annual basis to the EU Commission. To make the reporting of adverse reactions and events more streamlined, the MHRA has developed a web-based reporting portal, called the Serious Adverse Blood Reactions and Events (SABRE). Hospitals notify and confirm incidents that have occurred, and provide the MHRA with evidence that the incidents have been discussed within risk-management structures and that 'corrective and preventative actions' (CAPA) have been put in place to lessen the likelihood of recurrence. This web portal is also used to submit reports to the SHOT scheme, and hospitals can print a summary of reports submitted to use as evidence of participation for compliance with NHS Litigation Authority (NHSLA) standards.

The SHOT confidential reporting scheme was launched in 1996 following growing concern amongst UK transfusion specialists, haematologists, and other clinicians that there was little information on the safety of the transfusion process. It collects a wider scope of data than that of the MHRA, extending into the professional and clinical areas of transfusion practice, as well as the part of the transfusion process under the control of the hospital laboratory or blood establishment. SHOT is a professionally led, confidential, voluntary organization that aims to collect anonymized reports from across the UK on adverse events related to transfusion of blood and blood components (RBCs, platelets, FFP, cryo, and granulocytes), and more recently anti-D immunoglobulin and cell salvage.

All cases reported to SHOT are subject to expert scrutiny, to ensure that the data reported are accurate and comprehensive. An annual report and a separate summary leaflet have been published each year by SHOT since 1998 (based on 1996/7 data) in which several general and specific recommendations are made with the aim of improving transfusion safety. Recommendations are targeted at all relevant professional groups, from the four UK Chief Medical Officers, through to each and every member of hospital staff involved in transfusion, as there is the opportunity for everyone to influence the safety of the process.

Serious adverse reaction

An unintended response in a donor or in a patient that is associated with the collection or transfusion of blood or blood components that is fatal, life-threatening, disabling, or incapacitating, or which results in, or prolongs, hospitalization or morbidity.

Serious adverse event

Any untoward occurrence associated with the collection, testing, processing, storage, and distribution of blood or blood components that might lead to death or life-threatening, disabling or incapacitating conditions for patients, or which results in, or prolongs hospitalization or morbidity.

SHOT findings are used to:

- Aid the production of national clinical and laboratory guidelines for the use of blood.
- Improve standards of hospital transfusion practice.
- Educate users on the hazards of transfusion and their prevention.
- Inform policy within the four UK transfusion services and via the EU Commission.
- Identify new trends in adverse events and stimulate research.

What is reportable

- SARs are reportable to both the MHRA and to SHOT, regardless of where in the transfusion process the error originated.
- SAEs are reportable to the MHRA if they fall within the responsibility of the blood establishment or hospital transfusion laboratory quality system. Adverse events involving clinical staff, or involving a blood product, such as anti-D immunoglobulin, are not reportable to the MHRA, but should be reported to SHOT.

More reported incidents fall into the incorrect blood component transfused (IBCT) category than any other. This includes all reportable episodes where a patient was transfused either with a blood component or plasma product that did not meet the appropriate requirements, or which was intended for another patient. IBCT also includes inappropriate or unnecessary transfusions: cases where the intended transfusion is carried out, and the component itself is suitable both for transfusion and for the patient, but where the decision making is faulty. Handling and storage errors are cases of transfusion of a correct component to the intended patient, but where handling or storage errors may have rendered the component less safe for transfusion.

There have been some important trends in reporting since 1996. These include:

- A decrease in the number of ABO incompatible transfusions erroneously administered from a high in 1997–1998 of 41 ABO incompatible transfusions to 10 ABO incompatible transfusions in 2014.

CASE STUDY 7.4 Incorrect blood component transfused

- A unit of group A, D-positive blood was correctly checked and collected from the blood bank by a healthcare assistant.
- The blood was taken to the ward and handed to a staff nurse.
- The 'bedside' check was completed in the treatment room but unfortunately the nurse then connected the unit to the wrong patient, who was group O, D-positive.
- The patient suffered an AHTR, requiring supportive therapy and prolonged hospital stay but made a full recovery.

- The number of cases in which blood of the wrong group was transfused to a patient, or where blood was transfused that was intended for another patient has actually not increased over the years, fluctuating between 16–80 cases per year. Initiatives that have had an impact on the incidents of ABO incompatibility and wrong blood include the various *Better Blood Transfusion* publications, and the expanding role of hospital transfusion practitioners, the NPSA, now superseded by the Care Quality Commission (CQC), Safer Practice Notice 14 'Right Blood Right Patient', and data from the National Comparative Audit.

- Mortality and morbidity: overall, mortality rates have dropped, with only one case of mortality definitely related to a haemolytic transfusion reaction reported in 2014. Episodes of major morbidity have also gradually reduced.

- The incidence of TRALI peaked in 2003 with 36 cases, but only nine cases were reported in 2014. The steady fall in these cases has coincided with the introduction of male-only plasma for FFP, and for suspension of pooled platelets, where possible, in an attempt to reduce the number of TRALI cases.

- The incidence of TTI has also tailed off from 14 proven cases in 1996–1997 to just six between 2010 and 2014 (all of which were viral in nature) and no bacterial TTI since 2010. This is due to the cumulative effect of new generations of microbiological testing, as well as initiatives to reduce bacterial contamination, such as improved cleaning of the donor arm and diversion of the first 20 ml of blood at donation, which captures the skin plug.

- TA-GvHD has reduced in incidence from four cases in 1996–7, to one case in 2000–1 and no cases in subsequent years. This is likely to be the direct effect of universal leucodepletion, which was commenced in the UK in November 1999. It should be noted, however, that one of the cases occurred post-leucodepletion and that therefore leucodepletion cannot be considered as eliminating all risk of TA-GvHD.

- The incidence of ATR remained steady over the ten-year period until 2006–7, when the number of cases increased. This is likely to be a direct result of the influence of the BSQR, which require that all serious transfusion reactions are reported, and, in 2014, 343 cases of ATR were reported.

- The incidence of DHTR has not significantly altered over the entire reporting period from the original report to the 2014 report.

CASE STUDY 7.5 *Severe allergic reaction leading to cardiac arrest after platelet transfusion*

- 56-year-old given a dose of pooled platelets pre-operatively.
- Developed a rash and became hypotensive under anaesthetic, followed by cardiac arrest.
- Successfully resuscitated.
- Vital signs returned to normal after 30 minutes with treatment.
- Decided to use washed platelets in future.

- There has been an increase in the number of handling and storage errors reported (188 in 2014) that may also have been influenced by the BSQR in 2005.

- Inappropriate and unnecessary transfusions have also increased (175 in 2014) in the last few years. This may be the effect of increased awareness of this as a major risk for patients, which, previously, was probably often misdiagnosed as acute respiratory distress syndrome (ARDS).

The figures show that SHOT has been working effectively as a haemovigilance system; although it has seen an increased rate of reporting over the years, the rate of the most severe category of adverse events and reactions is dropping. This shows that there is an increased awareness of safety issues for patients and an improved culture of reporting. Although the advent of the BSQR may have been a slight setback, overall reporting to the haemovigilance systems, SHOT and MHRA, has increased, and SHOT anticipates an increase in reporting of true SHOT incidents in the coming years, as the value of haemovigilance becomes more apparent, and the web-based reporting systems enhance access for users. See Figure 7.2.

> ### Key points
> Haemovigilance is the systematic surveillance of adverse transfusion reactions and events, and collating data on these to improve safety throughout the transfusion chain from donor to patient.

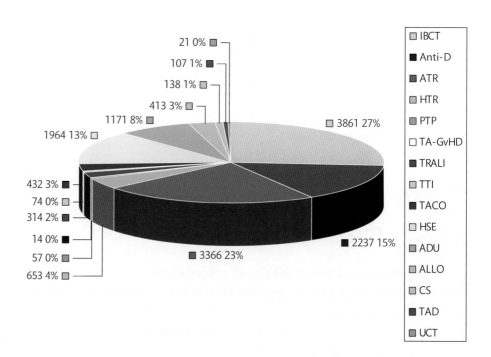

FIGURE 7.2
Cumulative numbers of cases reported to SHOT 1996–2014.

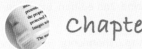

Chapter summary

- Compatibility testing ensures that the correct blood component is selected for a patient, and that the correct tests have been performed and compared with any historical results for that patient.

- Pre-transfusion testing consists of ABO and D grouping, plus an antibody screen.

- In the absence of atypical antibodies, both in the current samples and in an historical sample, then an ISXM can be used, or EI can be used as an alternative.

- If a clinically significant, or potentially clinical significant, antibody is present in the current sample, or has been identified in an historical sample, or the patient is disqualified in some other way from receiving blood by either ISXM or EI, then blood that is antigen compatible should be crossmatched by IAT.

- Even if the compatibility procedures have not identified any incompatibility, the recipient may have an adverse reaction when transfused; this could be immune or non-immune, immediate or delayed.

- Laboratory investigation of suspected reactions includes retesting pre-transfusion and post-transfusion samples, plus further tests, depending on the nature of the reaction.

- Reactions can be classified as either an SAR or an SAE.

- SARs are reportable to both the MHRA (SABRE) and to SHOT, regardless of where in the transfusion process the error originated. SAEs are reportable to MHRA.

- Since SHOT started collecting data in 1996, the overall trend has been towards safer transfusions, with fewer cases of death directly associated with transfusion, and an increased awareness of the pitfalls of the transfusion process.

- The aim is: right blood to the right patient, at the right time.

Further reading

- **Daniels GL. *Human Blood Groups*. Wiley-Blackwell, Hoboken (2013).**

  BSH (2012) Guidelines for pre-transfusion compatibility procedures in blood transfusion laboratories. **http://www.b-s-h.org.uk/guidelines/guidelines/pre-transfusion-compatibility-procedures-in-blood-transfusion-laboratories/**

  BSH (2009) Guideline on the administration of blood components. **http://www.b-s-h.org.uk/guidelines**

  BSH (Addendum August 2012) Guideline on the administration of blood components. **http://www.b-s-h.org.uk/guidelines BSH (2012)** Guideline on the investigation and management of acute transfusion reactions prepared by the BSH Blood Transfusion Task Force. Guideline on the administration of blood components. **http://www.b-s-h.org.uk/guidelines**

- **Klein HG & Anstee DJ *Mollison's Blood Transfusion in Clinical Medicine*. 12th edition. Wiley-Blackwell, Hoboken (2014).**

- **Murphy M & Pamphilon DH.** *Practical Transfusion Medicine*. **2nd edition, Blackwell, Hoboken (2005).**

SHOT (2014) Serious Hazards of Transfusion annual report. **http://shotuk.org**

SHOT (2014) Serious Hazards of Transfusion annual report—supplementary information. **http://shotuk.org**

Answers to the questions in this chapter are provided on the book's accompanying website:

 Go to www.oup.com/uk/avent2e

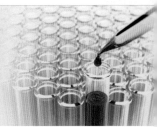

8

Immune-Mediated Red Cell Destruction

Malcolm Needs

Learning objectives

After studying this chapter you should be able to:

■ Describe the difference between intravascular and extravascular haemolysis.

■ Describe the role of antibodies and complement in red cell destruction.

■ Outline the clinical significance of red cell antibodies.

■ Describe the use of the direct antiglobulin test (DAT).

■ Outline the causes of haemolytic transfusion reactions.

■ Outline the types of autoimmune haemolytic anaemias and the problems associated with finding compatible blood.

■ Describe how red antibodies can cause hyperacute rejection in solid organ transplant.

■ Describe the phenomenon of passenger lymphocyte syndrome.

Introduction

In this chapter, we will look at how and why red blood cells (RBCs) are destroyed in the body, *in vivo*, by antibodies. This can happen in the following situations, and each will be considered after some general information about red cell-mediated haemolysis.

• Transfused RBCs destroyed by an antibody the individual has produced—a haemolytic transfusion reaction, which can be either acute or delayed.

• Patient's RBCs destroyed by an antibody in transfused plasma, for example anti-A,B in group O platelets given to a group A patient.

• An individual's RBCs being destroyed by an autoantibody they have produced—autoimmune haemolytic anaemia (AIHA).

- An individual's RBCs destroyed by an antibody derived from donor lymphocytes in a transplant, or transplanted donor RBCs being destroyed by an antibody from/in the recipient.
- Transplanted solid tissue destroyed by recipient antibody.

8.1 What is immune (antibody-mediated) red cell destruction?

The result of an interaction between an antigen on the red cell and an antibody can lead to the destruction of that red cell, but it is not the antibody itself that causes the destruction, rather it acts as a trigger for other mechanisms, such as the complement pathway *or* macrophages, mainly in the liver or spleen. The role of antigens, antibodies, and their interaction with the complement systems and macrophages was considered in Chapter 1. In summary, antibodies binding to their cognate antigen on a red cell (or, in certain circumstances, when the red cell antigen is also a histoantigen, on a tissue cell) can lead to the destruction of that cell by one of two ways; **intravascular haemolysis** or **extravascular haemolysis**.

Antibodies, usually IgM or the minority of IgG1 and/or IgG3, which activate the complement pathway and haemolyse the RBCs within the circulation (intravascular haemolysis), are mainly, but by no means exclusively, anti-A, anti-B, and, particularly anti-A,B. Most deaths resulting from the transfusion of incompatible blood are associated with these strongly haemolytic antibodies. Most IgG antibodies, however, bring about red cell destruction outside the circulation (extravascular haemolysis). The IgG antibody molecules on the red cell surface are recognized by macrophages, mainly in the spleen, and it is these cells that remove the antibody-coated RBCs from the circulation.

The binding of both IgM and IgG antibodies can lead to various immune mediators being activated, such as C3a (an intermediate peptide mediator of inflammation) and C5a (which can activate macrophages to ingest RBCs coated with complement), and it is these that cause most of the symptoms associated with increased red cell destruction. The clinical signs and symptoms that might be seen in a haemolytic transfusion reaction include some, or all, of the following:

- Fever (>1°C rise in temperature)
- Flushing of the face
- Lumbar back pain
- Hypotension (low blood pressure)
- Nausea

If the cell destruction is very brisk, such as in an ABO incompatible transfusion, other clinical symptoms might include:

- Haemoglobinuria (Hb in the urine)
- Anuria—renal damage (not passing urine)
- Unexplained bleeding, particularly at the infusion site, such as disseminated intravascular coagulation (DIC)
- A feeling of doom

The anaphylactic and chemotactic actions of the complement fragments, C3a and C5a, and the pro-inflammatory cytokines are the main effectors of these symptoms. C3a, for example, causes the constriction of the gut and bronchial smooth muscles that result in the classical

Intravascular haemolysis.
Red cells being haemolysed within the circulation by the classical complement pathway that has been activated by antibodies, especially ABO antibodies.

Extravascular haemolysis.
Immune-mediated red cell removal that takes place outside the circulation, usually in the liver and spleen.

symptoms of a haemolytic reaction of chest and lumbar back pain. C3a can also lead to tachy-cardia by constricting the blood flow to the heart. C5a, for example, is chemotactic for phago-cytes and neutrophils, as well as stimulating the pro-inflammatory interleukins IL-1, IL-6, IL-8, and tumour necrosis factor α (TNF α).

Rapid intravascular red cell destruction, due to ABO incompatibility, for example, rapidly stimulates the release of high levels of TNF α, followed by a more sustained production of interleukins (principally IL-1) and monocyte chemoattractant protein-1 (MCP-1). By acting to release histamine from basophils, and activation of both T and B lymphocytes, these molecules produce the effects of fever, hypotension, and shock.

The IgG antibodies that lead to extravascular haemolysis, also stimulate the release of IL-8, IL-1, and IL-6, but, again, in a sustained manner, with elevated levels still being detectable 24 hours after the original stimulus. IL-1 leads to a raised body temperature (fever) and hypotension, whereas IL-6 will activate T lymphocytes and induce B lymphocytes to become antibody-producing plasma cells. These cytokines can also activate the fibrinolytic pathway, which may lead to DIC, or cause the renal circulation to be reduced. If this is not treated quickly, it can lead to renal failure, one of the commonest clinical sequelae of haemolytic transfusion reactions.

If blood samples are taken soon after a haemolytic episode and analysed in the laboratory, the findings may include:

- A fall in haemoglobin (Hb)
- A fall in haptoglobins (Hp)
- The presence of spherocytes
- A raised reticulocyte count
- A rise in bilirubin levels
- A rise in serum lactate dehydrogenase levels (LDH).

These results are easily explained. As RBCs are destroyed or removed from the circulation quicker than they can be replaced, then the Hb level falls. Hb released into the circulation from the RBCs binds with the haptoglobins which carry it to the liver where it is broken down—the globin chains forming bilirubin, hence the increased levels of bilirubin. Raised levels of the enzyme LDH, produced in the liver, but largely carried in the RBCs, are associated with haemolysis, as the LDH carried in the RBCs is released into the plasma. Spherocytes are formed when IgG-coated RBCs bind to macrophages in the spleen, but instead of being fully ingested, the macrophage only removes part of the red cell membrane. The cell is then released back into the circulation as a spherocyte, but with a greatly reduced half-life. If haemolysis is very brisk, such as in intravascular destruction, the Hb may be found free in the plasma or urine. Once bound to albumin, it appears as the distinctively brown-coloured methaemoglobin.

Key points

When antibodies combine with antigens *in vivo*, they can activate complement and cytokines that, in turn, lead to the symptoms seen in haemolytic reactions.

SELF-CHECK 8.1

What is meant by 'intravascular' and 'extravascular' haemolysis?

8.2 Clinical significance of red cell antibodies

Do all antibodies cause red cell destruction? The simple answer is 'no', but most have that potential if the right conditions exist. In general, an antibody, if capable of causing red cell destruction *in vivo*, is considered to be clinically significant. There are a number of factors which contribute to the destructive potential of an antibody, including:

- Immunoglobulin class and subclass (IgM, IgG, and IgA)
- IgG subclass
- Complement activation
- Activity at 37°C
- Blood group antigen specificity
- Number of antigen sites per red cell
- Number of antibodies bound per red cell
- Equilibrium constant of the antibody
- Presence of blood group substances (antigens) in the plasma
- Activity of the recipient's reticulo-endothelium system (RES).

As a general rule, antibodies that are reactive at 37°C and are detectable by an antiglobulin test are considered to be 'clinically significant'. Those that fail to react at 37°C are considered to be clinically insignificant, but, as with any biological system, there are exceptions.

Alloantibody

An antibody that reacts with a 'foreign' antigen, usually either stimulated by red cells that have been transfused, or as a result of a feto-maternal haemorrhage.

The specificity of an **alloantibody** (e.g. is it anti-D or anti-Kn^a?) is the main indicator as to its potential significance, and this is based on reports in the literature of these antibodies having caused, or not caused, *in vivo* cell destruction, either by HDFN or transfusion reactions. Therefore, antibodies directed against the antigens of the major blood group systems (BGS), such as Rh, Kell, Duffy, and Kidd, and some of the antigens within the MNS BGS, are considered significant. Antibodies that react below 37°C to the Lewis, P1, and N antigens, for example, are not normally considered significant. There are, of course, some specificities that fall outside this broad definition, the most notable being anti-M; some rare examples react by the indirect antiglobulin test (IAT) at *strictly* 37°C, whilst most do not.

Most IgM 'naturally acquired', T cell independent, antibodies react only by direct saline agglutination techniques at temperatures below 37°C—some might react at 'room temperature', but few react above 30°C. The major exception are the ABO antibodies (although rarely anti-A$_1$), and the anti-H found in O$_h$ phenotype individuals.

Clinically significant antibody

An antibody capable of causing red cell destruction, albeit indirectly, *in vivo*.

Most **clinically significant antibodies** are, therefore, IgG, but they do not usually cause intravascular haemolysis. There are, however, four subclasses of IgG, 1-4, and only IgG1 and IgG3 are recognized by splenic macrophages, leading to extravascular red cell destruction. Although some antibody specificities are composed of a mixture of all four IgG subclasses, IgG1 and IgG3 predominating, some antibodies are composed of just IgG2 and/or IgG4, and these, therefore, are not clinically significant.

The rate of cell destruction is dependent on the number of antibody molecules bound to each cell, and this, in turn, is influenced by the number of antigens available on the red cell surface to which the antibodies can bind, and how well those antibodies do bind (the equilibrium constant). There is evidence that 100 IgG3 antibody molecules per red cell can lead to the recognition and removal of that cell by macrophages, whereas it takes 1000 IgG1 molecules per cell to produce the same degree of cell destruction.

Some antigens found on RBCs are also found in the plasma, for example Lewis, or, as in the case of antigens of the Chido/Rodgers BGS, associated with complement C4. If these are present in the plasma of blood being transfused to someone with the corresponding antibody, that antibody will preferentially bind to the non-red cell antigens. There will then be little or no antibody bound to the transfused RBCs, which will then not be destroyed.

As most IgG-coated RBCs are removed by the spleen, then in a patient who has an enlarged spleen, the removal and destruction of these RBCs can be increased above the normal expected rate. If the patient has a defective spleen, however, or the spleen has been surgically removed (splenectomy), then the major site for the removal and destruction of IgG-coated RBCs is absent, and they will have a longer survival time.

Sometimes, just knowing the specificity of the antibody, or mixture of antibodies, and that it/they react by IAT, is not sufficient to tell if it will be significant *in vivo*. In such circumstances, one or more of the following additional investigations can be performed:

- Determining the antibody's IgG subclass using monospecific antiglobulin reagents
- A titre to determine the antibody potency
- The thermal range over which the antibody reacts (e.g. does it react at strictly 37°C?)
- Cellular assays, using macrophages *in vitro*, to try to predict if the antibody will be recognized by macrophages *in vivo*
- *In vivo* red cell survival by injecting a small volume of radio-labelled RBCs, usually involving Cr^{51} labelling, and measuring how long these RBCs remain in circulation.

Key points

Although most antibodies have the potential to cause red cell destruction, those that do not react at strictly 37°C by an antiglobulin test are unlikely to be clinically significant.

Antibodies reactive at 37°C that are unlikely to be clinically significant

As stated above, the general rule is that red cell antibodies that do not react *in vitro* at strictly 37°C are regarded as clinically insignificant, as they do not normally lead to increased red cell destruction *in vivo*. But is the converse true—are all antibodies that react at 37°C significant? Clinical experience (supported by many publications) has shown that several alloantibodies reactive at 37°C do not cause haemolysis of serologically incompatible RBCs *in vivo*.

IgG antibodies that react with epitopes on the C4 component of complement are not uncommon, and are usually anti-Ch or anti-Rg. These antibodies can be neutralized by using inert, ABO compatible plasma. The term neutralized is slightly misleading, as it is not the antibody itself that is neutralized, but its apparent activity against RBCs is inhibited. As stated above, an antibody will more readily react with a non-cell bound antigen, in this case the C4 molecule that is abundant in plasma. RBCs take up C4 in a non-specific manner (it is not intrinsic to the red cell membrane), especially those stored *in vitro*. One way of assigning the specificity is using RBCs coated with C4 *in vitro*, which will react strongly with these antibodies. Inhibition, or neutralization, is a simple method for ensuring other alloantibodies present are detected and identified, and for crossmatching to be undertaken.

The CR1 (complement receptor 1, or CD35) protein on the red cell surface carries antigens of the Knops BGS. The antibodies usually exhibit so-called high titre, low avidity, or HTLA characteristics (although this term is now going out of favour, as not all these antibodies exhibit these characteristics), as the antibodies tend to react weakly, but when the serum is titrated, they tend to be reactive at quite high dilutions. Although the antibodies are invariably IgG, reacting by IAT, they are clinically insignificant.

The common feature of these IgG IAT reacting, but clinically insignificant antibodies, is that they react with the RBCs of almost all individuals; therefore, they 'get in the way' when investigating a blood sample for the presence of antibodies that are clinically significant. A variety of methods, such as inhibition with inert serum, or treating the RBCs with 0.2 M dithiothreitol (DTT) can be used to eliminate their activity.

A relatively new tool in the arsenal of blood transfusion is the availability of recombinant blood group proteins (rBGPs) to specifically inhibit, or neutralize certain alloantibodies, and, for example, one of these rBGPs is specific for the inhibition, or neutralization, of antibodies within the Knops BGS, allowing the detection and specificity of other, possibly clinically significant, alloantibodies underlying these antibodies.

Antibodies that react only with RBCs treated with a proteolytic enzyme, such as papain, are generally considered to be clinically insignificant for transfusion purposes (although rare exceptions have been reported in the literature) and, indeed, some examples of anti-E have been shown to be non-red cell immune, or 'naturally acquired'. Developing Rh antibodies, however, are often first detected only with RBCs treated with a proteolytic enzyme and examples have been reported where such antibodies have increased in strength, become reactive by IAT and have caused HDFN. For routine antibody screening, however, the use of such RBCs is not recommended in the UK.

Key points

Not all antibodies that react in the IAT at 37°C are clinically significant; knowing the specificity of the antibody will help decide which are likely to be significant.

SELF-CHECK 8.2

Why are some antibodies not considered to be clinically significant?

Direct antiglobulin test

If a case of immune red cell destruction is suspected, then the test most widely used is the direct antiglobulin test (DAT). In this test, the RBCs from the person being investigated are tested directly, without having to incubate RBCs and plasma, as in the IAT, with antiglobulin reagents to see if the RBCs have been coated, *in vivo*, with antibody (IgG, IgM or IgA) and/or complement (C3c or C3d). Column agglutination cassettes are available commercially for performing a DAT that includes monospecific anti-IgG, anti-IgA, anti-IgM, anti-C3c, and anti-C3d reagents, together with a control column that, if the test is to be valid, must remain negative. By using these, all the key players in red cell destruction are covered. A positive DAT in itself, however, is not diagnostic of an increased rate of red cell destruction *in vivo*, as there also has to be other evidence, such as a low Hb, a raised reticulocyte count, reduced Hp, raised bilirubin, and/or a raised LDH. Without this further evidence, even if a *de novo* antibody specificity is detected, the situation may be termed as a serological transfusion reaction, where there are no other clinical *sequelae*, other than a positive DAT and a new antibody specificity. Similarly, in rare cases, an increased rate of red cell destruction *in vivo* may be diagnosed, using these other parameters, even when the DAT remains negative.

8.3 Haemolytic transfusion reactions

Despite all the pre-transfusion tests that are performed to detect antibodies in the recipient's blood and to select compatible blood, some patients have a reaction to their transfusion, which can be haemolytic. Patients being transfused should be closely monitored for temperature, pulse, and blood pressure, and if there are any significant changes to any of these then a reaction should be suspected. See Chapter 7 for a more detailed account.

A patient might react to transfused blood from almost as soon as the drip has started to within 24 hours of the transfusion. In such circumstances the reaction is defined as an acute haemolytic transfusion reaction (AHTR). If symptoms commence after 24 hours of the transfusion, the reaction is defined as a delayed haemolytic transfusion reaction (DHTR).

AHTR are usually, but not exclusively, caused by ABO incompatibility, such as wrongly giving group A RBCs to a group O individual. There are also well-documented reports of these reactions occurring when group O platelets are given to a group A or B patient when the platelet preparation contains high titre anti-A/B. ABO incompatible transfusion reactions are usually accompanied by the classical symptoms, as detailed above, fever, lumbar pain, etc. Once suspected or recognized, the transfusion must be stopped and replaced by a saline drip, and diuretics administered, to help maintain kidney function. Further blood transfusion must not be given until the cause of the reaction is known.

DHTRs are often not noticed until 5–8 days after the transfusion has been given, when a fall in Hb is noted. Usually, there are no other signs to alert medical or nursing staff, although sometimes fever is reported. In these cases, an antibody stimulated by a previous sensitizing episode, a feto-maternal haemorrhage (FMH) or a transfusion, is present at the time of transfusion but at low levels, not detectable by the routine pre-transfusion testing. A secondary immune (anamnestic) response follows the transfusion and, as the antibody level increases, the incompatible RBCs become coated with antibody and are removed from the circulation. RBCs thus coated will give a positive DAT but as the transfused RBCs disappear, the DAT becomes negative and antibody appears in the plasma. Whilst the DAT is positive, but before there is free antibody in the plasma, it is usually possible to make an eluate (remove antibody from the surface of the RBCs) to test in order to find its specificity. Should the patient need a transfusion at this time, it is essential that the RBCs transfused are compatible with the antibody causing the haemolysis; the antibody eluted from the RBCs.

Over the years, reports sent to the UK Haemovigilance Scheme, the UK Serious Hazards of Transfusion (SHOT), show that anti-Jk^a is associated with DHTRs in 75% of cases; other antibodies implicated include anti-c.

Clinical correlation

Hyperhaemolysis is a rare complication of transfusion which has been mainly, but not exclusively, reported in patients with sickle cell disease (SCD). It has also been referred to as the sickle cell haemolytic transfusion reaction syndrome. It is characterized by the destruction of both the

Hyperhaemolysis
Characterized by post-transfusion Hb levels lower than pre-transfusion Hb levels, with marked reticuloctyopenia (a significant decrease from the patient's usual absolute reticulocyte level), hyperbilirubinemia, and haemoglobinuria.

transfused, usually serologically compatible, RBCs and those of the recipient. The condition is marked by the post-transfusion Hb falling to below that found pre-transfusion, together with a low reticulocyte count. The DAT is often negative and often no RBC antibodies serologically incompatible with the units transfused are identified. Further transfusion can exacerbate the haemolysis, or may even prove fatal; therefore, it is important that this condition is recognized early, and treatment with steroids, such as intravenous methylprednisolone, and/or intravenous immunoglobulin (IVIgG) started as soon as possible.

The exact pathogenesis of hyperhaemolysis is undoubtedly complex because of the destruction of both the transfused and the patient's own RBCs, but two have been postulated:

- Bystander haemolysis, in which an antibody, not necessarily a RBC antibody, but possibly an antibody directed against a human leucocyte antigen (HLA) activates complement which attaches to both the transfused RBCs and the recipient's own RBCs, leading to their destruction (Figures 8.1 and 8.2).
- Hyperactive macrophages in which both donor and recipient RBCs are destroyed by these cells. The theory for this is that HbSS RBCs and reticulocytes adhere to macrophages more readily than do HbAA RBCs and reticulocytes. Expression of vascular cell adhesion molecule 1 (VCAM-1) on endothelial cells is induced by cytokines and HbSS RBCs and reticulocytes adhere via integrin α4β1 to VCAM-1 on the vascular endothelium. VCAM-1 is also expressed on hyperactive macrophages, and thus these hyperactive macrophages destroy both HbSS RBCs and reticulocytes, and also HbAA RBCs (Figures 8.3 and 8.4).

Key points

Haemolytic transfusion reactions can happen immediately or within 24 hours of blood being transfused, usually because of ABO incompatibility, or may be delayed and not noticed for several days, as is mostly the case involving IgG antibodies.

SELF-CHECK 8.3

Define the terms 'immediate' and 'delayed transfusion reactions and give examples of both.

HLA	Frequency	RBC Antigen
HLA A2/A28	45%/9%	Bg^c
HLA B7	17%	Bg^a
HLA B17	10%	Bg^b

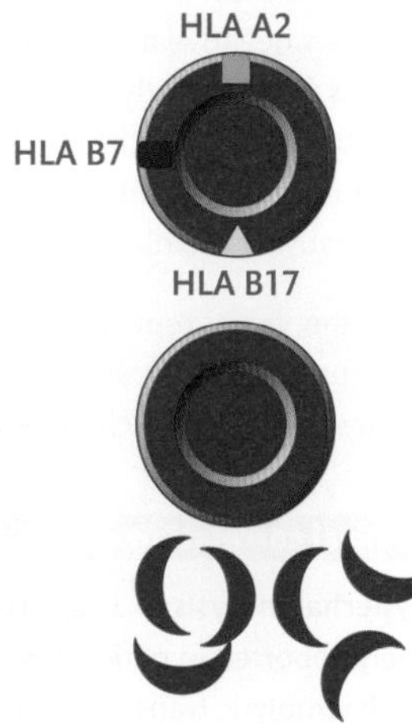

HLA A2

HLA B7

HLA B17

Other transfused RBC not expressing HLA antigens.

FIGURE 8.1
HLA antigens and the corresponding RBC Bg.

Patient's own HbSS cells.

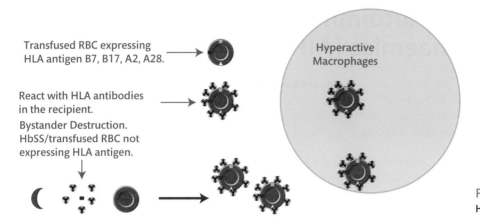

Transfused RBC expressing
HLA antigen B7, B17, A2, A28.

React with HLA antibodies
in the recipient.

Bystander Destruction.
HbSS/transfused RBC not
expressing HLA antigen.

Hyperactive
Macrophages

FIGURE 8.2
HLA-mediated RBC destruction.

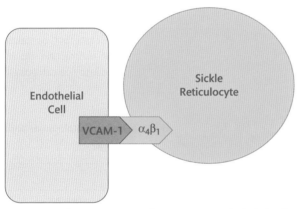

Endothelial
Cell

Sickle
Reticulocyte

VCAM-1 $\alpha_4\beta_1$

Cytokines induce expression of VCAM-1 on endothelial cells

FIGURE 8.3
VCAM-1/sickle reticulocyte
interaction.

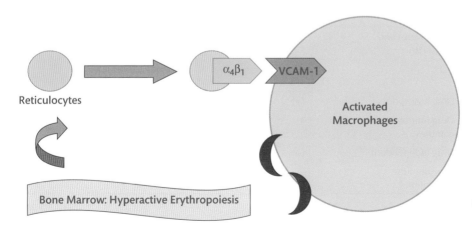

Reticulocytes

$\alpha_4\beta_1$ VCAM-1

Activated
Macrophages

Bone Marrow: Hyperactive Erythropoiesis

FIGURE 8.4
Destruction of reticulocytes/
sickle cells by hyperactive
macrophages.

8.4 Autoimmune haemolytic anaemias (AIHA)

Some patients produce **autoantibodies**, directed against their own RBCs, which can lead to an increased rate of RBC destruction—an AIHA. These differ from RBC alloantibodies, produced as a result of transfusion and/or an FMH, which do not destroy the individual's own RBCs, only those of a different blood group. Although the autoantibodies do react with antigens on the patient's own RBCs, the actual specificity of the antibody, or the exact antigen involved, is often difficult to determine, not least because the specificity of the antibody is usually directed against a high prevalence antigen, such as Rh17, Rh18 or Wr^b, but often mimic antibodies directed against polymorphic antigens within the Rh BGS, such as anti-E and anti-e. These antibodies not only react with the patient's own RBCs, but also the RBCs of most other people, thus presenting a dilemma when trying to provide compatible blood for transfusion.

AIHA is a relatively rare condition, usually found secondary to other clinical disorders, especially haematological malignancies. Patients with AIHA may present on admission with a very low Hb, sometimes <50g/l, and require an immediate transfusion to maintain their oxygen carrying capacity until other treatment has time to suppress the increased rate of RBC destruction. A positive DAT often helps with the diagnosis of these cases, but, as stated above, is not diagnostic on its own, as other indicators of increased RBC destruction should be present. In rare cases, the DAT may be negative. AIHA can be divided into five categories, see Table 8.1.

TABLE 8.1 Immunoglobulins and complement (C3) on red cells in cases of autoimmune and drug-related haemolytic anaemias.

AIHA type	IgG	C3	IgA	IgM	Notes
Warm AIHA	+	+	(+)	(+)	IgA and/or IgM sometimes present
Warm AIHA	+	–	–	–	
Warm AIHA	–	+	–	–	In 10% of cases
Warm AIHA; IgA	–	–	+	–	Very rare
Warm AIHA; IgM	–	–	–	+	Very rare
Cold AIHA	–	+	–	+	Usually high thermal amplitude reacting antibody
Mixed warm and cold AIHA	+	+	–	+	Very rare
PCH	–	+	–	–	Donath-Landsteiner antibody (IgG anti-P)
Drug adsorption	–	(+)	–	–	e.g. penicillin
Drug immune complex	–	+	–	–	e.g. phenacetin
Drug independent	+	(+)	–	–	e.g. methyldopa
Non-immune adsorption	(+)	–	(+)	–	e.g. cephalosporins

(+) may be present

- Warm AIHA
- Cold AIHA
- Mixed warm and cold AIHA
- Paroxysmal cold haemoglobinuria (PCH)
- Drug-induced/associated

Autoimmune cell destruction is not confined to RBCs. Both autoimmune and drug-associated immune destruction of platelets and other body tissues can occur.

Warm AIHA

Warm AIHA is the most common, so called because it is usually caused by an IgG autoantibody that reacts more readily at 37°C than at lower temperatures. Sometimes the C3 component of complement is also present on the patient's RBCs. The DAT, therefore, is positive with anti-IgG and sometimes with anti-C3 as well. If the RBCs are coated with IgG, destruction takes place in the spleen, but if complement has been activated, there might be some more rapid RBC destruction in the liver.

In some case IgM or IgG antibodies may be found in addition to IgG, and, very rarely, either IgA or IgM might be present on their own. It is only by using a monospecific anti-IgM reagent and a monospecific anti-IgA reagent that these cases are recognized. As suggested above, there have been cases reported where a patient has clinical AIHA but the DAT has been negative. On further full investigation with monospecific antiglobulin reagents, many of these have been shown to have IgA on the RBCs, but in others, it is assumed that either low-affinity auto-antibodies are involved, or there are low levels of IgG1 or IgG3 that are not detectable by the standard DAT.

The DAT has been reported positive (IgG and/or C3) in some patients with *Plasmodium falciparum* malaria. It is not clear to what extent RBC destruction is exacerbated when the DAT is positive, but there is evidence that mean Hb levels are lower in patients with a positive DAT than those without, and more transfusions are needed.

The autoantibodies found in the plasma of patients with warm AIHA usually react with all but the very rarest RBCs tested, but sometimes less strongly with some RBCs than others. These are likely to have a Rh-related specificity with, as suggested above, auto-anti-e or 'anti-e-like' being most commonly encountered. Although autoantibodies will probably lead to a decrease in the lifespan of any transfused RBCs, because they react with antigens found on most RBCs, any alloantibodies present may be much more significant, as these could cause the rapid removal of incompatible transfused RBCs. In addition to the adverse effects of the ensuing transfusion reaction, this might also exacerbate the underlying destruction of the RBCs coated with the autoantibody.

Although some cases of warm AIHA are idiopathic, occurring without any obvious underlying cause, most cases of positive DATs now seen in the UK are related to haematological malignancies. In a series of cases referred to an immunohaematology reference laboratory, only 5% were idiopathic AIHA, 16% were associated with cases of malignancy, and 10% specifically with myelodysplastic syndromes (MDS). With an increasing number of people being treated for these conditions, the number of positive DAT cases is increasing. Also, many of these patients presenting with a positive DAT and with 'warm reactive' autoantibodies present have been transfused. Figures show that about 75% of DAT-positive cases referred to reference laboratories have been transfused, and about 40–50% have alloantibodies present. The investigation and provision of blood for these patients is considered below.

Positive DAT without cell destruction

A number of patients and blood donors have a positive DAT with no evidence of increased RBC destruction; for donors the figures vary from 1 in 3000 to 1 in 15,000 in the UK (the large variation in numbers being explained by the technique used for the DAT testing, and whether clotted or anticoagulated samples were being used). The reason for the apparent lack of clinical significance might be that the cells are coated with IgG4 molecules that do not initiate RBC destruction.

Some patients with raised IgG levels can also have a weak positive DAT, presumably due to non-specific uptake of their IgG onto their RBCs. The use of the therapeutic immunoglobulin preparations, anti-lymphocyte globulin (ALG), anti-thymocyte globulin (ATG), and anti-CD38 can also result in a transient positive DAT, as the immunoglobulins 'stick' to the RBCs in a non-specific manner. In addition, some D-positive individuals with idiopathic thrombocytopenia (ITP) are given anti-D immunoglobulin. Most of these individuals also have a positive DAT as a result, with subclinical levels of RBC destruction, although, in some cases, there is a significant drop in Hb.

Key points

IgG antibodies are usually involved in warm-type autoimmune haemolytic anaemia, which can be either idiopathic, or, more likely, secondary to another disease, such as haematological malignancy.

Cold AIHA

These cases are rare. The antibodies associated with cold AIHA are not usually associated on the RBCs by the DAT unless a monospecific anti-IgM reagent is included in the battery of reagents used, but anti-C3d is often identified, indicating that an antigen/antibody reaction has taken place. This is because these cases are caused by a 'cold-reacting' IgM autoantibody, often with anti-I, anti-HI, anti-i, anti-Hi, or anti-H specificity, or a mixture of these specificities. The actual specificity, and, indeed, the titre of the antibody is largely irrelevant (for example, if the autoantibody has the specificity of anti-I, you would not transfuse the patient with very rare adult i blood, and there have been instances of clinically significant haemolysis by a low-titre autoantibody that has, nevertheless, got a wide thermal range/amplitude). The vitally important thing with cold autoantibody is, therefore, the thermal range/amplitude. If the antibody reacts *in vitro* at 30°C or above, it is clinically significant.

These antibodies are usually considered to be 'cold-reacting' and clinically insignificant, as they do not react at 'body temperature'. After some infections, however, such as glandular fever or mycoplasma pneumonia, the level of antibody can increase, together with its thermal range or amplitude, so that it becomes active at 30°C. The autoantibodies could then react with the individual's own RBCs in the peripheral capillaries (fingers, toes, nose, ears, etc.), where the blood temperature may drop to 30°C. At these lower temperatures, the antibody may bind to the antigens on the individual's RBCs, and initiate the complement cascade. As the RBCs return to the warmer parts of the body, the antibody dissociates from the antigen, but, as the complement cascade has been started, it can go to completion (the membrane attack complex, or MAC), resulting in intravascular haemolysis or rapid destruction of the C3d-coated red cells in the liver. When this happens, the patient can present with haemoglobinuria and an extremely low level of Hb after exposure to cold, and the EDTA sample will show evidence of gross (*in vivo*) haemolysis. In less extreme cases, the complement cascade is halted at the C3 stage (actually, C3dg) and C3d is detected on the RBCs that probably have a near normal half-life in the circulation. In such circumstances, transfused RBCs may be destroyed much more quickly than the autologous RBCs, as the C3dg coating 'protects' the RBCs from destruction, whilst the transfused RBCs will soon be coated with C3d, rather than C3dg, and so are more vulnerable to destruction.

In some disease states such as lymphoma, the malignant cells might form a single clone, producing an antibody with anti-I specificity. As the antibody comes from that single clone, each molecule will be identical—a monoclonal antibody. In some patients, the abnormal immunoglobulin produced might not have an antibody specificity, but can be produced in such large quantities that the total IgM levels rise so high that the patient suffers from effects of a raised plasma viscosity, affecting the circulation.

Mixed warm and cold AIHA

Mixed warm and cold AIHA is a rare condition, but its reporting is paradoxical. The laboratory investigations required to prove the condition in a patient are complex, and it is likely that true cases of mixed warm and cold AIHA are under reported, whereas false cases of the condition are almost certainly over reported. Treatment usually involves a course of corticosteroids, such as prednisone, but, if this fails, rituximab has been shown to be efficacious.

The laboratory investigations involved to resolve mixed warm and cold AIHA will be discussed later in this chapter.

Paroxysmal cold haemoglobinuria (PCH)

PCH is usually categorized as a cold AIHA, but unlike most examples of cold AIHA is not caused by IgM antibodies. The causative antibody in PCH is a bi-phasic IgG, usually with anti-P specificity, the so-called Donath-Landsteiner (DL) antibody. The antibody reacts in the cold, and activates complement in the warm, leading to haemolysis and haemoglobuinuria. The DL test is used to detect these antibodies. In this test, group O cells and the serum under test are first incubated at 0°C, and then at 37°C (Figure 8.5), while a control using the same reagents is incubated at just 37°C. In a positive test, haemolysis is seen in the tube incubated at both temperatures, but not in the one incubated at just 37°C. As complement has to be present in the test system, a clotted sample has to be used to provide the serum, and, as complement may be low in the patient's serum due to consumption, an indirect DL test, adding fresh inert serum as a source of complement, is the method of choice.

Although classically associated with the late stages of untreated syphilis, this condition is now almost always seen in children, and is often associated with a viral infection. Although it is self-limiting, that is, resolves after a few days, some patients do present with acute haemolysis that requires transfusion. P-positive units are usually well tolerated, especially if given through a blood warmer, rarely, these RBCs are rapidly destroyed, and very rare p RBCs are required for transfusion.

Key points

IgM cold-reacting antibodies, with an increased thermal range/amplitude, are associated with cold AIHA, unlike PCH, which is caused by a bi-phasic IgG antibody.

SELF-CHECK 8.4

How do the antibodies that cause warm and cold AIHA cause red cell destruction?

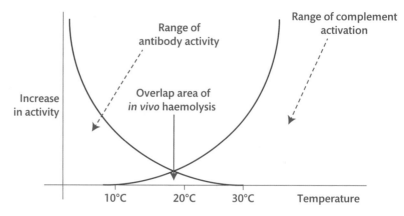

FIGURE 8.5
Haemolysis in PCH.

Drug-induced or -associated AIHA

Well over 100 drugs have been reported that are capable of binding to RBCs and initiating an immune antibody response. The exact mechanism is not known; however, it is likely that the drug, or the metabolite, interacts in some way with parts of the RBC membrane, and antibodies are stimulated that can react with the drug itself, to drug plus membrane components, or to the RBC membrane.

There are four possible mechanisms; the first two are drug-dependent, the third is drug-independent, and the fourth is non-immunological. It is possible that a drug might 'work' by more than one of these mechanisms.

- *Drug adsorption:* the antibodies react mainly against the drug coating the RBCs, rather than the RBCs themselves. The DAT in these cases is usually positive with monospecific anti-IgG and sometimes also with anti-C3d. The drugs mainly involved are the penicillins; haemolysis develops slowly, but can be life-threatening.

- *Immune complex:* the formation of drug–antibody immune complexes attached to the cell surface can result in acute haemolysis with haemoglobinuria and renal failure. Severe haemolytic episodes can recur, even with small doses of the drug. The DAT is usually positive with anti-C3d, but with some drugs that seem to complex poorly with RBCs, IgM or IgG can be detected. The antibody only reacts with drug-coated RBCs. Some of the newer cephalosporins have been implicated with this mechanism.

- *Drug-independent autoantibodies:* in some instances, the drug stimulates the production of an antibody that reacts with the RBC membrane, not the drug itself. This type cannot be distinguished from warm AIHA, as the RBCs react with anti-IgG and, in some cases, anti-C3d. The serum and eluate also react with normal RBCs without the drug having to be present. This type was more common when methyldopa was widely used as a drug to treat hypertension.

- *Non-immunological protein adsorption:* some cephalosporin drugs can alter the RBC membrane causing non-specific uptake of proteins, including IgG and IgM, which are detectable by the DAT. It is not clear if these RBCs have a shortened lifespan.

As cases of drug-associated AIHA are rare in the UK, investigation of these is usually performed by NHSBT-Sheffield Centre.

Key point

In some patients, RBC destruction can be caused by a drug which, in combination with red cells, can lead to the production of an autoantibody.

Investigation of, and crossmatching for, patients with autoantibodies

Transfusion should be avoided in these cases if other treatments can be employed. A transfusion is, however, sometimes required to correct a low Hb where the patient has symptoms of the anaemia.

Grouping of RBCs that have a positive DAT due to IgG can be performed using IgM blood typing sera, usually monoclonal, but those that require an IAT cannot easily be used, as the RBCs would react with the AHG regardless. Where possible, in addition to the standard ABO and D type, these patients should be typed, at least once, and as a minimum, for the Rh antigens C, c, E, e, and for the K antigen.

IgG coating the patient's RBCs can be removed by use of chloroquine diphosphate, but this reagent also denatures some antigens entirely, and weakens others, so this reagent should be used judiciously and the results carefully scrutinized.

Nowadays, CE-marked commercial kits are available that facilitate the genotyping of the patient's blood groups. More complex genotyping can be performed in specialized laboratories, such as the International Blood Group Reference Laboratory (IBGRL), but it must be remembered that results can only be used to predict likely expression of antigens. For example, an individual with acquired B will genotype as A, and individuals with the Fy(a-b-) phenotype may have the *FYB* gene, but the Fy^b antigen may not be expressed, if the individual is also homozygous for a mutation of a *GATA-1* gene, which prevents expression of the Fy^b antigen on the RBCs.

If the antibody screen is negative, but the DAT is positive, *and* the patient has been transfused within the previous three months, *and/or* has been pregnant within the previous three months, an elution should be performed to check that there is no alloantibody coating the RBCs. If an alloantibody is detected in the eluate, any units of blood crossmatched for the patient must *not* express the cognate antigen.

If the antibody screen is negative, but the DAT is positive, and the patient has not been either transfused, or pregnant within the previous three months, blood should be selected and crossmatched in the normal manner, but matched for Rh antigens and the K antigen.

If the antibody screening RBCs are positive, however, additional tests need to be employed to exclude the presence of alloantibodies which may be masked by unbound autoantibodies, free in the patient's plasma.

It is important to identify any alloantibodies that may be detected, as they are more significant when selecting blood for transfusion, than the autoantibodies. Specialist techniques involve adsorption of the autoantibodies onto either the patient's own RBCs—auto-adsorption—or selected reagent RBCs—allo-adsorption. The latter is used if the patient has been transfused within the previous three months, has been pregnant in the previous three months, or there are insufficient patient RBCs available for auto-adsorption. For usually warm AIHA, the plasma is split into several aliquots (depending upon the number of RBC samples used in the technique—usually two or three) and each aliquot has to be adsorbed at 37°C at least twice with each sample of RBCs, with double the amount of fresh or specially preserved, usually papain-treated RBCs, to remove the autoantibodies. Each aliquot of the adsorbed plasma is then tested by standard methods to detect and identify any alloantibodies present. It must be appreciated that although allo-adsorption with the selected RBCs will not normally remove alloantibodies directed against polymorphic or low prevalence antigens, these RBCs may well remove alloantibodies directed against high-prevalence antigens, such as anti-Vel, anti-Jr^a, etc. If at all possible, therefore, auto-adsorption is always the method of choice. Selection of blood for transfusion is based on the findings of these tests and the patient's phenotype, and adsorbed plasma might have to be used for the crossmatch. Blood crossmatched in this way is issued as being 'suitable for', rather than 'compatible with'.

For cold AIHA, adsorption can be performed in the same way but at 4°C rather than at 37°C.

As the cold autoantibody is usually an IgM, the autoantibody can also be denatured by treating the plasma with 0.01M DTT, which is a reducing agent that will break the J-chain holding the molecule together as a pentamer. Although the IgM molecule is now split into five monomers, and these are no longer able to cause direct agglutination of RBCs, these monomers are able to sensitize antigens on the RBCs, and so a monospecific anti-IgG reagent should be used for subsequent testing, including the crossmatch.

Finally, in the case of a cold autoantibody, rabbit erythrocyte stroma (available as a commercial preparation) can be used to adsorb out the autoantibody. These stroma, however, also adsorb out other antibodies, for example anti-B, and so, whilst plasma treated with this preparation can be used to detect and identify IgG alloantibodies, it must not be used for the crossmatch as an ABO incompatibility may be missed.

A case of mixed warm and cold AIHA should be suspected if the DAT is positive with anti-IgG, anti-IgM, and anti-C3d, and there is a reaction with all reagent RBCs whether treated with a proteolytic enzyme, such as papain, or not. Very often, the reactions by IAT at 37°C are comparatively weak, and the plasma may show signs of gross *in vivo* haemolysis. If there is a reaction at 30°C by direct agglutination, the plasma should be treated with 0.01M DTT, as this will denature any IgM autoantibody present (see above), but this treated plasma should then be tested by IAT at 37°C, using a monospecific anti-IgG reagent. If there are positive reactions by this technique there is a warm reacting IgG autoantibody present as well as a cold reacting IgM autoantibody of wide thermal amplitude, and a case of mixed warm and cold AIHA is proven. This is important for the clinician to provide the correct treatment.

Making and testing an eluate in any known case of AIHA is only performed if the patient has recently been transfused (and/or pregnant), has received a transplant, or there is an unexplained increase in the destruction of transfused RBCs, as this might be due to an unrecognized haemolytic transfusion reaction, rather than the underlying AIHA, or it could be a combination of the two, although transfusion in itself is known to exacerbate RBC destruction by autoantibody in some cases. Elution removes antibody bound to the RBCs, so that its specificity can be determined and its significance assessed. Obviously, of course, an elution will also remove any autoantibody bound to the RBCs and this will probably react with all reagent RBCs tested, so it is therefore vital that any reactions between these RBCs and the eluate giving stronger reactions are noted, as recognizing the presence of an alloantibody under such circumstances can be challenging. Obviously, as stated above, any units of blood transfused to the patient must not express the cognate antigen against which the alloantibody is directed.

Once it has been established that there are no detectable alloantibodies underlying the autoantibody, it is acceptable to crossmatch by the 'immediate spin' technique so that any ABO incompatibility can be detected, or, indeed, by electronic issue.

In a life-threatening situation, when there is no time to ascertain if there are any alloantibodies underlying the autoantibody, blood can be transfused that is ABO compatible, Rh and K matched, but only under the direction of a haematology consultant.

Key points

The presence and specificity of alloantibodies is more important than autoantibodies when selecting blood for transfusion in patients.

8.5 Haemolysis post-transplantation of bone marrow/stem cell transplant

The detailed description of haemopoietic stem cell transplantation and stem cell plasticity can be found in Chapter 10. In this chapter, only a description of RBC haemolysis post-transplantation of bone marrow/stem cell transplant will be described.

In stem cell or bone marrow transplants, although the donor and recipient are HLA-matched, they may be of different ABO and Rh blood groups, and this can cause problems post-transplant. Minor mismatches, where the donor is, for example, group O, but the recipient is group A, B or AB, can result in the production of antibodies to the recipient's RBCs, i.e. anti-A and/or anti-B. In major mismatches, as in an A donor and an O recipient, the converse situation arises; the recipient can produce antibodies (anti-A) to the donor RBCs.

If haemolysis occurs in ABO minor mismatches, it is usually 5–15 days post-transplant, often with an abrupt onset, a rapidly falling Hb, and possible renal failure as the result of the RBC destruction. Anti-A or anti-B are thought to be produced by B lymphocytes transfused with the bone marrow—so-called passenger lymphocytes, and there have been reports of fatalities due to the entire group A RBC volume of the patient being haemolysed by donor anti-A over a few days although this is a rare situation. In non-fatal cases, the haemolysis subsides as the patient's remaining incompatible RBCs are destroyed and replaced with those of donor origin. During the haemolytic episode, the DAT may be positive and the causative antibody eluted from the patient's RBCs. When investigating such cases, the eluate should always be tested, by IAT, with A or B RBCs, depending on the group of the recipient. Likewise, an IAT crossmatch must be performed post-transplant, even if no antibodies are detected in the antibody screen, so that IgG anti-A/B, if present, will be detected.

In cases of cord stem cell transplants, there is, of course, no such problem.

In major ABO mismatches, the recipient's ABO antibodies could destroy the donor's RBCs. These days, donor RBCs are depleted from the graft prior to infusion, and the recipient's ABO antibodies are depleted by such techniques as plasma exchange. However, the recipient's ABO antibodies can lead to the delay in erythroid engraftment of the donor RBCs, pure RBC aplasia or, as erythropoiesis increases, the residual antibodies might cause haemolysis of donor-derived RBCs. In these cases, the haemolysis is not usually noted until several weeks after the transplant; time periods of 30 to 100 days have been reported. The DAT is usually positive, with IgG anti-A/B being eluted from the RBCs.

Although ABO antibodies are most commonly implicated, other antibodies (Rh and Kidd) have been reported after stem cell transplants.

Transfusion post-bone marrow/stem cell transplant

As a general rule, group O RBCs are transfused to all patients, irrespective of their ABO, until all of the following criteria are fulfilled:

- No mixed-field reactions are seen when ABO grouping the patient's RBCs.
- Anti-A/B is no longer detectable by standard 'saline' reverse grouping and by IAT, using A_1 and B RBCs.

- The DAT is negative with polyspecific AHG.

When these criteria are fulfilled, then the patient's ABO blood group can be altered in their records, and further RBC transfusions are with the blood of the donor's group.

Where D *major incompatibility* exists, for example the donor is D-positive, the recipient D-negative, give D-negative blood until D-positive RBCs are detectable, then give D-positive blood. Where D *minor incompatibility* exists, for example the donor is D-negative, the recipient D-positive, then transfuse D-negative blood indefinitely.

Where fresh frozen plasma (FFP), cryoprecipitate, etc. is required, group AB should be given.

> ### Key points
>
> When haemopoietic stem cells are transplanted, there might be an immune antibody reaction between the recipient and donor RBCs, leading to RBC destruction.

8.6 Haemolysis post-solid organ transplant and hyperacute rejection

A detailed description of solid organ transplantation and xenotransplantation can be found in Chapter 9. In this chapter, only a description of RBC haemolysis post-solid organ transplant and one aspect of hyperacute rejection will be described.

With an increased demand for renal transplants, more patients are being transplanted with an ABO incompatible organ; in particular, A_2 renal donors to group B and O recipients. ABO antigens are histoantigens, and so are expressed on some tissues such as most epithelial cells (particularly glandular epithelia) and on endothelial cells, in addition to RBCs and some other blood cells.

It is important, therefore, that where a solid organ transplant is to be carried out and it is known that ABO antigens are expressed upon this organ, the ABO type of the donor and the recipient is serologically checked on more than one occasion to ensure ABO compatibility. Where a major ABO incompatible solid organ transplant is to be carried out, such as a kidney from A_2 donor to a group O recipient, it is vital that ABO antibody levels, particularly anti-A, are reduced by such methods as pre-, peri-, and post-operative plasma exchange, using plasma of the donor type, extra-corporeal immunoadsorption, use of IVIgG and anti-CD20 (rituximab). Failure to do this could result in hyperacute rejection of the kidney due to the recipient's ABO antibodies.

Where there is a minor ABO incompatibility, for example, a kidney from a group O donor being transplanted to a group A recipient, passenger lymphocyte syndrome (as discussed above) can occur. Essentially, ABO antibodies (in this case, anti-A) are produced by competent B lymphocytes derived from the graft.

The more lymphoid the tissue transplanted, the greater the risk. It is therefore more common in lung, and heart and lung transplantation, than in liver or renal transplantation, but it can and does occur with these tissue transplants too.

Key points

ABO antigens are expressed on some cells, other than RBCs, and so can play an important role in solid organ transplantation.

8.7 Haemolytic disease of the fetus and newborn (HDFN)

Although there is no doubt that the destruction of fetal/newborn RBCs by maternal antibody
comes under the heading of immune mediated RBC destruction, this subject is so important
that it is covered in a chapter of its own, see Chapter 3.

Chapter summary

- Despite, or perhaps because of, advances in clinical practice, immune-mediated RBC
  destruction still has to be considered in transfusion, transplantation, and pregnancy.

- Almost all RBC antibodies have the potential to cause RBC destruction if the right conditions exist. In general, an antibody capable of causing RBC destruction *in vivo* reacts at
  37°C by IAT, and is considered to be clinically significant.

- Some patients produce autoantibodies, directed against an antigen expressed on their
  own RBCs, which can lead to an increased rate of RBC destruction—an AIHA.

- As the population gets older, and as treatment improves, more people are treated for
  malignancies, and the number of patients with autoantibodies is increasing.

- Laboratory tests are employed pre-transfusion and transplant, and components selected
  to try to prevent *in vivo* RBC destruction, but an increasing number of stem cell and solid
  organ transplants are being given that are knowingly ABO and/or D incompatible and, of
  course, not typed for other RBC antigens.

- Although these problems are recognized and better understood, they have not been
  fully resolved, and so the need to investigate RBC antibodies, both allo and auto, will
  remain.

Further reading

- British Committee for Standards in Haematology. Guidelines for pre-transfusion
  compatibility procedures in blood transfusion laboratories. *Transfusion Medicine* 23
  (2013), 3–35.

- Daniels G, Poole J, de Silva M, Callaghan T, MacLennan S & Smith N. The clinical significance of red cell antibodies. *Transfusion Medicine* 12 (2002), 287–295.

- Klein HG, Anstee DJ. *Mollison's Blood Transfusion in Clinical Medicine*. 12th edition, Wiley-Blackwell, Hoboken (2014).

- Reid ME, Lomas-Francis C & Olsson ML. *The Blood Group Antigen FactsBook*. 3rd edition, Academic Press, Cambridge, MA (2012).

- Daniels G. *Human Blood Groups*. 3rd edition, Wiley-Blackwell, Hoboken (2013).

- Petz LD & Garratty G. *Immune Hemolytic Anemias*. 2nd edition, Churchill-Livingstone, London (2004).

Answers to the questions in this chapter are provided on the book's accompanying website:

Go to www.oup.com/uk/avent2e

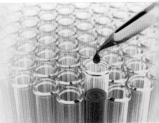

9

Human Leucocyte Antigens (HLA) and Their Clinical Significance

Neil D. Avent

Acknowledgements: the editor thanks Colin Brown who wrote an earlier version of this chapter in the book's first edition that forms the basis for this present update.

Learning objectives

By the end of this chapter you should be able to:

- Describe the HLA system.
- Outline the role of the HLA system in transplantation and transfusion.
- Explain the principles of matching for haemopoietic stem cell transplantation, solid organ transplantation, and platelet transfusion.
- Outline the common methods and technology for HLA typing and antibody testing used in the HLA laboratory.
- Understand the key immunological pathways targeted by immunosuppression.
- Have an understanding of the hurdles to overcome in xenotransplantation.

Introduction

Humans have a highly developed immune system that can distinguish self from non-self proteins and the principle molecules enabling this function are coded for by genes found in a region of the genome on the short arm of chromosome 6, known as the major histocompatibility complex or MHC. In fact many species have a MHC, even fish.

This ability to recognize cells from another individual of the same species or different species as foreign is a major barrier to transplantation and can cause some serious hazards of transfusion.

In this chapter you will learn about the human leucocyte antigens, the genes of which are found within the MHC, and how the detection and matching of the genes and gene products has contributed to the success of transplantation and the study of human disease.

9.1   A brief history of transplantation

- In 600 BC, Hindu surgeon Sushrutha experimented with autologous (see Box 9.1) skin grafting.
- In 1778 John Hunter first used the term 'transplant' when describing his work in transplanting ovaries and testes in animals.
- The nineteenth century saw a number of workers experimenting with autologous skin grafts.
- In 1910 Carrel and Guthrie developed methods for joining blood vessels together called 'anastomosis' that allowed many experiments on grafting kidneys, which all failed.
- In the 1930s Snell discovered the dominant histocompatibility locus in mice, the H-2.
- In 1933 the first kidney transplant in humans was performed by the Russian surgeon, Voronoy, but this transplant failed as the kidney was harvested approximately six hours after the donor had died.
- In 1937 Gorer developed the concept of self and non-self, following the observation that antigens on tissue cells are genetically determined and are involved in the destruction of foreign grafts.
- In the 1940s Medawar worked on the immunological problems of rejection when observing the problems associated with treating burn victims and injuries sustained as a result of the Second World War.
- In 1966 Kelly and Lillehei transplanted a kidney and pancreas into a patient suffering from end-stage diabetic nephropathy.
- In 1967 Dr Christian Barnard carried out the first human heart transplant.

BOX 9.1   Types of transplant

Autologous: the patient receives their own cell/tissues.

Syngeneic: the patient receives cells/tissue from a genetically identical donor, that is, an identical (monozygotic) twin.

Allogeneic: the patient receives cells/tissues from a non-identical donor of the same species.

Xenogeneic: the patient receives cell/tissues from a donor of a different species.

9.2 Human leucocyte antigens

The discovery of human leucocyte antigens

It was George Snell who showed that genetic differences were involved in the response to transplanted tissue. Snell bred **congenic** mice to discover the locus that was intimately involved in tumour graft rejection and named it 'H' for histocompatibility. Peter Gorer independently discovered an agglutinating antibody associated with rejection of tumour grafts and named it as the antigen II. It was later established that the antigen II was coded for by a gene located at the H locus described by Snell. The term H-2 was used to describe the murine MHC.

In the late 1950s three groups, in France, the USA, and the Netherlands were instrumental in the discovery of the human MHC. Jean Dausset (France) who identified a leucocyte agglutinating antibody in transfused patients recognizing an antigen he termed 'MAC'. This antigen was found in 60% of the French population and was subsequently found to be HLA-A2. Rose Payne (USA) found similar leucocyte agglutinating antibodies in the sera of multiparous women, and noted the pattern of reactivity of the sera with leucocytes of the newborn infant and their fathers and concluded that the offspring had inherited a paternal 'leucocyte factor'. Jon van Rood (the Netherlands) reported a systematic analysis of the reactivity of sera from patients that had undergone febrile transfusion reactions as well as sera from pregnant women. van Rood described the recognition of different leucocyte groups using panels of sera and speculated on the possible use in forensic medicine and bone marrow transplantation.

> **Congenic**
> Organisms produced as the result of specific inbreeding in an experimental setting so that they only differ in one gene locus.

Human leucocyte antigen gene location

The genes that code for HLA molecules are found within the MHC, which can be divided into two regions based on the structure and function of their products: the class I region where the HLA-A, B, and C genes are located; class II which contains the HLA-DR, DQ, and DP genes. There is also a class III region which does not contain any HLA genes, but genes encoding complement factors (C3 and factor B), tumour necrosis factor (TNF) alpha, heat shock proteins (HSP), and other genes involved in immune function. See Figure 9.1.

SELF-CHECK 9.1

What is the major histocompatibility complex and what is its function?

Human leucocyte antigen class I molecules

Human leucocyte antigen class I gene products consist of 45 kilodalton (kDa) glycopeptides folded into three extracellular domains called alpha 1, 2, and 3, a transmembrane region and a cytoplasmic tail; it is often called the class I heavy chain. The alpha 3 domain is non-covalently associated with beta 2 microglobulin, a ubiquitous plasma protein that is a product of a gene not within the MHC but on chromosome 15, and is also known as the light chain. The alpha 1 and alpha 2 domains of the heavy chain are folded to form a peptide binding cleft. The antigenic differences or polymorphisms of HLA-A, B, and C molecules are as a result of amino acid sequence variations in this region of the heavy chain. See Figure 9.2 and Box 9.2.

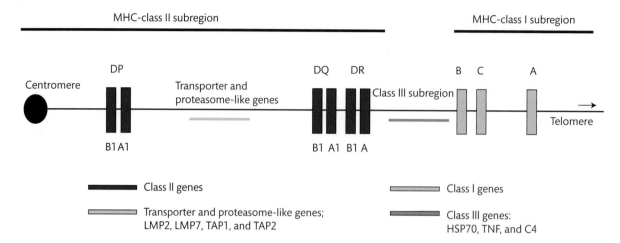

FIGURE 9.1

Map of the human major histocompatibility complex. The human MHC spans a region of approximately 9 Mb on the short arm of chromosome 6. This region of the genome is gene rich, containing 224 genes many of immune function and over half are predicted to be expressed. The MHC class I and II sub-regions contain the genes that code for HLA molecules.

FIGURE 9.2

Human leucocyte antigen class I molecule. The HLA class I molecule comprises a membrane bound heavy chain of ~45 kDa, folded into three extra-cellular domains α1-3, a transmembrane region, a cytoplasmic tail, and a water-soluble light chain known as β2-microglobulin. The peptide binding groove is formed by the α1 and α2 domains and β2-microglobulin non-covalently associated with the α3 domain.

BOX 9.2 Determining the structure of the human leucocyte antigen class I molecule

The structure of the HLA class I molecule was first visualized using X-ray crystallography (Bjorkman, 1987) and was a landmark discovery in the history of HLA. The peptide binding cleft was shown to consist of a beta-pleated sheet at its base and the sides were alpha helices. The size of the groove showed it was capable of binding peptides consisting of between eight and ten amino acids.

Human leucocyte antigen class II molecules

Human leucocyte antigen class II molecules consist of two chains, alpha and beta, and the genes coding for both chains are located within the MHC. The alpha chain is a 31–34 kDa glycoprotein non-covalently associated with a 26–29 kDa beta chain, and both chains have a transmembrane region and a cytoplasmic tail. Both the alpha and beta chain are polymorphic in HLA-DQ and DP molecules, but only the beta chain contributes to polymorphism in HLA-DR molecules. Human leucocyte antigens polymorphism will be discussed in more detail later in this chapter. See Figure 9.3.

Human leucocyte antigen expression

Human leucocyte antigen class I and II molecules can be distinguished by their distribution on different cell types. Human leucocyte antigen class I molecules are expressed on nearly all nucleated cells and platelets and are also found in a soluble form in plasma, where they can be adsorbed onto erythrocytes that do not normally express HLA molecules.

Human leucocyte antigen class II molecules have a more restricted distribution and are found on macrophages, dendritic cells, B lymphocytes, Langerhans cells, and thymic epithelium or so-called 'professional' antigen-presenting cells.

Antigen processing and presentation

The main function of HLA molecules is the presentation of foreign molecules, in the form of peptides, to the immune system. In this way, T lymphocytes, cells of the adaptive immune response, can be activated.

Pathogens that reside inside cells, such as viruses, can be recognized by HLA class I molecules. Viral proteins found in the **cytosol** are degraded by intracellular structures known as

Cytosol
The aqueous component of the cytoplasm in an intact cell.

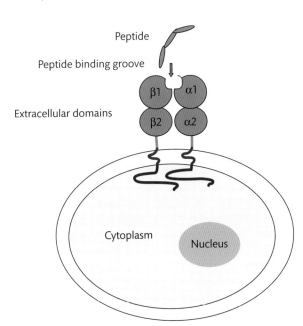

FIGURE 9.3
Human leucocyte antigen class II molecule. The HLA class II molecule comprises an α and β chain, both have two extracellular domains α1, α2 and β1, β2, respectively, a transmembrane region and a cytoplasmic tail. The α1 and β1 domains form the peptide binding groove for HLA-DR, DQ and DP molecules.

Proteasome

An intracellular proteolytic complex that degrades cytosolic and nuclear proteins.

Endosome

A membrane bound intracellular compartment providing an environment for material to be sorted before degradation by the lysosome.

proteasomes, some of the genes of which are located within the MHC. The peptides produced by this degradation are between eight and ten amino acids in length, just the right length to be loaded into the peptide binding groove of HLA class I molecules. However, the viral peptide will only bind if that particular HLA class I molecule has the correct binding groove for the viral peptide. These newly formed HLA class I molecules containing antigenic peptide are transported to the cell's surface via the Golgi apparatus and present their peptides to predominately CD8 positive (cytotoxic) T lymphocytes.

Pathogens that reside outside the cell, such as bacteria, can be taken up by phagocytosis or pinocytosis and degraded in the **endosome** normally by acid digestion. The peptides produced are of varying length and are loaded into the peptide binding groove of an appropriately complementary HLA class II molecule. These newly formed HLA class II molecules are transported to the cell's surface via the Golgi apparatus and present their peptides to predominately CD4 positive (helper) T lymphocytes.

This explains the biological role of HLA molecules and how they allow the immune system to recognize pathogens located inside or outside the cell. If an individual's HLA molecules are unable to bind to peptides derived from a pathogen, it can lead to infection and/or disease.

In normal circumstances, pregnancy (where the mother is exposed to the HLA molecules of the fetus inherited from the father) is the only natural situation when an individual would be exposed to another individual's HLA. However, transplantation and transfusion exposes the recipient to foreign (non-self) HLA which can cause powerful immune responses.

SELF-CHECK 9.2

What are the main functions of HLA class I and HLA class II antigens?

> ### Key points
>
> HLA genes are found within the MHC locus. This is divided into two regions, the class I region (HLA-A, B, and C genes) and class II (HLA-DR, DQ, and DP genes). Human leucocyte antigen class I molecules are expressed on nearly all nucleated cells and platelets, whereas HLA class II molecules have a more restricted distribution, being found on antigen-presenting cells.

Human leucocyte antigen nomenclature

Antisera

Blood serum containing polyclonal antibodies.

The different antigens of the HLA system were defined using antibodies from patients who had received multiple transfusions or pregnancies. Throughout the world, different laboratories used local names to define the reactivity of their HLA **antisera**. It was through collaboration at international histocompatibility workshops that a universal system of naming the different antigens was established. As a new antigen was found it was numbered sequentially, that is, the first three antigens to be named were A locus specificities A1, A2, and A3, followed by B locus specificities. New antigens that had not been officially named by the workshop nomenclature committee were distinguished by a 'w', for example Aw74, Cw3. The 'w' was removed following confirmation by the international workshop. However, the 'w' was retained for HLA-C locus antigens to prevent confusion with complement factors, particularly those whose genes are found within the MHC. Human leucocyte antigen Bw4 and Bw6 were found to be **public epitopes** on certain HLA-B locus antigens so they have kept their 'w'.

Human leucocyte antigen class II molecules were originally defined using cellular assays, the most commonly used was the mixed lymphocyte culture (MLC). When lymphocytes from two individuals are mixed in culture they can respond by the production of **cytotoxic** T lymphocytes directed against the determinant recognized as foreign. These were termed HLA-D. It was later shown that MLC reactivity could also be influenced by cell surface molecules that could be detected by antibody. These determinants were found on B lymphocytes but not T lymphocytes and named HLA-D related or HLA-DR molecules.

The naming of new HLA class II loci followed a different convention, going backwards through the alphabet. We now have HLA-DQ, DP, DO, and DM. There was originally an HLA-DN gene, but this was later shown to be a sub-unit of HLA-DO.

The application of DNA-based techniques in the late 1980s and early 1990s to HLA typing resulted in the definition of HLA polymorphism at the molecular level. Antibodies can detect differences at the protein level but molecular techniques allow the detection of nucleotide differences.

Human leucocyte antigen nomenclature has developed over the last 40 years to account for the high degree of polymorphism that can be detected using DNA-based techniques. The latest change to HLA nomenclature occurred in April 2010, and using HLA-DRB1*13 as an example, an explanation is shown in Table 9.1.

There are some alleles that end with a letter of the alphabet. This letter indicates some additional characteristics of the molecule:

A	Aberrant expression
C	Cytoplasmic expression only
L	Low expression levels
N	Null allele, no cell surface expression
S	Secreted, this molecule is only present in a soluble form

How many human leucocyte and alleles?–polymorphism

The number of serologically defined HLA molecules has remained constant for many years. However, the number of HLA alleles that have been described has increased rapidly and the statistics from October 2011 (www.ebi.ac.uk/imgt/hla/) are shown in Table 9.2.

The reason for this extensive polymorphism is apparent when we consider that the role of HLA is to present peptides from pathogens to the immune system. Human leucocyte antigen polymorphism is pathogen driven and HLA class I and II molecules have evolved to present peptides from a wide variety of pathogens. At a population level, it is important that there are many different HLA alleles to make it more likely that there will be individuals able to respond to a novel pathogen and maintain the survival of the species.

Public epitopes

A region of an antigen shared by many different antigens that is recognized by antibodies, B cells, or T cells.

Cytotoxic

The ability to kill cells either by loss of membrane integrity, necrosis, or programmed cell death, apoptosis.

TABLE 9.1 HLA nomenclature.

HLA	HLA region
HLA-DR	Identifies the HLA locus.
HLA-DR13	A serologically defined antigen.
HLA-DRB1*	Identifies the HLA locus and gene, the asterisk indicates the HLA allele(s) have been defined using DNA-based techniques.
HLA-DRB1*13	A group of HLA alleles with a common DRB1*13 sequence, termed **first field resolution**, that is, this is the field before the first colon.
HLA-DRB1*13:01	A specific HLA allele termed **second field resolution** as the numerals appear in the second field between the first and the second colon.
HLA-DRB1*13:01N	A **null allele**; there is no cell surface expression of the DRB1*13 gene product.
HLA-DRB1*13:01:02	An allele that differs by a synonymous (silent or non-coding) mutation.
HLA-DRB1*13:01:01:02	An allele that contains a mutation outside the coding region.
HLA-DRB1*13:01:01:02N	A null allele which contains a mutation outside the coding region.

When describing serologically defined specificities, they are not preceded by *.
Thus the serological HLA type of HLA-A1, B8, Cw7, DR3, and DQ2 would be reported as HLA-A*01, B*08, C*07, DRB1*03, DQB1*02 if typed using DNA techniques.

First field resolution

This is how a low resolution HLA type is described because the numerals describing the HLA molecule are in the first field before the colon, for example HLA-DRB1*12.

Second field resolution

This is how a high resolution or allele level HLA type is described because the second field after the first colon is populated, for example HLA-DRB1*12:01.

Null allele

A mutant gene that does not function like the normal gene. Many null HLA alleles lack cell surface expression and cannot present peptides to the immune system.

At an individual level HLA polymorphism is achieved by the following three factors:

1. Multiple loci—if we just consider the HLA loci important in transplantation (HLA-A, B, C, DRB1, DQB1, and DPB1), there are six different loci, increasing the potential number of peptides that can be bound by HLA molecules.

2. Multiple alleles—at each loci there are many different alleles so there is a low probability of two unrelated individuals having the same HLA type.

3. Co-dominant expression—each individual will inherit a set of HLA alleles on one chromosome from each parent and both sets will be expressed.

Studies of HLA polymorphism in different populations show that some HLA types are found almost exclusively in some populations, whilst other HLA types are found throughout the world (Table 9.3).

Key points

The extensive polymorphism of the HLA system enables peptides from pathogens to be presented to the immune system. The HLA nomenclature is agreed internationally and reflects the known HLA polymorphism at a molecular level.

TABLE 9.2 The number of human leucocyte antigen alleles and serological and cellular human leucocyte antigen specificities.

HLA locus	Antigens/specificities	Alleles
A	28	1,729
B	60	2,329
C	10	1,291
DRB1	21	1,051
DQB1	9	160
DPB1	6	150

TABLE 9.3 Examples of HLA types and distribution.

HLA-A*02	Throughout the world
HLA-A*01	European Caucasoid
HLA-A*25	European Caucasoid
HLA-A*36	Black African
HLA-A*36	Black African
HLA-A*43	Black African
HLA-A*08	European Caucasoid
HLA-B*54	Japanese
HLA-B*42	Black African
HLA-B*46	Chinese and Japanese
HLA-DRB1*03:02	Black African
HLA-DRB1*10	Indian/Middle Eastern

9.3 The detection and definition of human leucocyte antigens, alleles, and antibodies

Serological human leucocyte antigen typing

The first HLA typing methods were serologically based and relied on the detection of cell surface HLA molecules on lymphocytes isolated from peripheral blood (or spleen or lymph nodes in the case of deceased donors). Human leucocyte antigen typing laboratories maintained panels of well characterized HLA antisera obtained from multiparous women, patients immunized by transplantation or transfusions, and in some cases healthy donors given planned immunizations of HLA typed lymphocytes. The principle of the typing technique, termed the lymphocytotoxicity test (LCT) or complement-dependent cytotoxicity (CDC), has remained the same since the mid-1960s when Terasaki and McClelland pioneered the use of a microtitre plate format: the Terasaki plate (see Method box).

Serological typing had its limitations, which include:

- It requires viable cells that are sufficiently robust to withstand the LCT.
- Patients with low numbers of lymphocytes due to their disease or disease treatment may not be able to provide sufficient lymphocytes for typing.
- B lymphocytes are required for HLA class II typing, which constitute only 15% of peripheral blood cells and an additional B cell isolation method was required.
- Good quality typing requires large panels of well-characterized antisera, which are expensive to maintain as only about 15% of multiparous women produce HLA antibodies and a small proportion of these are useful typing sera.

Serological typing is still used as many commercial companies produce HLA typing trays and utilized monoclonal antibodies directed against different HLA specificities. Serological typing is also used in combination with typing using DNA-based techniques, to detect null alleles, where the gene for the allele is present but the protein is not expressed on the cell surface. The presence or absence of cell surface expression can have functional consequences, provoking alloreactions which are important when considering clinical transplantation.

DNA-based human leucocyte antigen typing

One of the main drivers for the introduction of DNA-based HLA typing was the limitations of serological HLA class II typing. DNA-based typing for HLA class II molecules was introduced before HLA class I typing.

Initially, the techniques involved treating DNA with restriction enzymes, which cut the DNA sequence at specific sites and the resulting fragments were of different sizes

METHOD Human leucocyte antigen typing: LCT/CDC

Each Terasaki plate contains 60 different antisera, including negative and positive controls and at least two plates (120 different sera) are used to obtain a basic HLA type.

In the standard LCT 1 ul of lymphocytes is added to 1 µl of antiserum already plated on the Terasaki plate, incubated for 30 minutes to allow antibody–antigen interaction to occur. Then 5 µl of rabbit complement is added to each well and the plate is incubated for a further 60 minutes before the reaction is stopped and the plate read. Where there has been specific binding of complement-fixing antibodies to the cells used in the test, the integrity of the membrane is disrupted, allowing the entry of dyes that allow the detection of dead cells. One of the most commonly used dyes is a mixture of acridine orange and ethidium bromide. Acridine orange is taken into the cytoplasm of live cells and, under UV light from a fluorescence microscope, these cells appear green. Ethidium bromide (EB) cannot cross the intact cell membrane, but when the cell membrane is disrupted, EB will enter the cell and intercalate with DNA and these cells appear red under UV light.

depending upon the HLA type, and visualized on a gel, usually involving radioactive markers. However, this technique was laborious and not sensitive enough for a highly polymorphic system such as HLA. The introduction of polymerase chain reaction (PCR) technology revolutionized HLA typing and currently the methods used by HLA typing laboratories all involve PCR.

1. *Sequence Specific Primer* (PCR-SSP): this approach requires the design of short sequences of DNA or primers specific for particular HLA allele or groups of alleles that can serve as templates for DNA synthesis when that particular allele is present. Patient or donor DNA, plus the building blocks for DNA synthesis, are added to a panel of primers, usually in a 96-well format, that cover all of the major HLA alleles groups, sufficient to obtain a basic HLA type. Each primer pair is tested for DNA amplification by performing agarose gel electrophoresis on the reaction mixture. If DNA amplification has occurred the product has a specific band on the gel of a specific molecular weight. The HLA type is determined by analysis of the reactivity with the panel of specific primers. Sequence specific primer is a rapid technique as the plates of primers can be stored frozen or freeze dried and be ready for immediate use, so this technique is commonly used for patient typing or situations where results are required rapidly, such as deceased donor typing. The resolution of PCR-SSP for rapid typing is usually first field or low to medium level (see Box 9.3), which is not satisfactory for stem cell transplantation but useful for solid organ transplants or matching for platelet transfusion.

2. *Sequence Specific Oligonucleotide Probes* (PCR-SSOP): this approach to HLA typing requires the design of strands of DNA that bind in the region of the HLA allele that is specific for that allele or allele group. The probe can be labelled with a fluorescent or radioactive tag so that specific binding can be detected. The patient or donor DNA to be HLA typed undergoes PCR amplification but the primers are not specific for a particular HLA allele group; they are usually HLA locus-specific. Originally, PCR-SSOP for HLA typing required DNA to be separated into its single strands, immobilized on suitable membrane, and reacted sequentially with probes of different specificity. Probes with the complementary sequence of the DNA under investigation would bind and be detected via its fluorescent tag. Since the late 1990s, the PCR-SSOP has been modified so that the probes are immobilized on nylon membranes or fluorescently labelled microbeads. The PCR amplification involves the incorporation of **biotin** into the amplicons so that it can be detected with a **streptavidin** coupled label, such as **phycoerythrin (PE)**. The HLA type is determined by analysis of the reactivity with the panel of specific probes. The resolution of typing by PCR-SSOP can be varied by the number of probes used and medium-to-high resolution typing can be obtained using this approach. Sequence specific oligonucleotide probes is not normally suited to rapid typing as required for deceased donor testing, but is well suited to typing large numbers of individuals, as required for donor registry typing.

3. *Sequence Based Typing* (PCR-SBT): this is currently the gold standard of HLA typing that can give allelic level typing but is more costly and time consuming than PCR-SSP or PCR-SSOP. The SBT approach to HLA typing involves determining the nucleotide sequence of the HLA alleles of an individual. However, to save time and cost, the sequencing is usually restricted to the region of greatest polymorphism, the peptide binding cleft, in HLA class I genes. Exons 2 and 3 code for this region of the molecule. In HLA class II molecules, exon 2 codes for the peptide binding cleft.

4. *Next Generation Sequencing* (NGS): in the past few years NGS has begun to impact on HLA typing (Hosomichi et al., 2015 Further Reading) and Chapter 2 for a description of NGS techniques.

Biotin

A water-soluble B complex vitamin, necessary for the growth of the cell, production of fatty acids, and metabolism of protein and fat. It is used in the laboratory because it interacts strongly with streptavidin. Thus molecules labelled with biotin can be detected with streptavidin conjugated to a reporter molecule.

Streptavidin

A bacterial protein purified from *Streptomyces avidinii* that has a high affinity for biotin.

Phycoerythrin (PE)

A red protein found in red algae and cyanobacteria. It is used as a fluorescent label for antibodies used in the laboratory for the detection of specific markers on cell surfaces, in the cytoplasm, or on DNA, by utilizing its ability to absorb blue green light and emit orange-yellow light (475 ± 10 nm).

Key points

The first HLA typing methods were serological detection of cell surface HLA molecules on lymphocytes. This has been largely replaced by DNA-based HLA typing using methods such as sequence specific primer (PCR-SSP), sequence specific oligonucleotide probes (PCR-SSOP), and sequence based typing (PCR-SBT).

Human leucocyte antigen antibody detection and definition

Human leucocyte antigen antibodies can be produced in response to pregnancy, blood transfusion, and transplantation. The route of immunization can affect the type of antibody that can be detected.

Human leucocyte antigen typing (LCT/CDC)

The LCT technique described for HLA typing is the same as was originally used for antibody screening but, in this process, the panel of well-characterized sera is replaced by a panel of HLA-typed donor lymphocytes, which is employed to detect antibody of unknown specificity. Many laboratories employ an extended incubation time to increase sensitivity, that is, 60 minutes for cells and serum followed by 120 minutes after the addition of complement. This extra time allows the detection of low-affinity or low-titre antibodies.

The procedure has remained popular because it is simple, reproducible, and relatively inexpensive, but cannot detect non-complement fixing antibodies that are also clinically significant, and is probably the least sensitive technique available. False positive reaction can occur when testing patients receiving antibody therapy such as anti-thymocyte globulin (ATG) or anti-CD3 therapy.

BOX 9.3 Human leucocyte antigen typing resolution

The level of typing used to discriminate between HLA molecules:

Low resolution typing; serological or antigen level typing HLA-DR12 or HLA-DRB1*12

Medium resolution typing; molecular typing that identifies a group or string of alleles belonging to the same antigenic group, for example HLA-DRB1*12:01/12:06/12:10/12:17

High resolution typing; molecular typing that identifies a single or group of alleles that share the same sequence of the peptide binding cleft that interacts with the T cell receptor, for example HLA-DRB1* 12:01/12:06/12:10/12:17

Allele level typing; molecular typing that identifies the specific HLA allele, for example HLA-DRB1*12:01

Enzyme-linked immunosorbent assay (ELISA)

In the ELISA technique, purified HLA antigen is immobilized on the surface of a 96-well plate. Patient serum or plasma is added to the plate and incubated to allow antibody–antigen binding to take place. Excess serum is washed off and an anti-human immunoglobulin conjugated to an enzyme, such as horseradish peroxidise, is added. This binds to any HLA antibody-antigen complex and when the enzyme substrate is added, the breakdown of the substrate is linked to a colour change which can be read in an ELISA reader.

The method of antigen preparation can determine whether the ELISA can be used for screening or antibody definition of specificity. Pooled antigen stripped from the surface of platelets or cells and purified has been used to manufacture antibody screening kits but will only indicate the presence or absence of HLA-specific antibody. Antigen isolated from individual cell lines, but not pooled, has been one approach used to manufacture antibody specificity definition kits and mimics the cell panel approach used in the LCT technique.

Enzyme-linked immunosorbent assay is also a relatively simple technique, with an objective readout and is amenable to testing large batches of samples. This technique can indicate the presence of HLA-specific antibody as it is not affected by non-HLA antibodies such as ATG. There is always the possibility with any technique that does not use antigen in its native form that the isolation, purification, and immobilization procedure may expose epitopes not normally seen in the native antigen.

Flow cytometry

The flow cytometry method uses the same principle of the LCT and ELISA methods; a panel of HLA typed lymphocytes or purified HLA molecules immobilized on beads is mixed with patient sera or plasma and incubated to allow antibody binding to take place. The detection of bound antibody is achieved using a fluorescently labelled anti-human Ig antibody. The most common labels used are fluorescein and phycoerythrin (PE).

In the flow cytometer, the cell suspension is passed through a laser, which excites the fluorescent tag on the cell surface. The excited tag emits light at a specific wavelength governed by the fluorescent label used and is detected and measured by the machine.

Luminex

A new type of solid phase technique using Luminex technology has been the most widely used technique for both HLA-specific antibody detection and definition of specificity. In this system, fluorochrome-dyed polystyrene beads are coated with specific HLA antigens, which are then used to detect the antibodies in the serum or plasma. The precise ratio of these fluorochromes creates 100 distinctly coloured beads, each of them coated with a different antigen. The beads are then incubated with the patient's serum and specific antibody bound to the beads is detected by the addition of a PE-conjugated antihuman IgG (Fc specific) antibody. The resulting positive or negative reactions are read using a Luminex analyser, which consists of two lasers. One laser can distinguish between up to 100 different beads sets in a single tube, and the other detects PE label bound to the HLA antibody-antigen complex.

Antibody detection using Luminex is now widely used and it has been shown to be more sensitive than either CDC or ELISA, although the clinical benefit of this increased sensitivity is not yet clearly defined, particularly in the transplant setting.

Key points

Human leucocyte antigen antibodies can be produced in response to pregnancy, blood transfusion, and transplantation. Techniques for antibody screening and identification include the LCT technique, the ELISA technique using purified HLA antigen, and flow cytometry using the same principle as the LCT and ELISA methods. A new type of solid phase technique using Luminex technology is now widely used.

9.4 Clinical significance of human leucocyte antigens in transplantation

The importance of the HLA system in transplantation was first seen in renal transplantation, where it was observed that graft survival was improved in transplants between siblings, when compared to unrelated stem cell or deceased solid organ donors. In solid transplants between parents and children where only one HLA haplotype is shared, graft survival was observed to be at a level between that seen in identical sibling and deceased donor transplants.

Data from all solid organ transplants in the UK are collated by NHSBT ODT (Organ Donation and Transplant). Internationally, bodies such as the Collaborative Transplant Study (CTS) based in Europe, or the United Network for Organ Sharing (UNOS) in the USA have all shown the benefits of HLA matching, through analysis of the outcome of thousands of transplants. Independently, many of these studies have shown a hierarchy in the effect of the different HLA loci on graft survival, where HLA-DR matching is shown to be the most beneficial when compared to HLA-A or B matching.

Solid organ transplantation

There is a significant shortfall in the number of available donor organs to recipients. This has necessitated research into the potential use of xenotransplantation from transgenic animals (see Section 9.7) In the UK, consent is required from relatives of the deceased to donate organs for transplant, but in July 2013 the government of Wales adopted a system of presumed consent, where an individual would need to opt out of organ donation should they so desire. See Table 9.4 for the numbers of different types of solid organ transplants in the UK. In many European countries (24 including, e.g. Spain, Belgium, Austria), the adoption of presumed consent has been highly effective in increasing the number of available organs for transplant. This chapter is focused on the laboratory management of organ mismatch, and the reader is referred to further resources (Watson & Dark, 2012, Further Reading) for greater details on the pathologies that require solid organ transplantation and resultant immunosuppression.

The importance of HLA in solid organ transplantation differs with the type of organs transplanted and is discussed later in the chapter. The immediate problem with transplanting an organ is the presence of pre-formed HLA and ABO blood group antibodies, which can cause the rapid rejection of the organ. Therefore, prior to transplantation every effort is made to detect and define donor-specific antibodies and, where possible, the HLA type of the donor and recipient is matched to limit graft rejection.

TABLE 9.4 Numbers of solid organ transplants in the UK 2014–2016

Transplant type	2015–2016	2014–2015
Kidney (total)	3265	3122
Pancreas	230	244
Kidney & pancreas	167	173
Pancreas islets	31	23
Heart	194	180
Lungs	182	185
Heart & lung	6	1
Liver	855	830
Intestine	15	24
Other	26	17
Cornea	3731	3343

Types of rejection

Organ rejection can be categorized as hyperacute, acute, and chronic. *Hyperacute rejection* occurs when there is irreversible damage to the transplanted organ within minutes or hours due to the presence of preformed circulating antibodies, primarily directed against ABO blood group antigens or HLA class I antigens on the endothelial cells of the graft. Antibody–antigen interaction can result in the activation of the complement system, leading to cell lysis, but also to the formation of clots, leading to ischaemia and infarction of the graft. The incidence of hyperacute rejection can be limited by performing extensive characterization of the patient's pre-transplant serum to detect the presence of donor-specific antibodies, and performing a crossmatch with the patient's serum against donor lymphocytes. A positive crossmatch, due to donor-specific IgG antibodies, would normally be a contraindication to transplantation for organs such as kidney and pancreas, but there are now methods to transplant organs in the presence of donor-specific antibodies. Human leucocyte antigen-specific antibody incompatible transplants (AiT) have been performed, but require the careful monitoring of antibody levels and specificity, in conjunction with a protocol to reduce antibody levels.

Acute rejection is primarily a cellular event where the mismatched HLA molecules on the graft serve as targets for cytotoxic T lymphocytes. Human leucocyte antigen molecules can be recognized by T cells directly or indirectly: direct allorecognition occurs when recipient T cells recognize peptides, derived from the graft and presented by donor antigen-presenting cells; indirect allorecognition involves the patient's own antigen-presenting cell processing and presenting peptides, derived from the kidney allograft, to alloreactive T lymphocytes.

Using kidney transplantation as an example, direct allorecognition occurs when donor antigen-presenting cells, such as dendritic cells, migrate from the graft to a local lymph node, where they stimulate alloreactive T cells. These T cells can mediate graft destruction if untreated.

Human leucocyte antigen-specific antibodies can also be associated with acute rejection as studies, which demonstrate plasma cells and T cells infiltrating the rejecting allograft have shown. The donor-specific antibodies are normally formed *de novo* following transplantation and can damage the graft via the activation of complement, or through antibody-dependent, cell-mediated cytotoxicity (ADCC), whereby the antibodies coat graft cells and immune effector cells cause graft damage via interaction with antibody Fc binding. Acute rejection usually occurs within the first three months following transplantation, but can occur within days, and can be limited by HLA-matching and the use of immunosuppressive drugs.

Chronic rejection can be caused by immunological and non-immunological factors and results in a slow deterioration in graft function, occurring months to years following transplantation. Both donor-specific antibody and T lymphocytes have been implicated in mediating this chronic deterioration in graft function. In kidney allografts, it is characterized by fibrous intimal thickening of the arteries, interstitial fibrosis, and atrophy of the renal tubules. Studies have also shown that an increased number and severity of acute rejection episodes is a risk factor for developing features of chronic rejection. Other non-immunological factors, which have been shown to be associated with chronic rejection, include how the organ is preserved and perfusion when the organ is harvested, recipient factors such as infection, hypertension and drug toxicity, donor age, and organ tissue quality.

SELF-CHECK 9.3

What is the importance of HLA typing in solid organ transplantation?

Renal transplant allocation

In the UK kidneys are normally allocated on the basis of blood group and HLA type, where priority is given to donor-recipient pairs showing no (0) mismatch at HLA-A, B, and DRB1, that is, 000 mismatched. Paediatric patients are given first priority, then the level of sensitization is taken into account. Other factors considered in the allocation algorithm are: waiting time, HLA match and age combined, donor-recipient age difference, location of the patient relative to the donor, HLA-DRB1 and HLA-B homozygosity, and blood group match. These factors are considered to, where possible:

- Prevent a patient waiting for a transplant for many years.

- Avoid an 'old' kidney being grafted into a young recipient.

- Reduce **cold ischaemia time**, which has been shown to be a risk factor in graft survival, by keeping a short distance between where the organs are harvested to where they are implanted.

Those patients that are HLA homozygous and, therefore, require a homozygous donor for a 000 mismatched graft are also given access to these very useful donors. Finally, although transplants should be blood group compatible, an effort is made to match blood group so that O group donors are given to O group patients, where possible.

Cold ischaemia time
During transplantation this time begins when the organ is cooled with a cold perfusion solution after organs are harvested and ends after the tissue reaches physiological temperature during the implantation procedure.

Pancreas transplant allocation

Blood group matching is a priority for the pancreas allocation. A number of clinically relevant patient, donor, and transplant-associated factors are used to award the patient points, resulting in an individual total points score (TPS). The number of points each patient has is used to rank them in terms of priority for transplantation. Matching at HLA-A, B, and DR, HLA sensitization, time waiting for a transplant list, and factors previously mentioned that are used for kidney allocation, all contribute to a patient's TPS.

CLINICAL CORRELATION

The HLA-matching scheme used in the allocation of kidneys in the UK initially takes into account polymorphism at the *HLA-A,-B,* and *DRB1* loci:

000   No mismatch at HLA-A, B, or DR

010   One HLA-B mismatch

100   One HLA-A mismatch

110   Two mismatches (1 × HLA-A, 1 × HLA-B)

Sensitization to HLA-A, B, C, DR, DQ, and DP is considered prior to crossmatching and transplantation.

Heart and lung transplant allocation

Retrospective studies have shown that HLA matching, particularly for *HLA-DRB1*, has a beneficial effect on graft survival. However, there are a number of factors that prevent the prospective HLA matching of hearts in the UK:

- Physical size of the heart compared to the recipient is important.
- Small donor pool.
- Relatively small patient waiting list.
- Short cold ischaemia time (hearts should be transplanted within four hours of harvesting).

Lung transplants have similar restrictions and organ allocation protocols that apply to heart transplantation. In some cases, the heart and lungs are transplanted as a block.

Liver transplant allocation

Livers are allocated on the basis of blood group compatibility and matching of O group donors for O group patients, where possible. Human leucocyte antigen matching plays no role in the allocation of livers for transplantation.

Cornea transplant matching

The eye is often described as an immunologically privileged site, being protected from the normal effects of the immune system. No HLA matching is performed for first corneal transplants, but, if the graft is rejected, HLA sensitization is taken into account for subsequent grafts as vascularization has usually occurred, meaning the cornea is accessible to the recipient's cellular and humoral immune system.

Crossmatching

The presence of donor-specific HLA antibodies has been shown to be important in hyperacute, acute, and chronic rejection and it is recommended that, where possible, a pre-transplant crossmatch be performed prior to transplantation. The logistical issues associated with cardiothoracic transplantation (see heart and lung transplant allocation) means that it is not always possible to perform a pre-transplant crossmatch in the laboratory. Instead, a 'virtual crossmatch' is performed, whereby the HLA mismatch between the patient and donor and the

HLA antibody screening history of the patient is formally assessed to avoid pre-formed donor-specific antibodies. This practice is also applied to a well-defined category of renal patients, namely, patients who are not sensitized to HLA and have a full and current sensitization history.

The crossmatch test is designed to partially reproduce, *in vitro*, what will happen *in vivo* when the organ is transplanted, by 'bathing' donor cells in patient's serum. The LCT and/or flow cytometry techniques are most widely used for solid organ transplantation. Patient serum samples, selected to represent the sensitization history of the patient, are mixed with donor cells, from peripheral blood in live donors (or prior to organ retrieval for deceased donors) and lymph node or spleen cells from deceased donors. The T and B lymphocyte populations can be isolated prior to the LCT crossmatch or labelled with lineage-specific conjugated antibodies as part of the flow cytometric crossmatch, and the patient's own lymphocytes can be tested to allow detection of autoreactive antibodies, which can aid interpretation of the crossmatch results. The techniques used are the same as described previously for LCT and flow cytometry.

Interpretation of the crossmatch is usually performed in conjunction with information from the antibody screening history and sensitization events. T cell-positive crossmatches could be due to HLA class I-specific antibodies or autoantibodies. B cell positive crossmatches can be due to the presence of HLA class II, but B cells also express high levels of HLA class I, which can detect antibody that are not detectable using T cells alone. Therefore, it is important to have an accurate antibody profile of the patient prior to embarking on crossmatching as this may prevent unexplained positive crossmatches, which could potentially increase the cold ischaemia time of the organ whilst another recipient is found for the organ.

Key points

Organ rejection can be minimized by HLA typing, matching, and crossmatching.

Rejection can be categorized as:

Hyperacute, occurring within minutes or hours of the transplant.

Acute, usually occurring within days up to the first three months following transplantation.

Chronic, slow deterioration of graft function, occurring months to years following transplantation.

Haemopoietic stem cell transplantation

Haemopoietic stem cell transplantation (HSCT) is the treatment of choice for a variety of haematological malignancies, primary immunodeficiencies, inborn errors of metabolism, and bone marrow disorders. Haemopoietic stem cells for transplantation can be derived from bone marrow, peripheral blood, or umbilical cord blood, and the source of stem cell used can be dependent on the disorder to be treated, which also can influence the type of donor used, for example HLA matched or mismatched (see Box 9.4).

Studies in Western Europe show that most patients have a 30% chance of finding an HLA identical sibling donor. Figure 9.4 shows that patients with siblings have a 1 in 4 chance of being HLA identical.It also shows the potential for the generation of new haplotypes due to crossing over or recombination. The best outcomes for HSCT in terms of overall survival are seen in HLA identical sibling transplants as they may also be matched for products of non-HLA genes. If no suitable family donor is available, a search for an unrelated donor is performed, first nationally, then, if no suitable match is found, internationally. See Figure 9.5.

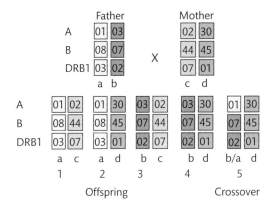

FIGURE 9.4

Human leucocyte antigen inheritance. Human leucocyte antigen genes are inherited en bloc and a set of genes on one chromosome are known as a haplotype. Each offspring inherits one paternal and one maternal haplotype, giving four possible haplotype combinations. However, there are rare occasions when there is reciprocal exchange of DNA between homologous chromosomes during meiosis or crossing over leading to a recombinant haplotype as seen in offspring 5.

In the UK, the National Registries include: the British Bone Marrow Registry (BBMR) (part of NHSBT), which recruits blood donors in England, Scotland, and Northern Ireland; the Anthony Nolan Trust, which is a charity that recruits donors throughout the UK; and the Welsh Bone Marrow Registry, which only recruits donors from Wales. Bone Marrow Donors Worldwide (BMDW) facilitates donor searches throughout the world by holding data of over 17 million donors from 64 HSC registries in 44 countries and 44 cord blood banks in 26 countries. More registries and cord banks are added every year.

The HLA matching requirements for adult unrelated stem transplantation are more stringent than those used for solid organ transplantation or platelet transfusions. Haemopoietic stem cell transplantation involves transfusing **immunocompetent** cells into an immunosuppressed recipient. Any HLA mismatches could be recognized as foreign by the donor lymphocytes and

Immunocompetent
The ability to produce an immune response following a challenge with an antigen.

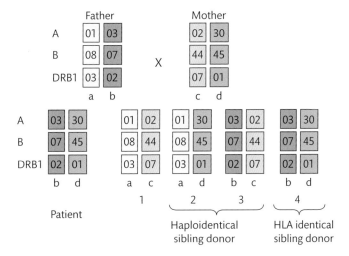

FIGURE 9.5

Human leucocyte antigen matching. An HLA identical sibling is the ideal donor as they share the same haplotypes inherited from their parents. Haploidentical transplants can be between parents or siblings that share one haplotype with the patient, in this example, siblings 2 and 3 and the parent share one HLA haplotype with the patient.

lead to graft versus host disease (GvHD), which can be fatal. Most centres would aim to match for both alleles at the five loci (*HLA-A*, *B*, *C*, *DRB1*, and *DQB1*), so they describe a fully matched donor as a 10 out of 10 match, and would aim to achieve at least a 9 out of 10 match. Human leucocyte antigen-DP is taken into account by some transplant centres where there is a choice between equally matched donors. Since HLA-DP is not in **linkage disequilibrium** with HLA-DR, it is often mismatched, but this HLA mismatch on the patient's cells may also serve as a target for the graft versus leukaemia (GVL) effect.

The lymphocytes present in cord blood are more naive and not as immunocompetent as adult lymphocytes and this has been used in part to explain the lower incidence and milder severity of GvHD seen in cord blood transplants compared to adult stem cell transplants. The two main factors influencing the outcome of cord blood transplantation are HLA matching and haemopoietic stem cell dose. The level of HLA matching is not as stringent for cord blood transplantation and Eurocord studies show that up to two mismatches at the *HLA-A* or *B* loci can be tolerated, but the cell dose must be increased where mismatching takes place. The minimum matching requirements are high resolution for *HLA-DRB1* and low-to-medium resolution for *HLA-A* and *B*. As more data become available, better outcomes are seen where high-resolution typing is performed for HLA class I in addition to HLA class II.

Human leucocyte antigen mismatching can have a crucial effect on transplant outcome so it is important that the HLA laboratory performs the appropriate level of typing, and that the reports and advice are relevant for the type of transplant.

Other factors influencing donor selection for HSCT include:

Cytomegalovirus (CMV) status:	match the CMV status of donor and recipient if possible.
Age:	transplant outcomes are better with young donors <30 years old.
Male donors:	as male donors have both X and Y chromosomes their T cells do not see sex chromosome products as foreign, but T cells from female donors can recognize male HY minor histocompatibility antigens as foreign.

Linkage disequilibrium
The tendency of certain alleles at different loci to occur on the same chromosome more often than expected by chance, for example HLA-A*01-B*08-DRB1*03:01 are in positive linkage disequilibrium as the observed frequency of this haplotype is greater than the expected frequency.

Post-transplantation chimerism testing

There are a number of ways to assess engraftment or disease re-occurrence following allogeneic HSCT. One of the most sensitive methods used by histocompatibility and immunogenetics laboratories employs the use of short tandem repeat (STR) markers with allele sizes that differ among individuals. The pre-transplant genotypes of the recipient and donors are established and samples taken from the recipient post-HSCT are tested to determine the presence of donor material. Where the recipient sample consists of 100% donor DNA, it is referred to as full donor chimerism, or mixed chimerism where both recipient and donor DNA are detected.

HSCT for malignant disease often involves myeloablative conditioning using total body irradiation and/or chemotherapy. In these cases, the aim is to achieve full donor chimerism as the presence of any recipient cells may potentially result in the malignancy returning. Mixed chimerism may be satisfactory if the haematological disorder does not require full donor chimerism. For example, in the case of some haemoglobinopathies or enzyme deficiencies, there may be a minimum number of donor cells required to produce enough cells carrying the corrected haemoglobin or enzyme to counteract the effects of the defect.

> **BOX 9.4** Human leucocyte antigen matching for haemopoietic stem cell transplantation
>
> Most adult unrelated stem cell transplant programmes match for: HLA-A, B, C, DRB1, and DQB1 and aim to achieve a 10/10 or 9/10 match using high-resolution HLA typing.
>
> Cord blood transplant programmes also aim to match for the same HLA loci as adult stem cell programmes, but the minimum requirement is to match for: HLA-A, B, DRB1 and aim to achieve a 6/6, 5/6, or 4/6 match using high-resolution typing for HLA-DRB1 and low-to-medium resolution for HLA-A and B.

9.5 Clinical significance of human leucocyte antigens in transfusion

Immunological refractoriness to random platelet transfusions

Many patients with haematological disorders and some cancers require transfusion support (red cells and platelets) due to the disease itself or the side effects of its treatment. A normal platelet count can range from $150 \times 10^9/l$ to $400 \times 10^9/l$ but, when the count falls below $30 \times 10^9/l$, there is a risk of bleeding. Patients with low levels of platelets are transfused with donor platelets until they regain the ability to produce their own platelets.

Both pooled or single donor platelets are leucodepleted and have the same average number of platelets. Therefore, stable patients transfused with either product should have a rise in platelet count of between 30 and $40 \times 10^9/l$. In approximately 30–50% of transfusion-dependent patients, there is not an adequate rise in platelet count following transfusion. These patients are described as **refractory** to random platelet transfusion. Platelet refractoriness is defined as the failure of the transfused patient to gain adequate platelet increments ($<10 \times 10^9/l$), one hour or up to 24 hours post-transfusion. The causes can be immune-related or non-immune.

Non-immune causes include:

- Old or badly stored platelets
- Sepsis
- Disseminated intravascular coagulation in the patient
- Drugs such as amphotericin B, ciprofloxacin

Immune causes include:

- Human leucocyte antigen class I specific antibodies
- Human platelet antigens (HPA) specific antibodies
- High titre ABO alloantibodies

Most cases of immunological refractoriness are due to HLA class I-specific antibodies, which will bind to transfused platelets that express the cognate HLA class molecules. Cells of the monocyte/macrophage system will, in turn, recognize the antibody complex via the Fc region and remove the platelets from circulation. Human platelet antigen antibody-mediated destruction follows the same mechanism. ABO-mismatched platelets transfused into allo-immunized patients can result in a 20% reduction in the platelet increments post-transfusion. Circulating immune complexes involving the ABO system have also been shown to decrease the survival of transfused platelets.

Laboratory investigation of refractory patients involves:

- Screening the patient's serum for the presence of HLA-specific antibodies
- Definition of HLA antibody specificity
- Human leucocyte antigen class I typing of patient and donors
- Provision of HLA selected platelets

Although platelets express HLA-class I, the expression of HLA-C is lower than HLA-A or HLA-B on cells and poorly expressed on platelets. Therefore, most laboratories only match for HLA A and B. In addition, HLA-B and C are closely co-located on the chromosome and, as such, are usually inherited together, so matching for HLA-B can often result in matching for HLA-C.

Serological crossreactivity
This is where antibodies react with a public epitope shared by different HLA molecules. These HLA molecules that share a public epitope are often described as cross reactive groups (CREG), for example anti-HLA-B7 antibodies, can crossreact with a shared epitope on HLA-B42, B55, and B56.

The provision of HLA selected platelets is based on the HLA type of the patient and their HLA antibody profile using a panel of HLA typed donors. The matching system used for the provision of HLA selected platelets is different to that used for solid organ or haemopoietic stem cell transplantation. The NHSBT matching criteria are based on two grades of matches, see Box 9.5.

- 'A' grade, where there is no mismatch between donor and recipient.
- 'B' grade, where patient and donor are mismatched, with the number of mismatches denoting the type of B match, for example B1 for one mismatch, B2 for two mismatches, etc. Mismatching is carried out on the basis of the known **serological crossreactivity** that exists between different antigens of the HLA-A and B loci.

Key points

Platelet refractoriness is the failure to gain adequate platelet increments ($<10 \times 10^9/l$), one hour or up to 24 hours post-transfusion. The causes can be non-immune or immune due to HLA, HPA, or ABO antibodies.

BOX 9.5 *Human leucocyte antigens matching for platelet transfusion*

'A' grade match:

Patient:	HLA-A*01, A*02; B*08, B*44	
Donor 1:	HLA-A*01, A*02; B*08, B*44	No mismatch
Donor 2:	HLA-A*01, A*01; B*08, B*08	No mismatch

'B' grade match:

Patient:	HLA-A*01, A*02; B*08, B*44	
Donor 1:	HLA-A*01, A*11; B*08, B*44	B1 match (one mismatch)
Donor 2:	HLA-A*01, A*11; B*08, B*49	B2 match (two mismatches)

Febrile non-haemolytic transfusion reactions (FNHTRs)

Febrile non-haemolytic transfusion reactions (FNHTRs) are some of the most common transfusion reactions and are characterized by fever, chills, and a rise in temperature of more than 1 or 2°C, occurring during or 30–60 minutes following the transfusion. Other symptoms, such as rigor, flushing, increased heart beat rate (tachycardia), nausea, and vomiting can also be present.

Febrile non-haemolytic transfusion reactions can be triggered by a variety of factors. Human leucocyte antigen or HNA antibodies, present in the recipient and reacting with white blood cells in the transfused product, have been shown to be the main immunological trigger of these reactions, and antibodies against white cells are found in 70% or more of patients who suffer from FNHTRs. In most cases, it is likely that the antibody–antigen complex may directly activate the cells to produce pyrogenic cytokines leading to the febrile reaction.

A number of studies have reported that the incidence of FNHTR is reduced when the white cells are removed from the transfused product by leucodepletion. The decreased number of leucocytes not only presents fewer targets for leucocyte-reactive antibodies, but also reduces the probability of sensitization in the non-sensitized patient.

Universal leucodepletion was introduced in England in October 1999, but cases of FNHTR have still been reported. It is likely that some of these reactions are due to an accumulation of cytokines released by the residual white cells in the stored blood component, especially in platelet concentrates.

Transfusion-related acute lung injury (TRALI)

Transfusion-related acute lung injury (TRALI) is a rare but life-threatening complication of blood transfusion where the patient experiences respiratory distress within 2–6 hours following a transfusion. Symptoms generally include fever, hypotension, chills, cyanosis, non-productive cough, dyspnoea, and sometimes severe hypoxia. Chest X-ray shows severe bilateral pulmonary oedema or perihilar and lung infiltration, without cardiac enlargement or involvement of the vessels.

The mechanism of action

Most cases of confirmed TRALI are associated with the presence of HLA class I or class II antibodies in the plasma of the transfused component, with specificities corresponding to the HLA antigen(s) present in the recipient. Granulocyte-specific antibodies, for example anti-HNA1, HNA-2, and HNA-3 have also been implicated (see Chapter 6). These antibodies are most commonly found in blood and blood components donated by women who have had multiple pregnancies.

Products that contain a significant proportion of plasma, such as whole blood, platelets and fresh frozen plasma (FFP), and even the small amount of plasma in red cells in optimal additive solution (e.g. SAGM), have been implicated in some TRALI reactions.

Transfusion-related acute lung injury cases have also been reported where no HLA or granulocyte antibodies have been detected. These reactions also appear to be mediated by a soluble lipid substance, which accumulates during the storage. Animal studies have shown that these soluble lipids are biologically active and can activate granulocytes to induce the release of anaphylatoxins, cytokines, and chemokines, which promote neutrophil chemotaxis and aggregation in the lungs. The resulting reaction causes endothelial damage and increased pulmonary vascular permeability, resulting in fluid leakage into the alveoli and an accumulation of fluid in the lungs (oedema).

Look-back studies have shown that products from donors implicated in TRALI reactions have been transfused into other patients with no reported serious clinical consequences, suggesting that other factors, such as the predisposing clinical condition of the recipient, may influence the initiation of TRALI. These observations have led to the proposal of the 'two hit' hypothesis for the development of TRALI. The first hit involves the action of antibodies or soluble mediators and the second hit involves the influence of the clinical condition of the patient.

Treatment of TRALI includes intensive respiratory and circulatory support. In almost all cases, oxygen supplementation is necessary, although mechanical ventilation may not always be required. The majority of patients improve both clinically and physiologically within two or three days with adequate supportive care and, once recovered, there is no residual damage in these patients. Mortality still remains at 6%, however.

Transfusion-related acute lung injury reduction

The English National Blood Service and other blood services around the world have introduced changes in the manufacture of blood components, with the aim of reducing the incidence of TRALI. These measures take into account that HLA and granulocyte antibodies in blood components primarily originate from female donors who have been sensitized by pregnancy.

The TRALI reduction measures include:

• The production of FFP from donations collected from male donors.

• The use of male donor plasma to re-suspend pooled platelets.

• The preferential recruitment of male apheresis donors such that, from 2008, 80% of all apheresis platelets collected by NHSBT were from male donors.

• Human leucocyte antigen and HNA antibody screening of all new female apheresis donors added to the panel.

Transfusion-associated graft versus host disease (TA-GvHD)

Transfusion-associated graft versus host disease (TA-GvHD) is a rare but fatal adverse reaction to transfusion. Acute GvHD, usually associated with allogeneic haemopoietic stem cell transplantation, and TA-GvHD share similar features, but there are important differences. Both types of GvHD result from the presence of viable lymphocytes in the allograft or transfusion recognizing the host mismatched HLA molecules. These donor lymphocytes must be immunocompetent and share one HLA haplotype with the host; the donor is commonly HLA homozygous and is not recognized by the host as foreign.

Clinically, the GvHD reactions are similar, affecting the skin, liver, and gut, but TA-GvHD differs in that it occurs much sooner (normally 8–10 days following transfusion) and over 90% of TA-GvHD cases are fatal, whereas HSCT GvHD can be treated successfully.

The diagnosis of TA-GvHD mainly depends on finding evidence of donor-derived DNA in the blood and/or affected tissues of the recipient, known as detection of chimerism. Using

DNA analysis allows a wider range of markers to be employed, including HLA genes or other genetic markers.

The chimerism test requires DNA to be extracted from recipient samples taken pre- and post-transfusion and from samples of the implicated donors. DNA can be extracted from skin (both affected and unaffected areas), hair follicles, or nail clippings. Post-mortem samples from the spleen or bone marrow, if available, can also be used as a source of DNA. If donor chimerism can be detected in the patient, it can be used to confirm the diagnosis of TA-GvHD.

As there is no effective treatment of TA-GvHD and the mortality rate is extremely high, a lot of effort is put into preventing its occurrence. Although the introduction of universal leucodepletion in the UK has been associated with a significant reduction in the number of reported cases of TA-GvHD, the residual lymphocyte numbers may still be enough to initiate TA-GvHD.

Irradiation of cellular blood components renders the donor lymphocytes non-viable and protects the recipient from potentially developing TA-GvHD. It is recommended that all cellular blood products for at risk patients should be irradiated with a minimum of 25 Gray (Gy), prior to transfusion. See Chapter 5 for more on irradiated blood components.

SELF-CHECK 9.4

What measures have transfusion services introduced to reduce the incidence of HLA-related adverse effects of transfusion?

Key points

Human leucocyte antigen antibody-mediated complications of transfusions include febrile non-haemolytic transfusion reactions, TRALI (caused by HLA antibodies present in the donor), and TA-GvHD (resulting from the presence of viable lymphocytes in the allograft or transfusion recognizing the host mismatched HLA molecules).

9.6 Immunosuppression

Immunosuppression treatment is the norm for patients receiving solid organ transplants, and for the treatment of certain autoimmune diseases (e.g. Crohn's, Systemic Lupus Erythematosus (SLE)). It is not the objective of this chapter to provide a comprehensive list of the various drugs licensed for immunosuppressive treatment, but to give a broad overview of their mechanisms of action especially relating to the key components of the immune system, both at cellular and molecular levels. Monoclonal antibodies directed against both cytokines released by immune cells (for example anti-TNFα; anti-IL1β) are licensed for use, as well as those directed against cell surface components (for example the IL-2 receptor, CD25, and anti-CD52 CAMPATH-1H). These monoclonal antibodies' mode of action is to blockade the binding of natural ligands (e.g. IL-2 binding to its receptor IL-2R), and to prevent the interactions of cells (e.g. binding to the T-cell receptor complex CD3). See Figure 9.6 for some examples. At the molecular level, a wide variety of immunosuppressive drugs are available whose mode of action is well characterized. Again, they are used to suppress the immune response by blockading intracellular pathways that lead to the production of immunostimulatory cytokines or the proliferation of these cells. Examples are shown in Figures 9.6 and 9.7.

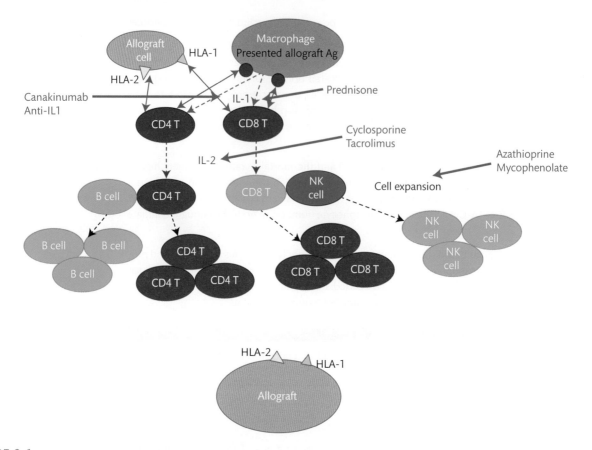

FIGURE 9.6
Cellular responses to antigens on allografts and their immunosuppression. Sites of action of selected immunosuppressants are shown in light blue. The HLA class 1 and 2 antigens on the allograft drive a cellular response via CD8 T cells (HLA-1) or CD4 T cells (HLA-2). This response leads to the synthesis of specific cytokines IL-1 and -2.

To briefly describe these intracellular signalling pathways, ligation of the T-cell receptor complex CD3 ($\alpha,\beta,\gamma,\varepsilon_2$) triggers the binding of immunophilins (e.g. the FK506 binding protein (FKBP)) to calcineurin, which in turns triggers the phosphorylation of NFAT (nuclear factor of activated T cells) which induces its translocation to the nucleus. Here phosphoNFAT drives the expression of a number of genes, including the major interleukin, IL-2, which when released from the T cell induces expansion of other immune cells. IL-2 binding to a T-cell receptor drives a sequence of signalling events through mTOR (mammalian target of rapamycin) following binding of an immunophilin (see Figure 9.7). This then pushes the cell to proliferate through the cell cycle, and requires a plentiful supply of nucleotides to do so.

All of these processes are targets of immunosuppressive drugs. Mycophenolate and Leflunomide suppress nucleotide synthesis and sirolimus binds to the immunophilin FKBP preventing its association to mTOR. In the calcineurin pathway cyclosporine and tacrolimus (further FKBP binding proteins) prevent the phosphorylation of NFAT, and thus its translocation to the nucleus and eventual switch on of key immune response genes (e.g. IL-2).

Immunosuppressive drugs are highly effective, but not without consequences as may be expected when the immune system is suppressed, as the individuals become immunocompromised. There is a higher incidence of cancer and infection due to the decreased immune surveillance, but these are the price to pay to enable the graft to be tolerated by the recipient.

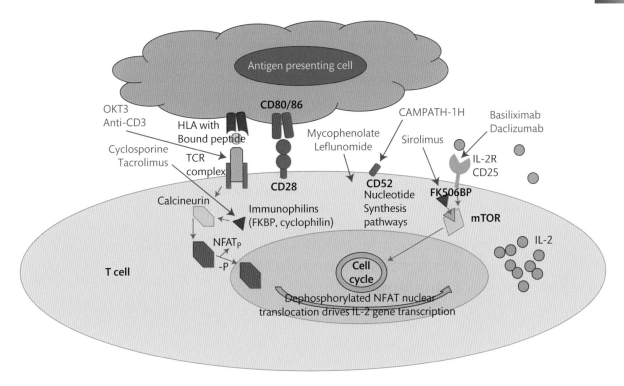

FIGURE 9.7

Cellular pathways of the T cell that are targeted by immunosuppression. The T cell interacts with an antigen-presenting cell via its T cell receptor (TCR, CD3). This leads to the stimulation of calcineurins, which in turn lead to the phosphorylation of nuclear factor of activated T cells (NFAT). This migrates to the nucleus and stimulates the expression of IL-2, a potent stimulator of T-cell proliferation. The sites of specific immunosuppressants are shown in red and described in the text.

9.7 **Xenotransplantation**

The strive to source alternate non-human organs for transplantation has been ongoing since the 1960s. This included several chimpanzee–human kidney and baboon–human heart transplants and were performed in emergency situations where there was chronic organ failure and total lack of suitable donors. All these experimental techniques resulted in failure within a year of transplant, but it was realized at this time that naturally occurring antibodies were the cause of rejection. With no further progress in the 1970s, xenotransplantation re-emerged (and with greater hope with the increased knowledge in immunology and immunosuppression) in the 1980s when baby Fae had a heart transplant from a baboon donor in 1984. Several further procedures were conducted in the 1990s including pig–human liver transplants (1995); pig islets to human transplants (1996); a baboon bone marrow transplant to a patient with AIDS (1996), and pig neural cells to 12 Parkinson's patients (1997).

For physiological compatibility, the xenografts obviously have to maintain the same functions as their human counterparts. But as we shall see there are many hurdles to overcome before this approach can ever be adopted. This area has given much impetus to the development of tissue engineering and stem cell biology using human sources. These physical obstacles, which are in themselves an illustration of the immunological challenges to any donor organ that must be overcome before there is successful engraftment, are discussed below. If the allograft were entirely successful, i.e if the following hurdles were overcome, there is still the issue of the consequential biosynthesis of the new xenograft of key hormones (e.g. the kidney is the main producer of EPO, the liver of thrombopoietin) which must also be addressed.

Hyperacute rejection—the α-galactosyl epitope

As previously mentioned, the rejection episodes observed in the 1960s were found to be due to antibody-mediated destruction of the xenografts. We can use the analogy to the transfusion reactions seen with ABO incompatibility, where naturally occurring anti-A and anti-B causes immune-mediated destruction of the transfused red cells. In all mammals except higher primates (including old world monkeys) ancestral α1,3 galactosyltransferase gene (α1,3GT) is inactivated, instead they possess the H-transferase (α1,2 fucosyl transferase, see Chapter 2). The α1,3GT produces a structure Galα1-3Galβ1-(3)4GlcNAc-R, the α-galactosyl epitope (α-Gal) at the termini of glycoconjugates in most mammals. Humans have naturally occurring anti-α-gal, and thus hyperacutely reject any xenograft that has this structure on its surface. One of the key developments of transgenic animals was to produce α1,3GT knockout pigs, in order to eliminate the α-Gal epitope on their surfaces.

Xenografts are unable to downregulate human complement

As discussed in Chapter 2 erythrocytes (and other cell types) possess a variety of complement control proteins (CCPs) that rapidly inactivate complement when it binds to their surfaces. These proteins include CD55 (decay accelerating factor, DAF), CD46 (membrane cofactor protein, MCP), and CD59 (membrane inhibitor of reactive lysis, MIRL) (see Figure 1.6). As xenografts have their species-equivalent versions of these complement control proteins on their surface they are unable to downregulate the effects of complement, and as a consequence human complement components will readily attack the xenograft. Transgenic animals thus have been produced that express human CCPs to prevent this effect.

Delayed xenograft rejection (DXR) or acute vascular rejection (AVR)

If hyperacute rejection can be avoided, then the next hurdle to overcome is DXR or AVR. This is essentially a type II endothelial activation episode, thought to be caused mainly by IgG anti-α galactosyl antibodies. This leads to the endothelial elevation of the following components: IL-1, ICAM-1, and E-selectin, which are in turn reacted against by natural killer (NK) cells and macrophages. Type 2 endothelial cell activation produces a pro-coagulant environment (increased expression of tissue factor and reduction in thrombomodulin) leading to thrombosis, which is normally physiologically controlled by tissue factor pathway inhibitor (TFPI), a component which is able to inhibit the action of coagulation component Xa. Here lies another problem for the xenograft; porcine TFPI is unable to inactivate human factor Xa, leading to inadequate control and resultant thrombotic events. Immunosuppressive therapy aimed at inhibiting the humoral B cell response is the only option here; however, α1,2GT knockout pigs should not produce anti-α galactosyl antibody responses.

Cell-mediated immune responses to xenografts

Once the barriers previously discussed (hyperacute rejection, DXR and AVR) have been overcome, then the major barrier of cell-mediated rejection of the xenograft will remain a significant hurdle. This is a very significant problem, and has not been widely studied due to the rejection episodes mentioned above. The xenograft will have a variety of different antigens (carbohydrate and protein) and HLA-1 molecules producing a wide repertoire of cellular responses (T cells to different peptide/carbohydrate antigens not found in humans; NK cells not binding appropriately to xenograft HLA-1 and not triggering their NK inhibitory receptors (KIRs)).

Xenotransplantation is therefore extremely challenging from an immunological perspective, and tissue engineering or stem cell plasticity (see Chapters 10 and 11) may represent much better alternative approaches. Despite its difficulties, xenotransplantation has given valuable information concerning the immunological processes of rejection.

SELF-CHECK 9.5

Why does xenotransplantation serve as an excellent model in our understanding of how our immune system responds to a foreign graft?

 Chapter summary

- The human leucocyte antigens play a pivotal role in the induction and regulation of immune responses as the main function of HLA molecules is the presentation of peptides derived from foreign molecules to T lymphocytes.

- A key feature of the HLA system is its extensive polymorphism which is advantageous to humans in enabling responses to a wide variety of pathogens, but presents a barrier to transplantation and some transfusions.

- The immunological complications of transplantation and transfusion such as allograft rejection, graft versus host disease, and platelet refractoriness can be limited by HLA matching. A higher degree of HLA matching is required for T cell-mediated complications such as GvHD in HSCT, compared with antibody-mediated complications such as immunological platelet refractoriness.

- The current technology used for the definition of HLA polymorphism is DNA-based molecular techniques, allowing the discrimination between different HLA alleles for HSCT or antigens for solid organ transplantation or platelet transfusion. The availability of purified single HLA molecules has revolutionized antibody detection and definition such that complex antibody reactivity can be defined in a single Luminex-based test.

- Advances in allele, antigen, and antibody definition are associated with challenges in determining the clinical relevance of this increased sensitivity.

- Immunosuppression is highly effective, but is a 'broad-brush' approach to downregulate the immune response. Side effects include increased incidence of cancer and infection.

- Xenotransplantation has taught us valuable lessons as to the interactions of grafts with all arms of the immune response from innate (e.g. inappropriate complement deactivation) to humoral and cellular responses.

Further reading

- Brown CJ & Navarrete CV. Clinical relevance of the HLA system in blood transfusion. *Vox Sang* 101 (2011), 93–105.

- Focosi D, Maggi F, Pistello M, Boggi U & Scatena F. Immunosupressive monoclonal antibodies: current and next generation. *Clin Microbiol Infect* 17 (2011), 1759–1768. Provides a comprehensive review on monoclonal antibodies used in immunosuppression.

- Hosomichi K, Shiina T, Tajima A & Inoue I. The impact of next-generation sequencing on HLA research. *J Hum Genet* 60 (2015), 665–673.

- Howell WM, Carter V & Clark B. The HLA system: immunobiology, HLA typing, antibody screening and crossmatching techniques. *J Clin Pathol* 63 (2010), 387–390.

  http://hla.alleles.org/antigens/recognised_serology.html

  http://hla.alleles.org/nomenclature/index.html

  www.ebi.ac.uk/imgt/hla/stats.html.

- Opelz G & Döhler B. Effects of human leucocyte antigen compatibility of kidney graft survival: comparative analysis of two decades. *Transplantation* 84 (2007), 137–143.

- Petersdorf EW. Optimal HLA matching in hematopoietic cell transplantation. *Curr Opin Immunol* 20 (2008), 588–593.

- Tait BD, Hudson F, Cantwell L, et al. Review article: Luminex technology for HLA antibody detection in organ transplantation. *Nephrology (Carlton)* 14 (2009), 247–254.

- Taylor C, Navarrete C & Contreras M. Immunological complications of transfusion. In: A Maniatis, P Van der Linden, & JF Hardy (eds) *Alternatives to Blood Transfusion in Transfusion Medicine*, Wiley Online Library, 2010.

- Watson CJE & Dark JH. Organ transplantation: Historical perspective and current practice. *Br J Anaesth* 108 suppl 1 (2012), i29–i42.

Discussion questions

9.1 Explain why HLA polymorphism is important to the human species.

9.2 Outline the methods available for HLA typing.

9.3 Outline the methods available for the detection of HLA antibodies.

9.4 What level of HLA matching is required for major solid organ and stem cell transplants?

Answers to the questions in this chapter are provided on the book's accompanying website:

 Go to www.oup.com/uk/avent2e

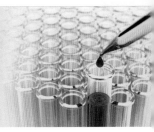

10

Haematopoietic Stem Cell Transplantation and Stem Cell Plasticity

Ruth Morse and Saeed Kabrah

Learning objectives

After studying this chapter you should be able to:

- Understand the biology of haematopoietic stem cells (HSC) transplants.
- Describe the various sources and methods of stem cell collection.
- Understand the clinical and laboratory requirement involved in stem cell transplantation.
- Understand the plasticity of haematopoietic stem cells and how this may be exploited for personalized medicine.

Introduction

The term 'stem cells' (SC) collectively (and sometimes inaccurately) describes a range of cell types with variable ability and functionality. It has been recognized that the initial all-encompassing SC is represented by the 'totipotent' SC which has the capacity to produce all the tissues of an embryo, including the supportive tissues of the placenta and amniotic sac. Such a cell can self-replicate maintaining the SC pool, differentiate down various lineages and retain a huge capacity for proliferation.

Perhaps the most well-known and utilized SCs are those of the bone marrow (BM), which early in the 20th century were shown to develop into a range of different blood cell

BOX 10.1 Conditions treated by HSCT

- Bone marrow failure syndromes for example fanconi anaemia, aplastic anaemia, Diamond Blackfan anaemia, congenital thrombocytopenia
- Haematological malignancy including leukaemia, lymphoma, myeloma
- Congenital diseases such as inherited metabolic disorders (e.g. inborn errors of metabolism), haemoglobinopathies (e.g. sickle cell anaemia, thalassaemia)
- Immunodeficiencies such as severe combined immunodeficiency, and severe autoimmunity
- Solid tumours requiring aggressive chemotherapy and/or radiotherapy such as breast, renal, ovarian, and testicular cancers

types including those of the myeloid lineage (red blood cells, platelets, and leucocytes) and lymphoid lineages (lymphocytes and natural killer cells). The first BM transplant was performed in 1968 where two siblings were treated for a condition known as 'combined immunodeficiency'. Since then transplantation of haematopoietic SCs has been used extensively for a range of different conditions related to compromized function of the BM and often represents the only curative option (see Box 10.1). Initially the transplants were performed using SCs from the BM; however, it was noted in 1978 that the blood in the umbilical cord was rich with haematopoietic SCs and so techniques were developed to harvest these cells and use them for transplantation. SC research has come a long way since these early observations, and there are now three recognized sources of haematopoietic SCs: from BM, umbilical cord blood (UCB), and peripheral blood (PB), as well as new ways to manipulate and use them in the best interests of the patient. Each patient is unique so clinical treatments are increasingly being developed to focus on personalized medicine to ensure the patient gets the best outcome for their condition.

10.1 **Stem cells**

The term 'stem cell' is often misunderstood in the general population as exclusively describing a cell from an embryonic source, and as such has suffered from ethical objections to research on them. However the term 'stem cell' encompasses a whole range of cell types which are distinguished by the terms used to describe their range of potential and proliferation capacity. True SCs are relatively rare in the population of cells; however, they all share some unique properties:

- Unspecialized: SCs do not have any specialized functions—they are unspecialized, but can form cells with specialized functions.
- Self-renewal: they have the capacity to proliferate and renew themselves almost indefinitely.
- Differentiation: SCs can differentiate into a range of cell types with functions and characteristics suitable for the organ or tissue they will become.

SCs can be wide or narrow in the range of cells they can make and early descendants of SCs can be classed as 'progenitors'. SCs and progenitors are distinguished by the fact that progenitors can differentiate but can no longer renew themselves. They are usually committed to a particular lineage, for example myeloid progenitors can only make myeloid blood cells. This distinguishes progenitors from 'adult' SCs; such cells are recognized to reside in organs of the body, and like embryonic SCs are unspecialized and able to proliferate and differentiate into the range of cells required for the organ from which they came. It is currently uncertain if adult SCs can produce cells of other tissues of the body, but evidence of this will be discussed at the end of the chapter. It can be confusing as to what level of ability a cell type may come from with respect to SCs or progenitors, so Table 10.1 has summarized the different levels of SCs and progenitors to help clarify the differences.

SCs seem to be present (as **adult stem cells**) in most tissues and organs of the body and appear to be there to protect the organ or tissue from extended injury or damage, by replacing worn out or dying cells. The ability of SCs to proliferate and differentiate into new cells is controlled by messages from the environment in which they live, so currently an interesting area of research is the ability to make stem or progenitor cells develop into lineages that they normally wouldn't become. The idea that SCs might be induced to develop down a completely different lineage depending on the environment in which they are placed is termed **plasticity**. Understanding how SCs might develop into different cell types would offer a new and exciting way to perform transplantation as well as correct diseased and damaged tissue. This chapter will discuss established approaches for using haematopoietic SCs for the purpose of correcting disease of the BM and will consider new ways of exploiting the plasticity of SCs for novel approaches to personalized therapy.

Adult stem cells
Undifferentiated cells that are found throughout the body and replace damaged or dying organs/tissues by cell proliferation.

Plasticity
The ability of cells to become cell types which they are not normally recognized to become.

Key points

Stem cells represent a range of types and potency and encompass both embryonic and adult stem cells.

TABLE 10.1 Definitions of stem cell potency and their levels of specialism

Cell name	Cell potency	Level of specialism	Self-renewal	Source	Differentiation capacity
Totipotent Stem Cells	Totipotent	Unspecialized	Yes	2-cell stage of developing embryo	Infinite; all cells of body including tissues required to support embryo (placenta, trophoblast, etc.)
Embryonic Stem Cell	Pluripotent	Unspecialized	Yes; theoretically immortal	Blastocyst of embryo	All cells of the body but not the placenta or amniotic sac
Adult Stem Cell	Multipotent	Unspecialized	Yes	Adult organs	Cell lineages of the organ of origin; unclear if cells of other tissues
Progenitor Cell	Multipotent	Partially differentiated	No	Many but not all tissues	Capacity limited to cell lineages of organ
Oligopotent Stem Cells	Oligopotent	Partially differentiated	No	Many but not all tissues	Limited cell lineages but not all lineages of the organ
Unipotent Stem Cells	Unipotent	Partially differentiated	No	Many but not all tissues	Low; limited to a single cell lineage (e.g. sperm)

Pluripotent

Is the ability of the human stem cell to differentiate or become almost any cell in the body.

Multipotent

Multipotent progenitor or stem cells can give rise to many but limited types of cell.

Haematopoiesis

The process that generates blood cells in the bone marrow.

SELF-CHECK 10.1

How do we differentiate **pluripotent**, **multipotent**, and unipotent stem cells?

10.2 The bone marrow microenvironment

The BM is a highly complex environment and consists mainly of two compartments, the stromal microenvironment and haematopoietic system. Both compartments have dedicated SCs which maintain the functionality of the BM:

- mesenchymal SCs (MSC): originally identified in the BM, but are present in many tissues, they can differentiate into various mesodermal lineages including osteoblasts, chondrocytes, and adipocytes. They maintain the stromal layer of the microenvironment and provide support for haematopoietic SCs.

- haematopoietic SCs (HSC): located in the red BM, these cells are responsible for generating all the cells of the blood system through the process of **haematopoiesis**. HSC are frequently defined as being the CD34+ fraction of SC collections.

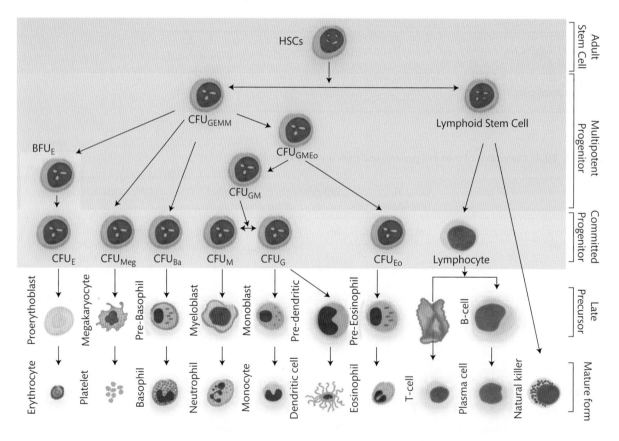

FIGURE 10.1

Haematopoiesis produces the different types of blood cells through stem cells with different plasticity capacity.

MSC are most common in the BM, but even there they are estimated to only represent about 0.001 to 0.1% of the total nucleated cells, and similarly the HSC are estimated to comprise about 0.01% of the myeloid fraction of the BM. Under the influence of cytokines and growth factors expressed by the MSC and stromal layer, the HSC are induced to proliferate and differentiate to ensure the blood is replenished appropriately and functioning correctly. HSC (considered multipotent) divide initially into myeloid and lymphoid lineages (oligopotent), which under further cytokine influence develop into the respective cells of the blood. As the cells become completely committed to a particular cell lineage, they lose their capacity to self-renew and so fully differentiate into the cell type they are intended to be. Cells of the blood system can be identified either microscopically by how they look (Figure 10.1) or using a machine called a flow cytometer which can count the number of cells that have surface markers specific to their lineage. HSC are identified by the presence of the surface marker CD34 (haematopoietic progenitor cell antigen CD34; part of the family of glycosylated type-I transmembrane single-chain glycoproteins), or by their ability to create colonies of cells (colony forming units, CFUs) in culture. Bone marrow comprises two stem cell types: HSC, which make the blood cells, and MSC, which make the components of the supportive bone marrow microenvironment.

SELF-CHECK 10.2

What is the difference between haematopoietic and mesenchymal stem cells? What different cell types do they make?

10.3 **Sources and collection of haematopoietic SCs**

HSC can be harvested from:

- Bone marrow (BM)
- Peripheral blood (PB)
- Umbilical cord blood (UCB).

The choice of the source of HSC can be influenced by several factors relating to the urgency of need for the patient to be transplanted. These include the patient's general condition, age, weight, disease status, and availability of a suitably HLA-matched donor. Each of the sources has advantages and disadvantages which will need to be considered on a case by case basis for each patient, including HLA matching requirement, cell dose, risk for acute and chronic graft versus host disease (see Table 10.2), and timescale for availability for the suggested source of HSC.

All patients and donors will be screened for bacterial and viral infection to prevent cross-infection, particularly where the donation may be infected and given to an immunocompromized patient. Any infections in a patient can become serious when the patient becomes immunosuppressed. For this reason only samples negative for these markers will be stored in the same freezing chamber to prevent cross-contamination, although the risk of this is very low. Tests carried out on the donation may include cytomegalovirus (CMV), human immunodeficiency virus (HIV) RNA and antibodies, human T-lymphotropic virus (HTLV), hepatitis B and C, herpes virus, and syphilis. Table 10.2 outlines the collection and transplantation of each of these cell sources, as well as associated complications.

TABLE 10.2 Bone marrow, peripheral blood, and umbilical cord as different sources of HSC.

Bone Marrow	Peripheral Blood	Cord Blood
Donor		
Potential donors may no longer be available or may have withdrawn consent. Donor must be found and retested to confirm the HLA typing and infectious disease results and to confirm that the donor is still willing and able to donate bone marrow. Significant donor attrition.	Potential donors may no longer be available or may have withdrawn consent. Donor must be found and retested to confirm the HLA typing and infectious disease results and to confirm that the donor is still willing and able to donate bone marrow. Significant donor attrition.	Once frozen, a cord blood unit is available until used. There is no donor attrition.
Donor may be available to give a second transplant or to donate blood for T cells if necessary.	Donor may be available to give a second transplant or to donate blood for T cells if necessary.	Donor is not available for a second donation.
Can be used for autologous (self) and allogenic (twin, sibling, unrelated donor, and parents) transplantation.	Can be used for autologous (self) and allogenic (twin, sibling, unrelated donor, and parents) transplantation.	Can be used for autologous (self) and allogenic (twin, sibling, unrelated donor, and parents) transplantation.
Donation		
No stem cell mobilization procedure.	Require stem cell mobilization regimens (growth factors and/or chemotherapy) for 4–8 days. Depending on CD34+ cell number on peripheral blood, donors receive either low dose (10 µg/kg/day) or high dose: (2×8 µg/kg/day).	No mobilization procedure.
By a surgical procedure under general anaesthesia using needles to withdraw liquid marrow from both sides of the back of the pelvic bone. Donors will be hospitalized for two days and may experience temporary discomfort and/or pain.	By apheresis procedures and donor may experience temporary discomfort and/or pain.	By draining blood from umbilical vein directly after the infant is born, no medical risk to mother or infant.
Single donation of 10–20 ml bone marrow per kg of donor's body weight.	Final donation volume is calculated by CD34+ cells number (2.5–4×10^6 per kg of donor's body weight, 70–250 ml). Usually is achieved in almost 68–87% of single apheresis, but less than 5% donors required more than two apheresis.	A small volume (40–150 ml) is collected.
Stem cells are purified and concentrated in lab. Final unit volume is 70–250 ml.	Stem cells are purified and concentrated in lab. Final unit volume is 70–250 ml.	Stem cells are purified and concentrated in lab. Final unit volume is 20 ml.
Bone marrow unit is used fresh (shelf-life is measured in hours).	Peripheral blood stem cells usually stored for short term (days to a few months).	Cord blood units are cryopreserved (stored in special freezers) and stored for up to 13 years.
Transplant		
After a formal search is started, it usually takes 2 or more months to transplant, if a donor is available.	After a formal search is started, it usually takes 2 or more months to transplant, if a donor is available.	When a match is found, it can take only a few days for confirmatory and special testing for shipment to the transplant centre (less than 24 hours in an emergency).

Bone Marrow	Peripheral Blood	Cord Blood
Generally requires a perfect match between donor and recipient for 8/8 HLA-A, -B, -C, and -DRB1 antigens. Additional HLA factors (HLA-DQ and -DP) increasingly used to improve prognosis.	Generally requires a perfect match between donor and recipient for 8/8 HLA-A, -B, -C, and -DRB1 antigens. Additional HLA factors (HLA-DQ and -DP) increasingly used to improve prognosis.	HLA-mismatched cord blood transplants are possible, making it easier to find a suitable match. Role of HLA-C, -DQ, and -DP are not yet known.
Patient must begin conditioning before the bone marrow is harvested. Coordination between donation and transplant is critical and complex.	Patient must begin conditioning before the peripheral blood harvest. Coordination between donation and transplant is critical and complex.	Cord blood graft can be shipped to the transplant centre before the patient enters the hospital and begins conditioning for transplantation. Coordination is simple. Cord blood units are shipped on demand.
		Cord blood units contain smaller numbers of stem cells. Slower engraftment may lead to prolonged hospital stay, and in certain cases, to serious complications. The number of cells needed depends on the recipient's weight.
Complications		
Latent viral infection in the donor is common (i.e. CMV > 50% in U.S. adult donors).	Latent viral infection in the donor is common (i.e. CMV > 50% in U.S. adult donors).	Latent viral infection in the cord blood donor is rare (i.e. CMV <1% in U.S.).
No risk of transplanting a genetic disease.	No risk of transplanting a genetic disease.	There is a small probability that a rare, unrecognized genetic disease affecting the blood or immune system of the baby may be given with the cord blood transplant.
Severe graft vs host disease (GvHD) is common with mismatched grafts.	Severe graft vs host disease (GvHD) is common with mismatched grafts.	GvHD less frequent, usually less severe and easier to treat.

Information from: Harvesting, processing and inventory management of peripheral blood stem cells by Aleksandar Mijovic and Derwood Pamphilon
https://www.ncbi.nlm.nih.gov/pmc/articles/PMC3168129/

Bone marrow stem cells

The BM comprises the soft tissue found in the centre of the long bones and the sternum. Here the haematopoietic SCs generate the blood cells of all lineages (red cells, white cells, and platelets). Blood cells when required develop under the influence of growth factors produced by the BM microenvironment, then pass through the marrow–blood barrier to enter the vasculature in order to perform their functions.

The BM is harvested under general anaesthesia in an operating theatre by a method developed by Thomas and Storb in 1970. The patient lays face down on the theatre table and BM is aspirated from the posterior iliac crest, which is the upper curved part on both sides of the pelvic

BOX 10.2 Cryopreservation

Cryopreservation is a mechanism to preserve living cells and tissues at very low temperatures, such that when resurrected they can continue to grow and proliferate. Unprotected cryopreservation is lethal to cells, partly because of the formation of water ice crystals internally in the cell (mechanical destruction) and as a result of this solutes in the cells become concentrated when the water freezes, which can also be toxic to the cells. As a consequence, cells are frozen in the presence of cryoprotectants which penetrate the cells and prevent water freezing internally by raising the solute concentration and binding to water molecules.

Typical, commonly used cryoprotectants include dimethyl sulphoxide (DMSO) and glycerol. These molecules are small enough to penetrate the cells and offer minimal toxicity. However, some cell death typically still occurs during cryopreservation, partly due to high densities of cells frozen in a limited volume, but also due to intrinsic toxicity of some cryoprotectants.

Cryopreservation usually involves mixing the cells with cryoprotectants and then slow freezing them—for mammalian cells, this is considered to be freezing at a rate of about 1°C per minute. In research laboratories this can be performed using portable benchtop freezing containers containing isopropanol which can be placed in –80°C freezers for a few hours. In clinical laboratories where cryopreservation needs to be strictly controlled, rate-controlled freezers can be used. Long-term storage of the cells involves placing the cryopreserved cells in the vapour phase of liquid nitrogen.

To resurrect cells, they are usually rapidly thawed at 37°C with agitation to encourage removal of cryoprotectants from the interior of the cells. In research laboratories it is possible to wash the cryoprotectants away from the cells, but for some clinical stem cell infusions this is not possible and patients comment on a 'taste' in their mouth from the eluted cryoprotectant; for DMSO this is described as tasting like garlic.

girdle, using a sterile BM harvest needle. The procedure takes about half an hour to perform. The harvested marrow is placed into a sterile collection bag containing a drug called ACD-A (citrate) which prevents the sample from clotting. A 5 ml sample is removed from the bag and sent to the laboratory in order to perform a total nucleated cell count, this allows for a calculation of how much BM needs to be harvested. However, in the UK, total nucleated cell dose is more typically used for selection of umbilical cord transplants (see 'Umbilical cord blood stem cells'). Once sufficient BM is harvested, the collection bag is sent to the laboratory to prepare the sample for transplantation. This usually involves concentrating the sample to remove unwanted red cells and increase the white cell population including the progenitor cells. This manipulated sample may be frozen by cryopreservation techniques (see Box 10.2) and stored ready for when the patient needs it.

BOX 10.3 Chemotherapy and radiotherapy mechanisms of action

Both chemotherapy and radiotherapy are considered to be 'non-specific' modes of therapy in that they target DNA to produce their toxicity to cells. As such they can be described as both genotoxic (DNA damaging) and cytotoxic (kill cells), and cells die as a result of exposure

due to the DNA damage exceeding the limit that cells can cope with and repair. Cells that survive, however, may be mutated and these can potentially form new cancers later on. Because every cell in the body (except red blood cells) contain DNA, every cell in the body is a potential target, thus giving the 'non-specific' description to this therapy and also explaining why patients get severe side effects from this therapy. Proliferating cells are particularly affected, explaining the characteristic symptoms of hair loss, gastro-intestinal disturbances (nausea, vomiting, and diarrhoea), and bone marrow suppression (anaemia and risk of infection).

Chemotherapy largely is split into four groups of drugs: the alkylating agents, antimetabolites, antibiotics, and plant alkaloids. Alkylating agents bind to the DNA leaving either alkyl groups that affect reading the DNA code, or cross-link the DNA so that it can't be separated for replication or gene expression. Antimetabolites look 'similar' to nucleotides in the DNA such that they either incorporate into the DNA helix, or they inhibit metabolic enzymes responsible for synthesizing nucleotides; either way they ultimately block further DNA replication. Antibiotics can slip between the bases in DNA (intercalate) and can create cuts in the DNA to break the helix, whereas plant alkaloids usually inhibit the spindle fibres that allow for chromosomes to be separated during mitosis. The vinca alkaloids (e.g. vincristine) inhibit the formation of spindles whereas the taxols (e.g. paclitaxel) stabilize the spindles so that they can't pull the chromosome apart. Other drugs like etoposide induce cuts in the DNA, and these breaks are also caused by radiotherapy directly hitting the DNA.

The ability to disturb the function of the DNA prevents cells from dividing; this is why it is a useful therapy to kill rapidly proliferating cancer cells, but also provides an easy mechanism to deplete haematopoietic cells that are proliferating in the bone marrow, in order to infuse new stem cells. These drugs are usually used in combination, selecting a few drugs from different groups to target as many cancer cells as possible.

Peripheral blood mobilized stem cells

Haematopoietic SCs can also be harvested from the peripheral blood and are currently the preferred source of SCs over BM harvests. HSC are about 10–100 times greater in the BM than the peripheral blood so can only be collected from the blood providing the donor has been given drugs or growth factors to 'mobilize' the SCs out of the BM and into the vasculature. Previously donors have been given G-CSF (granulocyte colony stimulating factor) alone or occasionally in the presence of chemotherapy drugs (only where the donor is also the patient!) to mobilize SCs (see Box 10.3). However, drugs such as plerixafor are now being used as well or instead. Plerixafor is an antagonist for the CXCR4 receptor on the surface of HSC. This receptor interacts with a chemokine called SDF-1α (stromal derived factor 1α) which is needed to retain the cells in the BM. By reversibly blocking this receptor the HSC are released into the vasculature. Plerixafor used in conjunction with G-CSF has been shown to be much more effective at mobilizing the HSC into the blood for harvest.

Where G-CSF is used alone, donors are given the growth factor typically for four days, then apheresis starts on day five with G-CSF continuously administered until the end of apheresis sessions. The target number of CD34+ cells is at least 2×10^6/kg body weight and anyone not achieving these numbers is considered a 'poor mobilizer'. Poor mobilizers are frequently seen in patients who will provide their own HSC (autologous transplant; see 'Autologous stem cells'), mainly because they may have already been given chemotherapy treatment for their disease which may be toxic to SCs. There are a few strategies available to improve cell numbers in poor mobilizers including: larger volume leukapheresis, re-mobilization, plerixafor, chemo-mobilization (patients only) with plerixafor and G-CSF, and finally BM harvest. The main aim is to achieve enough CD34+ cells for successful transplantation over several apheresis sessions, so daily blood counts are performed to determine the number of CD34+ cells in the blood in order to indicate when to start apheresis.

Apheresis is typically performed by placing a large bore catheter into one or both of the patient's antecubital veins; this may be placed each time apheresis is performed, or left permanently until apheresis and/or transplantation is completed. The apheresis equipment is a closed system, drawing the blood through one catheter into the machine which continuously centrifuges the blood to separate the components. The CD34+ cells are collected in the white blood cell fraction whereas other components like the red cells and plasma are returned to the patient. Each apheresis session may take anything from 2–5 hours to perform where up to 30 l of blood (about six times the average total human blood volume) is processed. It may be possible to collect enough CD34+ cells in one session, but several sessions may be required in order to collect enough cells. Depending on the patient and how they respond to the mobilization, apheresis sessions may need to continue for up to four days. Collected cells are frozen to protect them until they are needed for transplantation.

Umbilical cord blood stem cells

Umbilical cord blood is rich in HSC, with CD34+ cells estimated to be present at about 0.02–1.45% of the population of cells, which is close to the value of CD34+ in the adult BM. After the baby has been safely delivered, the umbilical cord usually pulsates for a short while to ensure that the child receives as much of the blood in the cord and placenta as it needs. Soon after the cord stops pulsating, the cord is clamped and cut—this usually, but not always, occurs before the placenta is delivered. The remaining blood in the umbilical cord can then be collected for transplant purposes. In some centres, the blood can be collected before the placenta is delivered, sometimes afterwards. Where the placenta is delivered, this can be placed in a 'sling' or 'hammock' with the remaining cord hanging below (Figure 10.2), so that gravity aids in blood collection. A needle is placed into the umbilical vein and the blood is drawn from the cord and placenta into a sterile collection bag, which takes only about five minutes to perform. The volume of collection is much smaller than that collected from BM or PB.

The sterile bag is sent to the cord bank for processing; a small aliquot is taken for infectious agent detection and the rest of the bag undergoes a 'slow sedimentation' technique which removes the red cells which are not needed, and concentrates the white cell fraction, which contains the CD34+ cells for transplantation. Although the initial volume collected

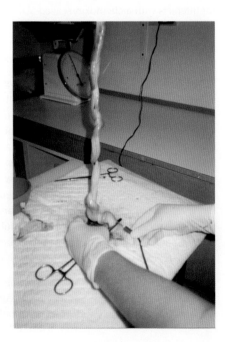

FIGURE 10.2
Collection of umbilical cord blood after delivery of the placenta.

may be about 120–150 ml, the final CD34+ fraction may only be about 30 ml but is rich in the HSC needed for the transplant. Samples are frozen in their bags until needed for transplantation.

Key points

Haematopoietic stem cells can be sourced from the bone marrow, the umbilical cord blood, and those mobilized into the peripheral blood.

SELF-CHECK 10.3

How do we harvest the different haematopoietic cells from the donor?

Cryopreserving haematopoietic stem cells

Any collected HSC need to be kept frozen until the time they are needed. Cells can become damaged when frozen unless they are protected by cryoprotectants. Typical reagents that are used are glycerol or dimethylsulphoxide (DMSO). The freezing process depends on the sample collected, but needs to be performed within a sterile environment such as a laminar flow cabinet in a clean room, in order to ensure the sterility of the product before it is infused into the patient. Cryopreservation usually involves a gradual slow freeze of the cells in the presence of cryoprotectant, followed by longer-term deep freeze in liquid nitrogen vapour at a temperature of –150°C to –180°C.

Stem cell donations in transplantation

SC donations (Table 10.3) can be:

- Autologous—originating from the patient who will receive them
- Allogeneic—donated from a family member or unrelated donor who is an identical or close tissue type (HLA) match
- Syngeneic—donated from a genetically identical twin.

Autologous stem cells

Sometimes the patient's own HSC can be used for transplant, but they need to be collected when the patient is in remission of their disease, and stored frozen until all chemotherapy has been completed. Whilst there will not be any complications of rejection of the transplanted cells, there is a risk that both the patient's blood and BM still contain malignant cells. The patient will need to go through rounds of chemotherapy to induce remission before HSC harvest, but this may lead to low HSC retrieval (for 'poor mobilizers' see 'Peripheral blood mobilized stem cells') and also immunocompromise in the patient, leading to a risk of infection. The collected HSC may also need 'purging' of residual malignant cells to prevent relapse of the disease by reinfusing it with the SCs; however, this type of transplant generally has a higher risk of relapse for this reason.

TABLE 10.3 The relative advantages and disadvantages of autologous, allogenic, and syngeneic transplants.

Comparison between autologous, allogeneic, and syngeneic stem cell transplantation

Type	Advantages	Disadvantages
Autologous	No need to identify donor if peripheral blood or marrow is uninvolved by tumour at the time of collection. No immunosuppression (low risk of infection.) No risk of GvHD. Dose-intensive therapy can be used for older patients (usually up to age 70). Low early treatment-related mortality (2–5%).	Not feasible if peripheral blood stem cells/marrow involved. Possible marrow injury leading to late myelodysplasia (either from prior chemotherapy or transplant regimen). No graft-versus-tumour effect. Not all patients can be mobilized to give adequate cell doses for reconstitution.
Allogeneic	No tumour contamination of the graft and no prior marrow injury from chemotherapy (less risk of late myelodysplasia). Graft-versus-tumour effect. Can be used for patients with marrow involvement by tumour or both bone marrow dysfunction, such as aplastic anaemia.	Dose-intensive regimen limited by toxicity (usually limited to patients < age 55). Time needed to identify donor if no sibling donor available/limited availability of donor for some ethnic groups. Higher early treatment-related mortality from GvHD and infection complications (20–40% depending upon age and donor source).
Syngeneic	No need for immunosuppression. No risk of GvHD.	No graft-versus-tumour effect

http://www.cancernetwork.com/cancer-management/hematopoietic-cell-transplantation
https://www.omicsonline.org/stemcell-transplantation-types-risks-and-benefits-2157-7633.1000114.pdf

Allogeneic stem cells

These are SCs collected from HLA-matched (tissue type matched) donors, who may be either family members (e.g. a sibling) or an unrelated donor. Because these donors are not genetically identical to the patient, it is important to HLA-match the donation as closely as possible to the patient to prevent graft rejection. A further complication in allogeneic HSC transplantation is a phenomenon called 'graft versus host disease' (GvHD) where the transplanted HSC recognize the patient as 'foreign' and attempt to reject the patient it has been infused into—this can be a life-threatening complication and needs to be controlled carefully. Both graft rejection and GvHD can be controlled with immunosuppressive drugs (Box 10.4). Thus, using a sibling donor is preferable to an unrelated donor as the genetic disparity will be less in a sibling so should represent lower rejection. Sometimes this genetic disparity can be helpful in fighting malignancy, however, as the transplanted SCs can recognize the malignant cells as foreign and will kill them; this is called 'graft versus leukaemia' (GvL) or 'graft versus tumour' (GvT) effect. This is more likely to occur in allogeneic transplants, but doesn't occur in autologous or syngeneic transplants because of genetic identity.

Syngeneic stem cells

Very few individuals have identical twins who may act as a donor of HSC for transplant. Here there are limited problems with the transplant itself because the two individuals are genetically

BOX 10.4 Immunosuppressive drugs

Immunosuppressive drugs can be used to reduce the immune system in patients receiving either stem cell or solid organ transplants, such that their new transplant is protected from being rejected by their own immune system. Patients are vulnerable on these drugs and administration needs to be tightly controlled and closely monitored to ensure that the drug concentration is not so low that rejection occurs, but also not so high that the patient is highly vulnerable to infection.

Underpinning graft rejection is the clonal proliferation of T cells in response to the graft so any drug that can prevent this is potentially useful. There are a range of drugs utilized for immunosuppression including the immunophilin binders (e.g. cyclosporine), the antimetabolites (e.g. mycophenolate mofetil), monoclonal/polyclonal antibodies, and corticosteroids.

Immunophilin binders tend to inhibit the signalling pathways that lead to cytokine release which promote T cell production. Antimetabolites, similar to those used in chemotherapy, inhibit DNA synthesis, but specifically target the pathways used in T cells. Antibodies raised against immune cells aid in the depletion of lymphocytes from the body. Glucocorticoids control the gene expression of a range of proteins known to control the development of the immune system, so as a result need to be used sparingly and for short periods of time as they can have extensive side effects. Clearly each of these drug groups act at different stages of T cell proliferation, so some can be used prior to a transplant to prevent the T cells from proliferating and causing rejection, whereas others can be used to 'rescue' patients by depleting already active T cells.

identical and therefore HLA identical, so graft rejection will not be a problem. However, the advantages of a GvL effect will not occur in a syngeneic transplant, so relapse of disease is more likely here than for an allogeneic transplant, but less likely than autologous where there is a risk of reinfusion of disease.

SELF-CHECK 10.4

What is the difference between autologous, allogeneic, and syngeneic transplants?

Donor leucocyte infusions

Choices of autologous, allogeneic, and syngeneic transplants will depend on the status of the patient, the disease they have, and the opportunities to find a suitable donor. Where an allogeneic transplant is performed and malignancy recurs, donor leucocyte infusion (DLI) may be performed with the aim of inducing remission by harnessing the GvL/GvT effect mentioned above. Here leucocytes are collected from the original donor and infused into the patient to augment an anti-tumour immune response, usually after the patient has had some chemotherapy to reduce the number of malignant cells. This effect needs to be carefully controlled so that the patient does not have too severe an immune response, but the approach has had success in a variety of haematological malignancies most notably chronic myeloid leukaemia (CML). DLI has also been utilized in non-myeloablative transplants (also called mini-transplants, see Box 10.5) which harness the power of the immune system to fight the malignancy instead of high dose chemotherapy; this may be used in elderly patients who are too old or ill to tolerate the high chemotherapy doses of standard procedures.

BOX 10.5 *Non-myeloablative or 'minitransplant'*

Haematopoietic stem cell transplants are usually associated with high-dose chemotherapy with or without accompanying radiotherapy prior to infusion of the stem cells. This therapy is called 'conditioning therapy' and is designed to remove all haematopoietic and cancer/leukaemia cells from the bone marrow. When it completely removes the cells it is termed 'myeloablative'. However, the majority of patients diagnosed with leukaemia are elderly, and this myeloablative conditioning therapy can be too dangerous for them, simply because they are too old or too ill to tolerate such aggressive therapy. Inability to tolerate the therapy means that they are not then eligible for stem cell transplantation, and myeloablative procedures are then kept only for the younger patients who will cope with the toxicity.

A recent procedure which has been called reduced intensity transplant or 'minitransplant' uses lower doses of chemotherapy, meaning that the haematopoietic and cancer cells in the patient are not completely removed, but make enough 'space' and immunosuppress the patient enough to allow for the infusion of donor cells. The process relies on the infused donor cells recognizing the cancer/leukaemic cells as 'foreign' and creating an immune response to the cells, resulting in a graft versus leukaemia effect. This effect can be increased by also infusing the patient with lymphocytes from the donor after the initial stem cell infusion. This procedure is less toxic to the patients, so is now offering a potentially curative therapy for older patients who normally would not be able to have a stem cell transplant.

Key points

Transplants can be autologous, allogeneic, or syngeneic. Before stem cells can be infused, patients need conditioning therapy (chemotherapy +/- radiotherapy) to remove their cancer cells.

10.4 Stem cell transplantation

Patient conditioning

Engraftment
When infused donor cells embed in the bone marrow and start producing new haematopoietic cells.

Myeloablation
Chemotherapy treatment given prior to a stem cell transplant that completely removes all haematopoietic and cancer cells.

Non-myeloablative
Chemotherapy treatment given prior to a stem cell transplant that does not completely remove haematopoietic and cancer cells, but instead depends on donor cells to kill the cancer.

Before the patient can be infused with the collected SCs, their own disease needs to be treated with chemotherapy and/or radiotherapy which generally serves three purposes:

- To deplete the marrow of the malignant or diseased haematopoietic system
- To make 'space' in the marrow for the incoming SCs
- To immunosuppress the patient to aid in the **engraftment** of the new SCs

This therapy is termed 'conditioning therapy' and may differ depending on the disease that the patient has. Usually the doses administered are high with the aim to 'myeloablate' the BM, this means that the haematopoietic cells of the BM are killed including the malignant cells. Usually **myeloablation** fully removes the haematopoietic system, but the microenvironment created by the MSC is relatively resistant to this therapy and remains in place so that it can support the new incoming cells. As described in Box 10.5, some protocols are of lower doses and are termed **non-myeloablative** conditioning and are used for 'mini-transplants'. Conditioning therapy typically uses drugs like cyclophosphamide, which is a nitrogen mustard alkylating agent. Cyclophosphamide can bind to DNA creating cross-links in the DNA preventing separation of the DNA strands and subsequent cell replication. Other drugs include busulphan, melphalan, etoposide, cytarabine and carmustine. Sometimes patients will also be treated with total body irradiation (TBI) which may be delivered as a single dose, or as smaller doses over a few days (fractionated).

This conditioning therapy is very toxic to the patient and needs to be administered carefully as depletion of the marrow can be fatal without support. Whilst it is important to remove the disease completely from the patient and conditioning therapy achieves this, the patient will die from BM failure without the newly transplanted SCs which aim to restore normal marrow function. Therefore it is also important to ensure that all chemotherapy has left the body of the patient before the new SCs are infused to protect the cells from the toxic effects. Usually the patient is allowed two days' recovery from conditioning therapy before the new SCs are infused.

SELF-CHECK 10.5

Why do patients need conditioning therapy before they receive their stem cell donation?

Reinfusion and engraftment

Once the patient has been conditioned and the decision has been made to infuse the new SCs, an authorized request is sent to the SC laboratory for the identified matched SC donation to be prepared for infusion. Some SC units will be delivered to the ward and the staff there will thaw the sample for reinfusion, in other units, a member of the lab staff will accompany the unit to the ward and perform the thawing there.

The patient's details are checked by two members of staff to ensure the correct patient is getting the correct sample, then the sample is thawed in a sterile water bath at 37°C. Thawing usually takes about 5 minutes and reinfusion should then occur within about 20 minutes of thawing. Reinfusion is relatively straightforward but needs to be infused in a controlled manner to maximize entry of the cells into the body. Infusion can be via a central vein over a period of a few hours, or may be infused via a 50 ml syringe attached to a port on a line inserted into one of the patient's veins. During the procedure the patient is checked for blood pressure, temperature, and pulse, and any other possible reactions. Sometimes the patient may have some side effects from the DMSO used to cryopreserve the SCs; these are usually mild such as facial flushing and a strong taste in the back of the mouth. Some side effects can be more serious though, such as bradycardia (heart rate <60 beats per minute), seizures, and renal failure, so if the SC volume is large, the cells are infused over a longer time period with a controlled flow rate.

SCs that have been reinfused into the patient traffic through the vasculature until they find the vicinity of the BM, then they adhere to the blood vessel walls, roll along the wall, and eventually pass through into the marrow space. Exactly how this is achieved is currently incompletely understood, but it is known that proteins called 'chemokines' which are expressed from the marrow act as attractants, persuading the HSC to cross into the marrow. A key chemoattractant is SDF-1α which interacts with the CXCR4 receptor on HSC, and it is this reaction which the mobilizing drug plerixafor antagonises to release HSC into the vasculature. Other suggested messengers include prostaglandins released from the cell membrane, G-CSF (used in mobilization), and various adhesion molecules. When the SCs enter the marrow, they engraft and under the influence of cytokines produced by the microenvironment, start to produce new haematopoietic cells.

Pancytopenia
Low numbers of blood cell lines
(RBC, WBC, and platelets).

The patient initially may have a period of 10–14 days of severe **pancytopenia**, but the first sign that the SCs have successfully engrafted is the presence of neutrophils and monocytes in the blood, followed by an increase in platelet counts. The patient will be monitored with regular full blood counts (FBC) to watch increases in white cell counts as well as further increases in neutrophils and monocytes.

Source of HSC and outcomes with engraftment

Depending on the source of the HSC, the outcomes for the patients can be very different. In order to achieve good engraftment, it is important to transplant enough CD34+ cells; PB achieve the highest numbers of CD34+ followed by BM, but yields from UCB vary from unit to unit. In general, higher doses of CD34+ cells ($> 2 \times 10^6$/kg body weight) result in better engraftment and survival, particularly in unrelated transplants; however, doses higher than 8×10^6/kg body weight are associated with higher chronic GvHD, particularly for PB samples.

As UCB represents a small sample generally, the total number of nucleated cells in a UCB unit is commonly used to help with sample selection alongside the number of HLA mismatches. It is recommended that where there is 6/6 HLA matches, more than 3×10^7 nucleated cells/kg body weight should be used, whereas with 5/6 and 4/6 matches, nucleated cells should be increased to more than 4×10^7 and more than 5×10^7 cells/kg body weight respectively. However UCB is immunologically naïve and so multiple samples can be pooled to ensure there are enough cells to transplant. It is recommended to match HLA as closely as possible for all pooled samples though.

Despite each of the sources all providing HSC, there are many studies that have compared the differences between HSC from BM, PB, and UCB during transplantation. It has been noted that UCB and BM have similar numbers of CD34+ cells but these are lower in PB. UCB also has a higher proliferative potential and can produce more colonies of haematopoietic cells than PB and BM, partly because they have longer **telomeres** so can replicate more times, and they also respond better to cytokines such as IL-3, IL-6, and stem cell factor (SCF). UCB is also less cytotoxic than PB or BM because it is immunologically naïve and has lower numbers of natural killer (NK) cells in the samples; as a result GvHD is a lower risk with UCB than with PB or BM. UCB is also less likely to be contaminated with viruses and tends to have the lowest risk of recurrence of leukaemia, so UCB seems like a great source of HSC. However, there are disadvantages to UCB that PB and BM do not have—mainly that UCB tends to be quite a small sample and can limit who can have cells from this source. Also HSC from UCB does not engraft as well as HSC from PB or BM. If it was possible to increase the size of the UCB and improve the engraftment, HSC from UCB could be the best option for most patients. There are other positives and negatives about using UCB over PB or BM, and these are summarized in Table 10.4.

Telomeres
Repeated DNA sequences at the ends of chromosomes that stabilize the DNA and chromosome structure. They are considered 'biological clocks' and control the number of times chromosomes can replicate.

Key points

Haematopoietic cells from different sources have subtly different behaviour in terms of ability to home to the bone marrow, how quickly they do this to make blood cells, and how likely they are going to cause immune reactions such as GvHD.

SELF-CHECK 10.6

Why might cord blood stem cells be considered superior to adult stem cells for transplantation?

TABLE 10.4 Comparing the advantages and disadvantages of umbilical cord blood over bone marrow and peripheral blood as a source of HSC.

Bone Marrow/Peripheral Blood	Cord Blood
Bone marrow donation requires surgery under general anaesthesia. Donors may experience temporary discomfort and/or pain. Long-term consequences of growth factors used in peripheral blood stem cell donations are uncertain.	When obtained from the delivered placenta and umbilical cord, cord blood donation poses no medical risk to mother or infant.
A transplant requires donation of 945 ml or more of bone marrow (mixed with blood).	A small volume (sometimes a few millilitres) can be used for transplantation. The number of cells needed depends on the recipient's weight.
Bone marrow and peripheral blood grafts contain large numbers of stem cells. Engraftment of neutrophils is rapid.	Cord blood units contain smaller numbers of stem cells. Slower engraftment may lead to prolonged hospital stay, and in certain cases, to serious complications.
After a formal search is started, it usually takes 2 or more months to transplant, if a donor is available.	When a match is found, it can take only a few days for confirmatory and special testing for shipment to the transplant centre (less than 24 hours in an emergency).
Potential donors may no longer be available or may have withdrawn consent. Donor must be found and retested to confirm the HLA typing and infectious disease results and to confirm that the donor is still willing and able to donate bone marrow. Significant donor attrition.	Once frozen, a cord blood unit is available until used. There is no donor attrition.
Donor may be available to give a second transplant or to donate blood for T cells if necessary.	Donor is not available for a second donation.
Bone marrow is used fresh (shelf-life measured in hours). Peripheral blood stem cells usually stored for short term (days to a few months).	Cord blood units are cryopreserved (stored in special freezers). Frozen cord blood has been transplanted successfully after up to 13 years in storage.
Patient must begin conditioning before the bone marrow or peripheral blood harvest. Coordination between donation and transplant is critical and complex.	Cord blood graft can be shipped to the transplant centre before the patient enters the hospital and begins conditioning for transplantation. Coordination is simple. Cord blood units are shipped on demand.
Latent viral infection in the donor is common (i.e. CMV > 50% in US adult donors).	Latent viral infection in the cord blood donor is rare (i.e. CMV <1% in US).
No risk of transplanting a genetic disease.	There is a small probability that a rare, unrecognized genetic disease affecting the blood or immune system of the baby may be given with the cord blood transplant.
Severe graft-versus-host disease (GvHD) is common with mismatched grafts.	GvHD less frequent, usually less severe and easier to treat.
Generally requires a perfect match between donor and recipient for 8/8 HLA-A, -B, -C, and -DRB1 antigens. Additional HLA factors (HLA-DQ and -DP) increasingly used to improve prognosis.	HLA-mismatched cord blood transplants are possible, making it easier to find a suitable match. Role of HLA-C, -DQ, and -DP are not yet known.

Cord blood transplants, as all unrelated hematopoietic stem cell transplants, can be associated with serious complications, severe organ toxicity, and, in some cases, death.

Outcomes and complications for SCT

It is currently estimated that every 20 minutes someone in the UK is diagnosed with a blood cancer meaning that around 2000 people per annum require a SCT in order to survive. As the majority of these do not find donors within their families, donations are procured from altruistic donors of SC which are banked at various facilities throughout the UK. About 90% of donations are from PB sources; however, tens of thousands of UCB samples are banked ready for treating patients.

Collaborative efforts between establishments such as the NHS Stem Cell Registry, NHS Blood and Transplant Service, and Anthony Nolan have vastly increased the likelihood that patients will be quickly and successfully treated for their BM disease or malignancy. Currently there are about 60,000 young volunteer donors (up to 30 years of age) who have been typed to high resolution, there are close to 50,000 UCB samples banked, over 1000 transplants performed per annum, and the time to procure a suitable donation so that patients get treated early in their disease has significantly reduced. The chances of ethnic minorities finding a suitable donor has also significantly increased. All these collaborative efforts lead to an improved patient outcome. Children fare particularly well post-transplant with a 70% and 69% overall five year survival whereas adults demonstrate 41% and 34% overall five year survival (unrelated adult versus UCB donations respectively). However, SCT is not without its difficulties and patients may suffer from a range of side effects or complications which can be classified into short or long-term complications or may bridge both timelines, such as GvHD (acute versus chronic).

Short-term complications

Very early complications that may be observed in the patient may be related to the chemotherapy used to produce conditioning prior to the transplant and as such patients will have the usual range of symptoms including feeling nauseous, having gastro-intestinal disturbances, loss of appetite, as well as issues like tiredness, anaemia due to reduced red blood cells, and bleeding or bruising (due to low platelet counts). Patients may be at increased risk of infection until their new haematopoietic system establishes and so may need to have antibiotics to protect them.

It is essential to monitor the patient for signs of SCT engraftment, where there is evidence that the SCs have homed to the BM and are now starting to produce new blood cells. A major complication is graft rejection, defined as failure of the patient to recover from **neutropenia**, resulting in pancytopenia and an urgent need for re-transplantation. Graft failure may occur for several reasons including immunological rejection, suggested to be due to ABO blood group mismatches, HLA mismatches, and recipient T or NK cell rejection. Failure may also result due to drug toxicity, inadequate SC numbers, septicaemia, and virus infections, such as herpes virus, CMV, and parvovirus. Where graft failure occurs, patients may urgently need a re-transplant in order to survive, except where autologous recovery occurs (usually seen when donor cells initially engraft but then later fail). Particularly where the patient has had an autologous transplant, there is also a higher risk for disease relapse; typically disease relapse does not respond well to cytotoxic chemotherapy alone, and extra measures such as a second transplant potentially with a donor lymphocyte infusion (DLI) may be required with mixed outcomes depending on the individual patient.

If there is successful engraftment, patients may succumb to GvHD which is a particular risk for transplants with non-genetically identical donations and is estimated to affect 50–80% of patients (see allogeneic transplants: sibling or unrelated donors). GvHD may be acute or chronic and is distinguished according to the timing of when they occur (acute is <100 days post-transplant, chronic is >100 days post-transplant). GvHD is potentially life-threatening and needs to be carefully controlled. Acute GvHD affects the skin, liver, stomach, and intestines whereas chronic GvHD affects the same organs but also affects various glands (salivary and tears), the connective tissue, mouth, oesophagus, and vagina. The two conditions seem

Neutropenia
Low numbers of neutrophil leucocytes.

to occur due to different processes in the immune system. Acute GvHD has risk factors of HLA mismatch, unrelated donor, sex mismatch of donor and recipient (especially where a female donor for a male recipient), intensity of the conditioning regime, and source of SC (PB or BM > UCB). All these factors infer a T cell-mediated reaction to genetic disparity between donor and recipient. As noted above, however, GvHD may be beneficial to the patient in producing a GvL/GvT response such that allogeneic transplants benefit from reduced disease relapse; clinicians would then be careful about considering how to control the GvHD to protect the patient both from morbidity/mortality from the GvHD versus mortality from relapsed disease.

Long-term side effects/complications

Chronic GvHD may be considered a longer-term complication and may manifest in a single organ or may be disseminated throughout the body, having a significant effect on overall quality of life. The symptoms of chronic GvHD resemble an autoimmune condition with the pathophysiology involving inflammation, fibrosis, and cell and humoral immunity. The condition usually occurs in the first two years post-transplantation.

Similar to the shorter-term complications, many symptoms in patients are cumulative effects of the chemotherapeutic conditioning. Patients often have difficulty in conceiving a child and infertility can be a significant problem. Patients can be offered the option to cryopreserve germ cells prior to any conditioning therapy to protect the precious germ cells from DNA damage and subsequent risk of mutation. However, depending on the age of the patient, further difficulties in conception may be apparent where women can succumb to a much earlier menopause post-transplant, as well as hormonal complications such as thyroid problems, which can make conception and carrying a fetus difficult. Other genotoxic damage includes induction of cataracts, but potentially the most difficult problem is the occurrence of therapy-related and donor cell leukaemia (DCL).

Therapy-related leukaemia (TRL) results directly from exposure to the DNA-damaging agents used for conditioning therapy, and is highly associated with the use of alkylating agents (such as the nitrogen mustards including cyclophosphamide), the topoisomerase II inhibitors (such as etoposide) and irradiation therapy. Of all the therapeutics used, these groups are by far the most DNA damaging and it is easy to see how mutational events could occur during the conditioning process. It is clear that transplant patients are at a greater risk of new primary malignancies related to the therapy, but it is suggested that this occurs for only around 0.4–13% of individuals surviving their first cancer dependent on the type of therapy they have had. Chemotherapeutics pose a much higher risk of TRL than exposure to irradiation therapy, but may take up to 15 years post-treatment to be observed. TRL typically manifests as either therapy- related acute myeloid leukaemia (t-AML) or myelodysplasia (MDS), and can equally occur from chemotherapy for a solid tumour or for conditioning for a haematological malignancy and SCT.

Intriguingly the recognition of a DCL opens new questions about the complications of SCT. This leukaemia is recognized to occur in cells originating from the donor who usually stays healthy. Why the donor cells become malignant in the patient but the donor remains healthy is largely unknown, but several theories have been put forward including radiation effects, bystander theory, occult/smouldering leukaemia in the donor, viral integration, defective BM microenvironment, and residual effects of the chemotherapy. DCL has increasingly been observed in recent years due to advanced genetic identification of the cells involved. Early testing was able to distinguish the source of the leukaemia as being from the donor where there was sex disparity between donor and recipient (XX versus XY chromosomes), but where donor and recipient were sex matched, many DCL occurrences were probably missed as being a 'relapse'. DNA satellite and polymorphic markers can now be used to distinguish the source of the leukaemia accurately as being a DCL. With better recognition, it may be possible to better understand the aetiology of DCL, but at the moment it is estimated to only occur in about 1 in 20 cases (~5%) or less of SCT and may be closer to about 1% post-UCB transplant, so it seems to represent a fairly rare complication.

Such genetic testing has allowed researchers to understand that HSC demonstrate significant plasticity and in this capacity may have the ability to be used therapeutically in novel ways for diseases other than those related to the BM; these will be discussed towards the end of the chapter. It is clear that there are significant life-threatening complications with SCT, despite it often being the only curative option available, so clinicians may decide on therapies that control disease rather than cure it until all other options 'run out'.

Key points

Complications in SCT can be short term or long term, with graft-versus-host disease being the main cause of graft failure.

SELF-CHECK 10.7

What are the range of complications we see with HSCT and when do they typically occur post-transplant?

10.5 Novel approaches to personalized medicine and stem cell plasticity

We have already noted that HSC and MSC have the potential to create a wide range of cell types comprising the haematopoietic system and BM microenvironment which work in collaboration to replace dead and dying blood cells and control our immune capacity. Such BM-derived SCs have also been noted for their beneficial therapeutic effects and future potential in various clinical disorders, although there are differing applications in their use as well as varying amounts of understanding in how they achieve this therapy. The additional identification of adult SCs in organs other than the BM offers the potential to utilize healthy cells from one organ in a patient, to treat other ailments if the cells can be encouraged to behave differently when placed in an alternative environment. This approach would avoid some of the obvious complications associated with transplanting 'foreign' healthy tissue from one individual to another and the subsequent requirement for immunosuppression due to HLA mismatch. It is believed that the development of the use of SCs in these ways could revolutionize therapy beyond what is currently possible.

At the moment, there appears to be two strategies for using SCs for clinical therapy; firstly in the context of simply transplanting the BM-derived SCs with their own functionality as described earlier in this chapter, or alternatively harnessing the plasticity of SCs with the aim to change their phenotype and functionality. Both approaches aim to correct fundamental deficiencies in diseased or injured tissue and currently have different degrees of success, especially in the hands of different researchers and clinicians. These differences appear to be linked to the multitude of ways in which the SCs are harvested, purified, administered, and maintained, as well as hampered by the different ways in which researchers can track their movement, differentiation and subsequent activity and proliferation. Inconsistencies in data are most likely influenced by the lack of a standard way to perform these techniques; however, as research and technology progresses, there is excitement regarding the potential to cure conditions that previously had limited options. The next section summarizes the approaches to therapy and benefits noted to date.

Key points

Bone marrow-derived stem cells can be used to replace malfunctioning tissues/cells either by direct replacement or by harnessing stem cell plasticity.

BM-derived stem cells for transplantation

Transplantation of SC for their intrinsic functionality has applications for BM failure syndromes, haematological malignancy and metabolic deficiency as well as autoimmunity. Transplantation is a well-developed and standardized procedure, but there are subtleties in the application of the procedure dependent on the clinical condition to be treated. For example, in malignancy there are choices to be made about the source of SC to be used and subsequent patient care. Where the underlying condition is a leukaemia, utilizing a HLA-matched sibling or unrelated donor may be the best course of action in order to achieve GvL affect; however, this needs careful maintenance to control GvHD with immunosuppression. SCT has benefitted from co-transplanting MSC alongside HSC infusion by increasing the homing capacity of HSC, reducing graft failure and GvHD. The immunosuppressive properties of MSC were suggested to contribute to all these outcomes; however, animal models of autologous transplantation, where immunosuppression was not an issue, also showed improved HSC migration and homing in the presence of MSC, though it was not clear as to the mechanisms involved.

Similarly with an intrinsic deficiency in the BM (e.g. Fanconi anaemia) or perhaps an inherited metabolic disease such as Hunter's or Hurler's syndrome, replacement of genetic defects with SCs harbouring the fully functioning missing gene(s) requires the source to be from a healthy donor, who is closely/completely HLA matched. Novel therapeutic approaches in this 'gene replacement' setting have described techniques where the patient's own SCs are utilized and fully functioning genes have been inserted into the cells via gene therapy methods. This would theoretically correct the genetic deficiency whilst avoiding being rejected due to the HLA on the SC being 'self'; this autologous gene therapy approach would have obvious benefits of not requiring immunosuppression and low risk of rejection to maintain the new functioning gene. However, gene therapy approaches are still not fully developed and maintaining long-term gene expression, as well as getting optimal insertion into the SC is still limited. Furthermore, it is difficult to dictate where in the genome the gene may be inserted and if this incurs a mutagenic event; this may lead to further malignancy or other genetic expression complications, which being a 'self' cell would have limited recognition and clearance (if any) from the body by the immune system.

For some solid tumours, such as breast cancer or neuroblastoma, chemotherapy with/without radiotherapy needs to be aggressive, and this therapy can destroy the patient's own BM. In these cases the patient's own BM will be harvested and cryopreserved prior to aggressive therapy, ready for reinfusion afterwards to reconstitute the blood and immune system. In this case, collection of BM from the patient, (providing there is no evidence of metastatic disease to the BM) may be the best option with respect to subsequent care and reduced need for immunosuppression.

Autologous BM SC transplantation has also been utilized for a range of autoimmune conditions such as multiple sclerosis (MS), systemic sclerosis, Crohn's, and systemic lupus erythematosus (SLE). The principle of this approach is that HSC are mobilized from the BM using regimes involving genotoxic chemotherapeutic drugs like cyclophosphamide followed by G-CSF. These are used in preference to drugs like plerixafor (CXCR4 antagonist) because the cyclophosphamide can reduce disease flare-ups from the G-CSF, as well as reduce the number of autoreactive T cells in the graft and perform a beneficial reduction in immunoreactivity and active inflammation, through cytotoxicity of the autoimmune lymphocytes. Frequently steroids can also be used to reduce immune reactivity and disease reactivation resulting from release of cytokines which occurs during conditioning therapy. Once the mobilized HSC are collected through leukapheresis, they can be purified to select for CD34+ cells, as well as depletion of the graft of autoreactive T cells causing the autoimmune condition. Before reinfusion of the graft, patients undergo aggressive immunosuppression therapy to deplete the patient of the autoreactive immune cells, which may mean cryopreserving the collected graft for a few weeks (40–60 days). There are several treatments adopted to immunosuppress the patient prior to reinfusion, including total body irradiation, antithymocyte globulin, and a range of chemotherapeutic agents. For some patients less aggressive therapy is appropriate and may involve removal of lymphocytes using monoclonal antibodies such as alemtuzumab (Campath; targets CD52 present on B lymphocytes). The hope is that by depleting the lymphocytes that are self-reactive and then reinfusing the harvested mobilized CD34+ cells, the patient's immune system will be reset and this will reduce progression of the disease.

Transplantation as described above, aims to use the intrinsic properties of the BM SC themselves to simply replace a diseased or poorly functioning BM compartment. Whilst SC transplantation is well defined, optimized, and widely performed, the procedure can still be life-threatening due to the procedural complications. As a result SC transplantation may be used as a 'last resort' when other therapies are available to allow the patient good quality of life. Thus SC transplant may only be used where the status of the disease is severe enough to warrant the risk, and where the patient is otherwise fit and healthy enough to tolerate the procedure. For example, for patients with chronic myelogenous leukaemia (CML) with **Philadelphia positive status** (~95% of patients are positive), the preference is to control their disease with drugs like imatinib, dasatinib, and nilotinib as initial therapy. This only controls and does not cure the disease, however; the only consistently successful curative treatment of CML is an allogeneic SC transplant. But whilst the drugs give good quality of life for extended periods (may be up to 10 years or more), these are used in preference to a curative option like SC transplant that has life-threatening complications.

Philadelphia positive status

Leukaemic cells that show the presence of a translocation between chromosomes 9 and 22 to create the BCR-Abl (tyrosine kinase) fusion protein. The derivative chromosome 22 is much smaller than usual and is termed the 'Philadelphia' chromosome.

Key points

The normal function of haematopoietic stem cells can be harnessed in transplantation to treat diseases such as leukaemia, autoimmunity, bone marrow failure, and replace failed bone marrow post-aggressive cancer therapy.

Use of stem cell plasticity for clinical application

The alternative, but less established use for SC in clinical practice, exploits the perceived **transdifferentiation** of SC. The premise is that when placed in a different tissue environment, SC will develop into the cell types consistent with that tissue because of growth factors or

Transdifferentiation

The ability of cells to change into a completely different cell type of another tissue.

signalling molecules that are specific to the environment. This approach in theory could work with any adult SC, not just those originating from the BM. After isolation and purification of SC, research has debated the relative merits of either transdifferentiating cells *ex vivo* into the required cell type prior to reinfusion, or alternatively simply placing the SC into the required location and hoping that the surrounding milieu of signalling molecules will instruct the cells to become the cell type they need to be.

The relative advantages of using HSC and MSC in these approaches over alternative adult SCs are that HSC and MSC are relatively easily isolated and purified, they are well defined in their functionality and phenotype, and are easy to inject into the right places, as well as having the intrinsic ability to mobilize and home to sites of injury. Indeed there appears to be a basic requirement that tissue injury is present in order to mobilize the HSC/MSC from the BM. However, even with HSC and MSC, it is rare to be able to produce a completely pure preparation of SCs, and there is still some controversy over therapeutic benefits being due to actual SC plasticity and differentiation versus their intrinsic immune-modulatory effects.

There is evidence that both HSC and MSC have capacity to transdifferentiate into other cell lineages within their main repertoire; for example lymphoid progenitors appear able to switch to myeloid lineages and vice versa, as well as MSC-derived adipocytes, chondrocytes, and osteocytes being able to interchange given the appropriate stimuli. However, the most interest comes from the suggestion that these cells can escape the usual range of cell lineages and become cells of different organs within the body. There is much controversy in the literature as to whether these observations are either experimental artefacts or also take place physiologically; clearly the best evidence comes from animal models of transdifferentiation, but this does not guarantee it also occurs in humans.

Evidence of HSC and MSC trafficking to sites of injury

The BM is naturally an hypoxic environment and it has been intriguing to note that both HSC and MSC travel to sites of hypoxia elsewhere in the body during ischaemic injury. For example, research has noted that both cardiac arrest and stroke episodes can induce HSC and MSC mobilization and it would be exciting to suppose that they do so in order to help repair the injury or replace dead or dying cells. Indeed evidence suggests that the trafficking of donor infused HSC to the BM may be induced by the naturally hypoxic conditions of the BM coupled with conditioning therapy-induced injury creating a release of chemokines and other factors to signal the HSC where to go to. Factors such as SDF-1α, IL-8, as well as release of prostaglandins and leukotrienes from the damaged cell membrane have all been implicated in attraction of HSC to the BM. Indeed hypoxic conditions and chemotherapy exposure have been shown to increase the levels of SDF-1α expression in the BM, as well as induce the expression of genes suggested to maintain the 'stemness' of HSC and MSC. Furthermore, hypoxic conditions due to injury in the brain and heart have demonstrated a similar release of the same homing molecules which naturally might induce HSC and MSC to migrate to this site of injury.

Whilst MSC theoretically have the widest range of cell lineages, there is controversial evidence of MSC effectively transdifferentiating into replacement cells in injured tissues, rather their immunomodulatory and immunosuppressive properties appear to play a bigger role in tissue repair. MSC appear to originate from a wide variety of tissues with those from the BM arguably being the best described; MSC have been sourced from skeletal muscle, adipose tissue, synovium, the circulatory system, umbilical cord, amniotic fluid, dental pulp, liver, and lung, in addition to the well-recognized MSC from BM and fetal blood. However, MSC from all these sources are not equivalent functionally with respect to their differentiation capacity and therefore may not be equally therapeutic in this setting. Furthermore, a potential bottleneck in MSC therapy is the capacity to expand enough cells in culture for infusion, without losing the natural 'stem-ness' as well as differentiation capacity of the MSC.

Applications of stem cell plasticity to therapy

More interesting is the novel testing of HSC and MSC in a range of clinical conditions to replace diseased tissue. Early observations of SC trafficking were demonstrated by Y chromosome markers of male origin SCs in female hosts which showed movement of BM or blood cells to hepatocytes and the epithelial layers of the skin and gut. Similarly, using fluorescence *in situ* hybridization (FISH) to track the Y chromosome, male mouse cells expressing normal male dystrophin gene were shown to be present in female host muscle fibres in a model of Duchenne muscular dystrophy. Similar observations have been seen in mouse models of cardiac arrest.

A key element of the possibility of SC plasticity in these settings seems to be the need to implant the cells into an appropriate microenvironment expressing the necessary signalling molecules for differentiation and functional response. Transplantation of suspensions of cells such as HSC or MSC has had more success in suggesting plasticity into different cell lineages than early models of transplanted tissue or organ fragments, because cell suspensions are surrounded by different cell types, whereas the fragments are still surrounded by similar cellular neighbours. Thus where tracking of sex-disparate transplanted cells has been performed in mouse models, it has been suggested that BM cells can develop into astrocytes and skeletal muscle. Similarly in both mouse and humans there is evidence of differentiation into hepatocytes, endothelial and myocardial cells, cells of the central nervous system, and glial cells.

MSC that were injected into newborn mice were shown to move through the brain and were able to adopt the morphology and phenotype of astrocytes and neurons. However, proteomic and microarray approaches showed differences in the gene expression of these cells compared with native MSC or native astrocytes and neurons. Further exploration of the 3D architectural microenvironment in which these migratory MSC resided suggested that alterations in the cellular cytoskeleton was more likely to give the appearance of neuronal cells and change the gene expression, rather than result in true transdifferentiation. Thus this would question the application of such SC in treating neurological disorders or spinal cord injury in the absence of a clear neural phenotype.

Where there is a question over differentiation into neural cells, there are a range of publications supporting epithelial cell development from MSC. Evidence suggests transdifferentiation into all lung cell types, skin, sebaceous ducts, retinal pigment, corneal keratocytes, tubular epithelial cells, and muscle cells. Unfortunately, although MSC are also suggested to become hepatocytes, administration failed to show the ability to regenerate liver tissue or rescue a range of enzyme-deficiency conditions. Currently in the UK, the five biggest clinical killers are coronary heart disease, stroke, cancer, lung disease, and liver disease which are estimated to cause more than 150,000 deaths per annum in the under 75s. The use of SC to help alleviate the symptoms and/or cure these conditions would have massive economical and clinical benefits. The following section summarizes what is known about the use of SC in cardiovascular disease and type I diabetes as examples of key potential applications of SC therapy.

Stem cell therapy in cardiac ischaemia

Coronary heart disease causes about 74,000 deaths per annum in the UK making it one of the biggest killers of under 75s. Whilst the death rate from cardiac ischaemia has significantly improved over the last few decades, there is still a need for new approaches to both improve the overall health of the population as well as to correct damage post ischaemia. Ischaemic heart disease is characterized by death and loss of cardiomyocytes due to a sudden loss or decrease of blood perfusion to the cardiac tissues, eventually resulting in scarring, heart wall thinning, cardiac overload, and ultimately heart failure and death. The heart has repair mechanisms including proliferation of cardiomyocytes in response to arrest, and mobilization of BM SC to the site which promotes angiogenesis and aims to repair lost cardiac tissue and restore functionality. However, these are insufficient to replace the damaged tissue.

Hypoxia in heart tissue can induce the release of SDF-1α and IL-8 (promoting mobilization of MSC/HSC), and hypoxia inducible factor (HIF-1α) leading to upregulation of vascular endothelial growth factor (VEGF) and CXCR4. Collectively these events promote angiogenesis, erythropoiesis, and vascularization, as well as induce MSC to be more responsive to hypoxia, improving MSC function and fate. The hypoxic environment appears to control gene expression in MSC through epigenetic changes including methylation status of the genes, and control of gene expression via miR expression. Furthermore MSC are able to not only express myocardial genes, but also demonstrate contractility and excitation-contraction coupling to become functional cardiomyocytes, which offers an exciting prospect into repair post-myocardial infarction.

Infusion of CD34+ cells also promotes therapeutic angiogenesis, although the mechanisms are not fully understood. There is evidence that CD34+ cells can become incorporated into the vasculature, can transdifferentiate into cardiomyocytes, and also have the ability to fuse with them. However, there is some confusion about whether clinical benefit is due to true transdifferentiation versus cellular fusing, because the vascular endothelium highly expresses the CD34 molecule and may be confused for transdifferentiated HSC. Overall, the use of HSC, CD34+ or MSC in cardiac ischaemia is to repair and replace damaged tissue as well as quickly re-establish blood flow. SCs can be delivered to the damaged heart tissue via invasive or non-invasive routes. SC can be directly injected into the tissue injury via an invasive epicardial injection during heart surgery or non-invasively via catheter infusion.

During invasive injection, the SCs are either injected into the damaged tissue itself or into the healthy tissue surrounding the site of damage. The relative advantage of direct injection is that cardiac ischaemia typically occurs because of blocked blood vessels around the heart, making delivery of the cells via the vasculature virtually impossible. Furthermore, direct injection guarantees that the SC get to the actual site of injury. Catheter-based approaches address the current trend towards non-invasive approaches and involves penetrating the skin and insertion of a catheter to infuse SCs. This would possibly require intra-arterial stents to ensure the SC get to the site of injury so catheter-based approaches are currently limited. Other non-invasive approaches harness the natural signalling processes of chemokine release that we have already considered. It is currently unknown if HSC/MSC become released from the BM in response to these messages, or if they are already circulating in the vasculature and then exit into the tissues at the injury site.

Several clinical trials have been performed, with evidence to suggest an improvement in exercise ability as well as reduced tissue damage, reduced scar tissue size, and noted improved cardiac wall flexibility and motion post-infusion of BM SCs in comparison to control subjects. There has been some conflicting evidence in the clinical trials, but it is suggested that this reflects the different approaches to SC purification, with some researchers using purified cell fractions and others using heterogeneous mixes of BM mononuclear cells. Exactly which cell types produce the therapeutic outcomes is unclear, but overall the outlook is of cardiac improvement in these patients.

Islet cell transplantation

Autoimmune attack of the β-islet cells in the pancreas leads to a destruction of the cells and consequent loss of insulin production leading to type I diabetes mellitus. The UK is currently placed fifth globally for incidence of type I diabetes in 0 to 14 year olds (24.5 per 100,000) and this is becoming an increasing problem, with the number of people living with diabetes doubling since 1996. The lack of insulin in the body leads to abnormally high levels of sugar in the blood and a range of symptoms including excessive thirst and passing of urine (especially at night), tiredness, muscle loss, blurred vision, and slow healing of wounds. Patients are managed by regular insulin injections to control their blood sugar levels. Recent research has developed new technology like biosensors or insulin pumps that can monitor blood sugar levels in real time with the ability to infuse insulin at appropriate levels. Poor glucose control can lead to significant long-term complications such as damage of vasculature, organs and nerves, a reduction in skin elasticity giving an aged appearance, cataract development, and life-threatening complications such as coronary artery disease, stroke, and atherosclerosis. Most of these complications result from glycation of proteins in the body tissues due to being 'bathed' in high glucose levels frequently, which reduces the functionality of the proteins.

In principle, real-time biosensors offer a good option for control, but there are limitations in that they need to be small enough in order to be worn without difficulty, be highly sensitive and reliable, be easily maintained, have a low risk of infection, and be as non-invasive as possible, as well as being unlikely to be rejected (if implanted) or compromised due to bodily functions. Whilst much progress has been made in the development of biosensors, the use of SC differentiated into β-islet cells would offer a 'biological biosensor' capable of replacing the damaged pancreas. In the past, transplantation of allogeneic islet cells from cadavers has been performed, but this is limited due to the numbers of islets available and the requirement for immunosuppression.

Initial studies injecting fluorescently labelled male mouse cells into female mouse models of diabetes were contradictory; some claimed evidence of fluorescence, Y chromosome markers and expression of genes such as *insulin*, *Glut2*, and *Pax6* in the β-islet cells, whereas others showed none. BM transplants in mice also showed that HSC which engrafted into the pancreas were expressing haematopoietic markers not insulin and this was supported when autopsy pancreatic samples from humans who had received HSC transplants did not show any HSC in the pancreas. However, there was no doubt that diabetic patients were showing benefit from HSC infusion.

Whilst there is much controversy, mechanisms of action of this clinical benefit of HSC appear to reside with their revascularization and immunomodulatory capabilities which help to regenerate the lost β-islet cells. Infused HSC seem to reside around ductal and islet structures without actually producing any insulin, but all the evidence shows an improvement in pancreatic regeneration and insulin expression. It has been suggested that autologous BMT in type I diabetes may improve the condition in the same way as for other autoimmune conditions by reducing the auto-reactivity and resetting the immune system. Furthermore, MSC infused into diabetic patients showed improved wound healing with a significant reduction in ulcer size; it was suggested that MSC differentiated into epidermal cells and vessel forming endothelial cells which contributed to neovascularization, and to the supply of oxygen and nutrients.

Allogeneic transplantation of islet cells suffers from the problem of immunosuppression and possible rejection, leading to eventual loss of islet function and return to insulin injections. Intriguingly a new approach to allogeneic islet transplantation has utilized the BM niche itself;

to host transplanted islet cells because it offers a vascularized environment which is protective and capable of supporting islet cell function and development. Preliminary experiments in mouse models have shown promise in using the BM as a site for islet cell transplantation.

Key points

Plasticity of bone marrow-derived cells has been used to correct damaged tissues elsewhere in the body, and either occurs naturally through stem cells trafficking, or can be performed clinically.

SELF-CHECK 10.8

What are the two novel approaches to the use of stem cells for personalized therapy?

10.6 Concluding remarks

HSC and MSC are cells showing a high degree of plasticity, besides the known capacity to fully replace the haematopoietic and immune systems. However, it is currently undetermined the full scope of cellular lineages that can be produced. What is clear is that the signalling from the surrounding microenvironment, particularly where there is hypoxia and injury, can promote mobilization of HSC and MSC as well as their differentiation into certain cell types with therapeutic implications. This signalling plays a role in both 'replacement' therapy via transplantation as well as the ability to either develop into different cell types or to act in a supportive role. However, limitations with tracking cells, sensitivity of techniques, and standardized methods means that we are still unsure as to how exactly HSC and MSC effect their therapy. There is conflicting literature claiming transdifferentiation into different lineages, evidence of immunomodulatory capacity, and fusion with neighbouring cells.

As techniques develop and methods become more reproducible, so our understanding of the full scope of the potential of SC both biologically and clinically should unfold to improve therapies. For the moment it is exciting to know that SC offer potential respite for chronically ill patients. Certainly for the patient it may not be currently necessary to understand the mechanisms by which they work, as long as we can safely control their activity.

 Chapter summary

- Haematopoietic stem cell transplantation is a well-established procedure which has developed significantly since it was first performed in 1968.

- There are three main sources of haematopoietic stem cells, originating from bone marrow, umbilical cord blood, and peripheral blood, which have slightly different advantages and limitations during the transplant procedure.

- Stem cells can be harvested from the patient (autologous), an identical twin (syngeneic) or an HLA-matched individual who may or may not be related to the patient (allogeneic).

- Harvested cells are processed, cryopreserved, and stored for transplantation at a later date.

- Cells are identified by surface markers such as CD34 and are enumerated to ensure enough cells are harvested for transplantation; for some transplants like umbilical cord blood, this is particularly important.

- Patients require conditioning therapy comprising chemotherapy with or without radio-therapy to prepare their bone marrow for infusion of donor cells, this can be reduced in intensity for particularly old or ill patients.

- Whilst a life-saving curative option for many haematological malignancies, it is also a life-threatening procedure that may be performed when there are no other options; stem cells transplants also have several short and long term complications with graft failure and GvHD representing significant problems.

- Stem cells can be used for transplantation to correct malfunctioning cells in several conditions including cancer, but plasticity of stem cells has offered novel personalized therapies in other conditions like cardiac arrest, ischaemic brain injury, and treatment for diabetes.

 ## Further reading

- Anthony Nolan Users operations guide available at: https://www.anthonynolan.org/clinicians-and-researchers/services-transplant-centres/using-anthony-nolan%E2%80%99s-services-guide

- Catacchio I, Berardi S, Reale A, De Luisi A, Racanelli V, Vacca A & Ria R. Evidence for bone marrow adult stem cell plasticity: Properties, molecular mechanisms, negative aspects, and clinical applications of hematopoietic and mesenchymal stem cells transdifferentiation. *Stem Cells International* (2013), Article ID 589139. Available from: http://dx.doi.org/10.1155/2013/589139

- Goyal G, Gundabolu K, Vallabhajosyula S, Silberstein PT & Bhatt VR. Reduced-intensity conditioning allogeneic hematopoietic-cell transplantation for older patients with acute myeloid leukemia. *Therapeutic Advances in Hematology* 7 (2016), 131–41.

- Hordyjewska A, Popiołek L & Horecka A. Characteristics of hematopoietic stem cells of umbilical cord blood. *Cytotechnology* 67 (2015), 387–96.

- Horwitz ME & Chao N. Non-myeloablative umbilical cord blood transplantation. *Best Practice & Research Clinical Haematology* 23 (2010), 231–236.

- Rojas-Rios P & Gonzalez-Reyes A. Concise review: The plasticity of stem cell niches: A general property behind tissue homeostasis and repair. *Stem Cells* 32 (2014), 852–859.

Answers to the questions in this chapter are provided on the book's accompanying website:

Go to www.oup.com/uk/avent2e

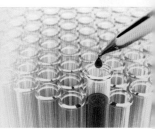

11

Tissue Banking

Richard Lomas, Neil D. Avent, and Vehid Salih

Learning objectives

After studying this chapter you should be able to:

- Describe the types of grafts that are currently used.
- Know what tissues are banked and how are they used.
- Outline how donors are selected, screened, and consent is obtained.
- Outline how tissues are procured from living and deceased donors.
- Outline how the collected tissue is processed.
- Outline how that tissue is preserved.
- Outline how tissues are stored and distributed.
- Be aware of the requirements of the UK Human Tissue Act.
- Have an appreciation of how regenerative medicine may impact on tissue transplantation.

Introduction

Tissue damage resulting from disease or trauma is a significant medical problem and many different ways have been tried to correct the damage, or to enable the patient to live with the problem. One of the earliest was the use of an artificial graft or a prosthesis, such as a metal plate to hold a fractured bone in place. But there are alternatives available. In other chapters, transplantation of cellular organs and stem cells have been considered along with the need to HLA match the donor and recipient to prevent rejection of the transplanted organ. However, there are other tissues (e.g. bone) that can be used as grafts, whose effectiveness is not dependent on a good HLA match. This chapter describes how tissue grafts are used clinically, and discusses the process by which tissue grafts are collected and treated to improve their clinical efficacy, make them safer, and render them suitable for long-term storage.

11.1 **Types of graft**

There are many strategies for replacing or repairing damaged tissues, a significant one of which is the use of tissue grafts. There are three basic types of tissue graft:

- Xenografts (grafts prepared from animal tissue)
- Autografts (tissue grafted from another site on the patient's body)
- Allografts (tissue donated by another person, and the focus of this chapter).

Occasionally, biological grafts may be combined with prosthetic materials to form a composite, **bioprosthetic graft**. Prosthetic grafts (made from artificial materials) may also be used.

Autografts are universally agreed to be the gold standard for tissue grafting from a clinical performance viewpoint. The use of the patient's own tissue obviates any risk of disease transmission or immune rejection, and allows transplantation of a living graft, with the requisite biological and structural properties, to facilitate tissue repair and regeneration. For example, autograft obtained from the **iliac crest** is used in many bone grafting procedures, and autograft skin is essential for the repair of deep burns. Autografts do, however, have significant and insurmountable differences. First, any operation using autograft requires a secondary procedure to procure the graft, resulting in additional morbidity at the donor site. Second, the amount of tissue that can be safely taken for autografting is limited. Bone graft taken from the iliac crest may suffice for sinus reconstruction, but may be insufficient in volume for a spinal fusion, or hip revision, and a patient with 80% burns will not have sufficient undamaged skin available to graft the entire burnt area.

Prosthetic grafts address the deficiencies of autografts in that there are no restrictions on graft size or availability, but they also come with disadvantages. A general disadvantage with all grafts made of non-biological material is that they do not integrate well with the patient's own tissue, and are much more prone to infection than biological grafts. Prosthetic grafts placed in the cardiovascular system may also be **thrombogenic** and require the recipient to take prophylactic anticoagulants, with the attendant risk of side effects.

The principle advantages of using allografts is that as a biological material they do not have the drawbacks of prosthetic grafts, and also much better approximate the complex biomechanical properties of human tissue—it is generally better where possible to replace 'like with like'. They can also, to a limited degree, replicate the biological properties of an autograft. Whilst the cellular content of an allograft will be rejected if exposed to the recipient's immune system, grafts placed in immunocompromised areas such as the cornea or **articular cartilage** may retain the viability, and hence maintenance and reparative properties, of the donor cells. Even short-term retention of graft viability can be beneficial, for example in the case of non-HLA-matched skin allografts which can temporarily engraft to a burn wound-bed, and promote regeneration of the recipient's own skin. The main drawback of allografts from a surgeon's viewpoint is the perceived risk of disease transmission from the graft to the recipient, originating either from the donor or from contamination acquired during procurement or preparation. If correct donor selection, testing, and tissue decontamination procedures are followed, the risks of disease transmission are very low or negligible. However, allograft transmitted infections have been recorded and are a source of concern to clinicians.

Xenografts are prepared from animal material; the most commonly used in surgery are porcine (pig) heart valve grafts. Other types of xenograft include bovine and equine pericardium, commonly used in cardiac surgery, and bovine bone-derived grafts used in orthopaedic and maxillofacial surgery.

Bioprosthetic graft
A composite graft comprising both prosthetic and biological materials.

Iliac crest
Part of the pelvic bone, often used as a source of bone autograft.

Thrombogenic
Material which causes blood to clot on contact.

Articular cartilage
Hard, smooth cartilage that lines bone in joint surfaces.

Key points

There are three types of graft available: xeno-, auto-, and allografts, plus prosthetic grafts. Although autografts are the most effective, allografts are becoming more widely used.

SELF-CHECK 11.1

What are the advantages and disadvantages of synthetic, xeno- auto-, and allografts?

11.2 Which tissues are banked and how are they used?

Most tissue allografts are donated by deceased donors, although some tissues may be donated for grafting by living donors following surgical removal during routine operations. The clinical requirement for different types of allograft varies both temporally and geographically. As certain types of graft are shown to perform well or less well, requirements fluctuate accordingly. There are additionally geographical variations in allograft usage, which may result (for example) from a lack of suitable local banking services. Perhaps the most widely and commonly banked tissues are those of the musculoskeletal system. The repair of damaged bones with prosthetic grafts has been performed since prehistoric times, and there is a major demand for bone allografts in many surgical areas, principally orthopaedic (spine and joint surgery) and also in oral/maxillofacial surgery. There are many different forms of bone allograft, ranging from massive **osteochondral grafts** used in trauma repair and following excision of large bone tumours, to fine, **morsellized bone grafts** used in joint and dental surgery. See Figure 11.1.

Tendon and ligament allografts are also commonly used, principally in knee surgery for the repair of ruptured or damaged **anterior cruciate ligaments**. There is also a growing use of more specialized musculoskeletal allografts, such as osteochondral grafts for the treatment of focal lesions of the joint surface, and allografts for repair of knee injuries. See Figure 11.2.

Skin allografts play a major role in the treatment of serious burn injuries. Whilst they do not permanently engraft they can be combined with small amounts of autograft, providing

Osteochondral graft
A composite graft, comprising bone plus an intact articular cartilage surface.

Morsellized bone graft
Bone graft milled to granules or powders of different diameters.

Anterior cruciate ligament
A ligament located within the knee joint that plays a crucial role in stabilizing the joint and a commonly damaged in sporting injuries.

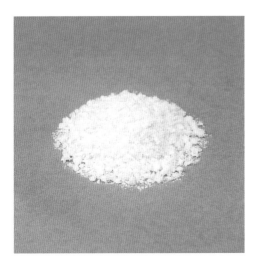

FIGURE 11.1
Morsellized cortico-cancellous bone graft.

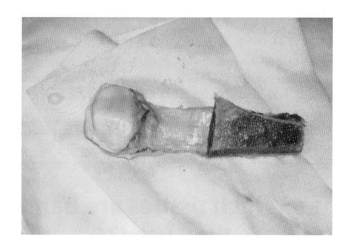

FIGURE 11.2
Patellar ligament graft, with patella bone and tibial bone block attached.

protection and cover to the wound-bed while the autograft induces the formation of new skin. Generally, a cadaveric skin graft comprises the epidermis and upper layer of the dermis. The allograft closely adheres to the recipient's wound-bed, covering exposed nerve endings and reducing pain and infection, whilst the presence of the intact epidermis reduces fluid and heat loss. There is also evidence that viable grafts are able to temporarily engraft to the recipient, further enhancing healing.

Other tissues that are banked include heart valves, blood vessels, pericardium, eye corneas and sclera, and amniotic membrane (used as a dressing in the treatment of eye and burn injuries). See Table 11.1.

> ## Key points
>
> The most widely and commonly banked tissues for engraftment are those from the musculoskeletal system, such as bones, tendons, and ligaments. Skin, corneas, and heart valves are also collected and banked.

TABLE 11.1 Types of tissue allograft used in different surgical specialities.

Surgical specialty	Types of graft used
Cardiac	Heart valves, vascular patches, pericardium
Orthopaedic (knee surgery)	Tendons, ligaments, meniscus, bone
Orthopaedic (hip)	Morsellized and structural bone
Orthopaedic (spine)	Morsellized and structural bone, demineralized bone matrix
Ophthalmology	Cornea, sclera, amnion
Burns	Skin, dermis
Plastic and reconstructive	Dermis
Oral and maxillofacial	Demineralized bone matrix
Vascular	Blood vessels

11.3 **How are donors selected, screened, and consented?**

The banking of tissues for therapeutic use is a multi-step process, the first stage of which is obtaining valid, informed consent for donation to take place. This section addresses the legal framework under which this consent must be obtained, and explains how this is accomplished by NHS Blood and Transplant Tissue Services (NHSBT-TS), the largest therapeutic tissue bank in the UK.

NHSBT-TS obtains tissues for therapeutic purposes and for ethically approved research projects. These may be obtained from living donors, where the tissue is removed following elective surgery (e.g. femoral heads donated following hip replacement), but most tissues are obtained from deceased donors.

It is crucial that when consent is obtained for tissue donation for any reason, be it for therapeutic or research purposes, it is both informed and valid. For the consent to be valid, it must be taken from the appropriate person in a manner that complies with legislative requirements. It also requires that the person giving consent is fully informed of all aspects of the donation process. Where the donor is deceased and consent is taken usually from bereaved relatives, there is a further challenge in ensuring that the process does not cause additional distress, whilst complying with legal and ethical requirements.

The primary legislation covering tissue donation is the Human Tissue Act. This was enacted in 2004, following well-publicized cases of organ retention following post-mortem examination without the knowledge or consent of relatives. Accordingly, the Human Tissue Act makes consent the fundamental guiding principle covering the use of donated tissue for any purpose, and provides for financial and custodial penalties for breaches of its requirements. It also established a regulatory body, the Human Tissue Authority (HTA), with a remit to license and inspect all establishments procuring and storing human tissue.

The HTA provides guidance and direction, through the publication of codes of practice, the first of which deals specifically with consent. This clarifies that the removal, storage, and use of relevant material from deceased donors, and the storage and use of relevant material from living donors requires consent. The HTA defines the term 'relevant material' as 'material other than gametes, which consists of, or includes, human cells'. Certain tissues, such as hair and nail clippings, are not classified as relevant material and are not covered by the Act.

As already mentioned, for consent to be valid, it must be given by the appropriate person. With a living donor, this is generally the donor themselves. However, for deceased donors the situation is often more complex. The HTA defines a 'hierarchy of consent', specifying in order of relevance who can give consent in these cases. The highest priority is given to the wishes of the deceased themselves if expressed in life, for example through the organ donor register. If this was not done, then priority is given to the deceased's nominated representative, a person who was appointed in life by the deceased to make these decisions. If neither of these situations is the case, consent must be sought from a person who was in a 'qualifying relationship' with the deceased. This may be (in order of priority) a spouse or partner, blood relation, or friend.

It is also important for consent to be considered valid, that the person giving consent is fully informed with regard to all aspects of the donation process, including how, where, and when the donation will take place, how much tissue will be removed, and the purposes for which the tissue may be used. The scope of the consent must be defined as closely as it is practical to do; it is recognized that when tissue is donated for research purposes, a generic consent may be appropriate as the specific nature of the research for which the tissue may be used may not be known at the point of donation. However, where the tissue is donated for a specific purpose, such as a defined research project, or for transplantation, this information must be provided to the person giving consent.

The duration of the consent must also be specified; this may be enduring, that is, it remains in force unless it is specifically withdrawn, or time limited. The person giving consent may also withdraw it at any point before or after donation (providing that the tissue has not already been used), and it is important that they are informed of this right.

With the exception of anatomical examination or public display, where written consent is required, the Human Tissue Act does not specify the format in which consent should be recorded. Verbal consent, documented either by audio recording or in the patient's notes, is also valid. The Act recognizes that in itself, a signed consent document does not make the consent valid; it must be shown that all the information necessary for the person to give appropriate consent was given prior to the decision being made.

The procedure by which the NHS Blood and Transplant Tissue Services (NHSBT-TS) obtains consent for tissue donation was developed following consultation with a number of interested parties, including donor families and donor transplant co-ordinators, and has been ratified by the HTA. Indeed, during a recent inspection by the HTA the procedures in the National Referral Centre (NRC) were described as exemplary and are now used as an example of best practice in their *Code of Practice for Consent*.

Consent for tissue donation within NHSBT-TS is handled by a dedicated National Referral Centre (NRC), based in Liverpool. This unit is staffed by nurse practitioners (NPs) who are specially trained to assess the suitability of potential donors, and obtain valid consent for donation. The centralization of this service allows for rapid training of the NPs taking consent, quick dissemination of best practice, peer support for staff who need to undertake delicate and sensitive conversations with bereaved families on a regular basis, and also enables the application of lean working principles to maximize the efficiency of the unit.

Consent for tissue donation within the NRC is done by telephone, using a defined protocol. This is beneficial to donor families as it can be done at a pre-arranged time, in the surroundings of their own home with family members present for support. It also allows the option of donation to families of donors who have died outside a hospital environment. The NP must ensure that the conversation takes place in a quiet area without risk of disturbance, and a designated room is made available for this purpose. They then contact the donor family, and ensure that they are speaking to the appropriate person as defined in the hierarchy of consent. As the consent is verbal, the conversation is recorded to provide a record of the information that was provided by the NP, and what was agreed to by the person giving consent. The conversation requires that the NP provides appropriate information in order for the person giving consent to make an informed decision. This information includes:

- What the donor's expressed wishes in life were (if known). They establish this by checking if the donor is registered on the organ donor register prior to contacting the family.
- Which tissues may be donated.
- The timeframe under which donation will take place.
- How tissues are removed, and how the donor body is reconstructed afterwards.
- What is the clinical requirement for the donated tissues.
- How the donation process may affect the appearance of the donor.
- That viewing of the donor after donation is possible.

- That tissues may be stored in a tissue bank for a prolonged period of time before use.

- Sometimes, donated tissue is not suitable for transplantation; in these cases it may be used for ethically approved research, providing they so consent.

- That the donor's GP will be contacted to obtain medical history.

- That a blood sample will be taken to test for transmissible diseases, including HIV and hepatitis. If any of these test results may have significance for the health of other family members, they will be contacted and offered appropriate advice.

- Their right to withdraw consent at any time prior to use of the grafts, and an explanation of how to do so.

This is very much a two-way conversation, and the family are given the opportunity to ask questions and request further information about any aspects of the donation process. During the consent process, a detailed medical and behavioural history of the donor is also obtained from their family using a structured questionnaire to ascertain the medical suitability to donate. This is necessary to ensure the safety of the donated tissues. It must be considered that tissue grafts are in almost all cases used for 'life-enhancing', rather than 'life-saving' procedures; there are generally alternative treatments available (e.g. the use of inorganic bone substitutes in place of bone allografts, or the use of porcine heart valve grafts in place of allografts). The risk–benefit analysis for tissue allografts is therefore skewed more towards the risk side of the equation. Tissue donors are therefore carefully selected to minimize the risk of either transmitting diseases from the donor to the recipient, or transplanting a tissue that may perform poorly. This selection process takes the form of physical testing, and a review of the donor's medical and behavioural history. The donor's relatives, and or friends are interviewed to elicit any lifestyle factors that may render the donor a higher risk for disease transmission, and the donor's GP and any other medical practitioners treating the donor are queried to obtain as accurate and complete a medical history as possible. Significant lifestyle factors that preclude donation are intravenous drug abuse, high-risk sexual behaviour, and even the presence of recent tattoos. There are many medical conditions that either restrict or preclude tissue donation. Common reasons for total medical deferral include malignancy and sepsis, due to the potential risk of disease transmission. Other conditions may result in the deferral of tissues for physical reasons, for example the genetic condition **Marfan's syndrome** results in weakened connective tissue. Musculoskeletal and cardiovascular allografts would not be donated by a donor with Marfan's, but skin grafts would be acceptable. A comprehensive list of donor selection guidelines is maintained by the UK Blood and Tissue Transplantation Services, accessible online at: www.transfusionguidelines.org.

Marfan's syndrome
A genetic disorder, causing weakness of the connective tissue. A contraindication for donation of soft tissue allografts.

Screening of blood samples from potential tissue donors is also mandatory. Blood samples are screened for markers of a range of microbiological infections by using the same screening assays as used for testing blood donations. This screening includes the markers defined as mandatory, and any discretionary testing determined by the donor's medical or travel history, for example malaria and *T. cruzi*. All donors are screened for syphilis antibody, HBsAg, anti-HCV, anti-HIV, anti-HTLV, anti-HBc, and also by HCV-PCR, HIV-PCR, and HBV-PCR. The supplementation of routine serology testing with the new generation of nucleic acid tests serves to reduce the risk of false negative results, where a donor has only recently been exposed to a pathogen and not mounted sufficient immune response to trigger antibody tests. Nucleic acid testing is capable of detecting infection at a much earlier stage than the equivalent antibody test. However, serology screening still has the advantage of being able to detect a past exposure that may speak to lifestyle risks. This combination is especially important for testing of deceased tissue donors, where only a single blood sample can be taken at the time of donation. With donors of living tissue, it is possible to take a second blood sample at a time post donation to reduce the risk of these 'window period' infections. However, if PCR testing is used on the initial sample too, this is not now considered necessary.

A key limitation with serological testing is that it is only possible to test for diseases which are known about, and for which a validated test is available. It will take some time for the presence of novel transmissible diseases to become apparent, and even after a novel disease has been identified, it may be some time before a test is developed. A contemporary example of this problem is new variant Creutzfeldt–Jakob disease, which is known to be present in the donor population, especially in the UK. There is as yet no reliable blood test for this disease, and this screening must rely solely on assessment of a donor's medical history (did they show any clinical indications or dementia, etc.) and of any lifestyle risks (use of human growth hormone, etc.).

Assessment of donor safety is therefore a multi-step process, designed to investigate and identify any potential risks that might result from implantation of the tissue.

Key points

Before any tissue can be used, the donor, or in the case of a deceased donor, the nearest relatives, must have given consent; the donor's medical history must be reviewed and a sample of blood from the donor tested for the same microbiological markers as a blood donor.

SELF-CHECK 11.2

What is the role (in the UK) of the HTA?

11.4 How are tissues retrieved?

When a donor has been accepted for tissue donation, the next stage is to physically retrieve, or procure, the tissue from the donor. This is a very different procedure for deceased and living donors, and these will therefore be addressed in different sections. Irrespective of the type of donor, the overall objective of tissue procurement is to obtain the tissue to as high a standard as possible, minimizing or eliminating all risks to the tissue associated with the retrieval process.

Deceased donors

Warm ischaemia time
The time elapsing between death and a body being placed into a refrigerated environment.

With deceased donors, a key factor in ensuring the quality of the tissue grafts is the time post-mortem that the tissue is procured. Following death, the integrity of the intestinal walls deteriorates, and intestinal microflora begin to migrate throughout the body, contaminating other tissues. Additionally, autodegredation of all tissues commences as cells die and release lytic enzymes into the tissue. The rate of both these processes is critically dependent on temperature; therefore, it is crucial that the **warm ischaemia time** is minimized and the body is cooled as soon as possible after death. The permitted time for post-mortem retrieval varies between different countries. However, generally a maximum post-mortem time of 48 hours is permitted, subject to an acceptable warm ischaemia time. The optimal time and place to procure tissues from deceased donors is in the operating theatre, immediately post-mortem. However, the availability of these facilities for tissue donation is limited, and is generally restricted to tissue grafts that can be obtained during routine organ procurement procedures, such as removal the heart for valve donation. In the UK, the large majority of tissue donations are performed in hospital mortuaries, or on rare occasions in funeral homes.

Retrieval of tissue in a mortuary, which is not designed for aseptic operations, is challenging. It is necessary to perform tissue retrievals once routine post-mortem examinations have been completed, to reduce the risk of cross contamination. It is crucial that prior to any retrieval activities commencing the donor is correctly identified. This involves checking the information given with the referral with information physically present on the donor, on a wrist band or toe tag. The cardinal rule here is that at least three points of identification (such as name, date of birth, address, or hospital number) must coincide. Once the retrieval team is satisfied that these requirements have been met, tissue retrieval can commence. Before any dissection activities take place, the donor is cleaned using surgical detergents, alcohol wipes, and sterile water. Any areas of the skin where incisions will be made, or where skin grafts will be retrieved from, are also shaved. The donor is then placed on a sterile field and the retrieval team will don sterile clothing to commence removal of tissues.

Generally, skin grafts (if consented for) will be retrieved first to prevent the skin becoming contaminated by internal body fluids following incisions to remove internal tissues. The areas of the body from where skin is retrieved are dictated both by aesthetic considerations and practicalities. Skin will not be retrieved from areas of the body that may be visible during an open casket funeral, such as the face, neck, hand, or lower arms. Additionally, given that the primary requirement for skin grafts is in burn surgery where large sheets of skin are required, skin is not retrieved from areas where this is not practical. In practice, skin grafts are retrieved from the back of the torso and the back and front of both legs. Skin is retrieved using an instrument called an electric dermatome that can be adjusted for cutting depth and width so that skin is taken in long strips of nominal thickness 0.3 mm. This results in a split skin allograft, which comprises the epidermis and the upper layer of the dermis—in practice the thickness of the skin varies considerably depending on the person performing the procurement, the donor, and the anatomical area it is being taken from. Care is taken to avoid taking skin grafts where the skin is excessively blemished (for example, the presence of raised moles), and where the donor is tattooed. There is no clinical reason why tattooed skin is unsuitable for donation, but if the tattoo is considered to be identifiable to the donor it will be avoided. Following retrieval, the skin is transferred immediately to a cooled, buffered transport solution and transported to the tissue bank on wet ice. To prevent seeping of blood or other internal fluids from the body surface following retrieval, a dilute bleach solution is applied which seals the exposed dermis.

Other tissue grafts are located internally and must be retrieved by incision. If retrieving heart, pericardium, and thoracic aorta, the chest cavity must be exposed. This is accomplished by making an incision from the throat down to the bottom of the sternum. Care must be taken not to expose the abdominal cavity as this will significantly increase the risk of contamination. The skin is then retracted, and the ribcage cut away in an inverted 'V' shape. At this point, **costal cartilage** may be retrieved from the ribcage. With the ribcage removed, the pericardium can then be dissected away to expose the heart and great vessels (if required, the pericardium may be stored for subsequent banking). The heart is then removed, together with the associated ascending aorta, and pulmonary trunk and arteries. It is good practice to remove a significant length of these vessels, associated with the pulmonary and aortic valves, as it gives the surgeon more options when implanting the graft. Long vessel lengths (conduits) can also serve as grafts in their own right, or be opened up to create a vascular patch graft. Normally, the entirety of the heart is removed even though only the outflow valves are required. This allows the delicate valve dissection process to be performed under controlled conditions. Some tissue banks may remove the apex of the heart following procurement. This

Costal cartilage
Hyaline cartilage, located between the ribs. Utilized as a graft material in reconstructive surgery.

Intercostal arteries

Small arteries, branching off the thoracic aorta and supplying blood to the intercostal space.

Anastomosis

The connection of two structures, for example a blood vessel graft to a native blood vessel.

Meniscal cartilage

Crescent-shaped fibrocartilage structures within the knee joint, which distribute weight and reduce friction during movement.

Cortical bone

Hard, compact bone forming the external part of all bones and providing strength and stiffness to the skeleton.

Cancellous bone

Open 'spongy' bone, mostly present in the ends of long bones.

exposes the ventricles, and permits the heart to be flushed with sterile, buffered saline following procurement, as a means of reducing contamination. A further graft that may be procured from the chest cavity is the descending portion of the thoracic aorta. This is easily accessed following removal of the heart, but must be carefully procured so as to retain sufficient lengths of the branching **intercostal arteries** to permit the creation of stable **anastomoses** on implantation. The chest cavity can then be reconstructed using absorbent padding material to replace lost tissue mass and soak up fluids, followed by replacement of the ribcage and suturing of the initial incision.

Many other tissue grafts are obtained from the lower limbs, including bone (femur and proximal tibia), tendons and ligaments (patellar, Achilles, and hamstrings), **meniscal cartilage**, and femoral arteries. Bone grafts may also be obtained from other anatomical areas depending on clinical requirements. However, the leg bones offer a large mass of easily accessible **cortical** and **cancellous bone** that can be processed into a variety of different grafts, and permits straightforward reconstruction after donation.

When retrieving tendons and ligaments, the first step is to make a shallow incision to just below the level of the subcutaneous fat layer. The tendon/ligament connective tissue is located very close to this layer, and care must be taken not to damage it during the initial fibrocartilage incision. The incision will be made to a generous length, to permit ease of access. Fine dissection is not required at this stage—during initial procurement the emphasis is on reducing the exposure of the tissues to environmental contamination, so excess connective tissue will be left attached to the graft. Where the tendon/ligament has a bone insertion point, a generous bone block is cut. In most cases, the whole length of the extensor mechanism will be exposed prior to dissection, although for hamstring tendons it may be possible to use tendon strippers to remove the tendon through a smaller incision.

Femoral arteries may also be procured from the legs. These can serve as lower limb bypass grafts, and may be obtained to a length of up to 30 cm, through an incision stretching from the groin to behind the knee. As with tendons, fine dissection is not performed in the mortuary, rather the whole vascular bundle containing the femoral vein (which may also be used as a graft) and sciatic nerve is retrieved for later fine dissection under controlled conditions. With careful dissection, the same incisions may be used for tendon, vascular, and bone graft retrieval.

For bone grafts, the whole femur is removed either as a single bone or cut into two or three separate sections. If meniscal cartilage grafts are being procured, the entire knee joint is dissected as an individual unit to permit later fine dissection. The distal femur, proximal tibia, and femoral head contain large quantities of good quality cancellous bone that may be used for structural grafting, and the femoral shaft is composed of thick cortical bone that may be used as strut or cylinder grafts, or dissected into more complex shapes. Again, fine dissection is not essential at this stage, the emphasis is on removing the grafts as quickly as possible, securely packaging them and getting them into a temperature controlled environment.

Following retrieval of bone grafts, the legs are reconstructed. This may be done with anatomically formed prostheses, but may also be accomplished just as effectively with plastic or wooden rods and padding materials, prior to suturing of the incision sites. It is important that the prosthetic reconstruction is secure, so that the prostheses do not become dislodged when the donor is moved subsequently. When all retrieval activities have been completed, and the tissues safely packaged for transportation, the donor is cleaned and the cadaver restored to as normal appearance as possible. A toe tag is affixed to the cadaver to notify mortuary technicians and undertakers that tissue donation has taken place, and that they should take special care when moving the donor so as to avoid damaging incision sites and dislodging prostheses.

Once finished, the retrieval team return the donated tissues to the tissue bank as soon as possible. Water ice in an insulated container is ideal for this purpose, as it can be packed around the graft to quickly dissipate heat. The use of other cooling mechanisms, such as freezer packs, should be approached with caution as close association with the tissue may cause it to freeze, which will damage viable tissue grafts.

Key points

With deceased donors, it is important to ensure the quality of the tissues removed. This can be affected by the time post-mortem that the tissue is procured and the way it is removed so that contamination is minimized. A large number of different, useful tissues can be retrieved from one donor, including skin, heart and heart valves, bone, tendons, ligaments, and arteries.

Living donors

Tissue retrieved from living donors is generally classified as 'waste' material removed during surgical procedures, with very occasional exceptions (such as the donation of skin to treat a severely burned patient by relatives and friends). Another tissue that may be donated by living donors is the amniotic placental membrane following childbirth. The tissue most widely donated by living donors is bone, specifically the femoral head removed during hip replacement operations. In these cases, the articular cartilage on the surface of the bone has deteriorated, but the underlying bone is still usually of good quality. The femoral head provides a significant volume (up to 100 cm^3) of cortico-cancellous bone that is of use to surgeons performing impaction grafting to replace lost bone stock during hip revision procedures. Bone removed during knee replacement operations has also been utilized for the same purpose in the past, but in practice is found to contain too high a proportion of cortical bone to be optimal for impaction grafting. Due to an ageing population, and the increasing incidence of hip replacement, this material is available in large quantities.

Obtaining tissue from living donors has many advantages from a tissue banking perspective. First, it must by necessity be retrieved in an operating theatre by surgeons rather than by the tissue bank staff. As the tissue is taken from living donors under aseptic conditions, the risk that it may be contaminated is greatly reduced, and a greater surety of safety with regard to transmissible viral diseases is possible as medical and behavioural history may be obtained directly from the donor themselves, and blood tests may be performed on fresh, good-quality samples rather than post-mortem samples as is often the case with deceased donors.

Operationally, the tissue bank will set up a donation programme, usually with hospitals performing large numbers of hip replacements. This is a genuinely collaborative arrangement, as these hospitals will also have a need for the allograft to treat patients undergoing hip revisions and thus have a vested interest in the success of the programme. The hospital takes responsibility for screening and consenting patients, and retrieving the femoral heads, bacteriology testing samples, and blood samples using kits supplied by the tissue bank. The grafts and blood samples are then collected by the tissue bank who arrange for the blood and bacteriology samples to be tested by accredited laboratories, and store the grafts in quarantine until all the results are known. Depending on the surgeon's requirements, the grafts can then be issued as unprocessed, fresh frozen femoral heads, sterilized with gamma irradiation, or processed to remove donor marrow prior to issue—see Section 11.5.

Amnion
The innermost of the two membranes surrounding the placenta.

Donation of amniotic membrane is in principle a very similar process. The **amnion** is utilized as an ocular surface graft, and occasionally to treat burn wounds. It is donated by mothers undergoing elective Caesarian deliveries, whereby the placenta is removed surgically under aseptic conditions, exposing it to less risk of contamination than a vaginal delivery. The whole placenta is collected, and sent to the tissue bank for further processing.

Key points

Tissues from living donors are regarded as being 'waste' material. As they are retrieved in the aseptic environment of an operating theatre this greatly reduces the risk of contamination.

SELF-CHECK 11.3

What steps are taken when retrieving tissues to reduce the risk of bacterial contamination?

11.5 Tissue processing and preservation

The major activity of a tissue bank is the processing of donated tissues. Whilst there are multiple ways in which tissue grafts can be processed, there are perhaps three core reasons why they are processed:

- To make them safer; for example, by the use of decontamination protocols
- To make them more clinically effective; for example, by the removal of donor cells to reduce immunogenicity and improve incorporation
- To make long-term storage (banking) possible; for example, the use of lyophilization (freeze drying) or low-temperature storage.

A fourth reason, which relates more to operational considerations, is to make tissues easier and cheaper to store and transport, for example a lyophilized graft can be stored and transported at ambient temperature, which reduces operating costs and the need for specialist low-temperature storage facilities.

The methods by which a graft can be processed depend on the properties of the graft that need to be retained. Whilst it may be desirable to sterilize a graft to increase safety, this is not practical where retention of donor cell viability is needed. This also affects the timescales under which a graft is processed. When grafts arrive at the tissue bank, they are still in quarantine, as much of the donor information required to release them for clinical use is not yet known. It is therefore best to hold them in quarantine until this information is obtained, to avoid the risk both to personnel and the facility from handling tissue that may contain pathogens, and to avoid committing resources to processing grafts that may need to be discarded. This is achieved by deep freezing the grafts in their original packaging. However, this is not possible if tissue viability is an essential attribute for the graft, as deep freezing will render donor cells non-viable on thawing. Where this is required, as is the case with skin, heart valve, cardiovascular, and meniscus grafts, the tissue must be processed immediately on arrival at the tissue bank. Whilst individual protocols for different tissues may vary, the core methodology by which viable tissues are processed is broadly the same, comprising of dissection, decontamination by antibiotic cocktail, and cryopreservation. This methodology is discussed in detail by considering the procedures for banking the two most widely used viable grafts: skin and heart valves.

Skin

Skin grafts are utilized principally in the treatment of severe burn wounds, although they may be used to treat conditions with similar pathologies, such as **toxic epidermal necrolysis** and **necrotizing fasciitis**. There are conflicting opinions as to whether the grafts need to be utilized as viable grafts. As in many cases with tissue banking, good-quality clinical data comparing different types of graft are scanty at best, and the bank is led by the requirements of individual surgeons. In the UK, it is the opinion of many burns surgeons that viable skin grafts, when applied to a wound bed from which all necrotic tissue has been excised, will temporarily 'take' to the wound, (the blood vessels in the graft anastomose to blood vessels in the wound bed) providing a blood supply to the graft and allowing the donor cells to assist the healing process. This is not a permanent engraftment, but is assisted by the fact that burns victims are naturally immunosuppressed. The graft will be rejected after a period of up to six weeks, but during this period it contributes actively to the healing of the wound.

The earliest method for the banking of skin was to place it in a refrigerator in a nutrient solution. This had the advantage of retaining cell viability, but only for a short period (up to two weeks) and was thus of limited practicality for tissue banking. The only feasible method for preserving viability long term is to cryopreserve the graft. The skin grafts are transported to the tissue bank in buffered, isotonic transport fluid which is essential to prevent acidification of the medium due to the metabolism of the donor cells. On arrival, the grafts are transferred to a decontamination solution, which comprises a range of broad spectrum antibacterial and anti-fungal antibiotics, prepared in a buffered nutrient medium. The use of antibiotics permits the selective targeting of microorganisms whilst minimizing damage to cells, and the use of a base buffered nutrient medium helps maintain cell viability during the incubation. The incubation may be performed at refrigerated, ambient, or normothermic temperatures, generally for a period of up to 24 hours with agitation. Prior to commencement of the decontamination, samples of tissue for microbiology testing are obtained ('pre-process' samples). It is necessary to test the tissue both pre- and post-process as residual antibiotics from the decontamination step may bind to the tissue and compromise post-process testing.

Following decontamination, the tissue is dissected and prepared for cryopreservation. All of these activities must be performed in a grade A environment within a grade B clean room. The strips of skin are laid flat, and trimmed so that the edges are flush. Any sections with perforations are discarded, as are any that are thought to be too fragile. Skin allografts do not require great mechanical strength, but must be able to withstand routine handling. The grafts are rinsed thoroughly to elute residual antibiotics from the decontamination step (although as mentioned previously some traces remain) and immersed in a cryoprotectant solution. This solution usually contains dimethylsulphoxide (DMSO) or glycerol dissolved in a buffered nutrient solution to a final concentration of 10–25%, depending on the bank. The grafts are incubated in the cryoprotectant solution for a short period to allow the cryoprotectant to fully permeate the skin; post-process microbiology samples are taken and the graft is spread onto a gauze or other supportive framework, and packaged. Given that the grafts will be stored cryopreserved at low (<–180°C) temperatures, appropriate packaging materials must be used; there are several plastic materials formulated for this purpose. When the grafts are sealed,

Toxic epidermal necrolysis
A serious life-threatening condition, usually caused by reaction to medication, resulting in the detachment of the epidermis from the dermis.

Necrotizing fasciitis
A serious infection of the skin and subcutaneous tissue, requiring aggressive debridement of infected tissue.

using two layers of packaging, they can be removed from the clean room environment and cryopreserved. The grafts are maintained in a quarantine location pending satisfactory review of the processing paperwork, acceptable microbiology results, and release of the donor. They are then made available for issue.

Key points

Skin for transplant should ideally be a viable tissue. It is commonly used to treat burns, where it will temporarily 'take' to the wound, providing a blood supply to the graft and allowing the donor cells to assist the healing process, but is not a permanent engraftment and will in time be rejected.

Heart valves

Heart valve allografts are used principally for the repair of congenital defects in younger patients, and for the replacement of diseased or damaged valves in older patients. As with skin grafts, there are conflicting opinions as to whether the grafts need to be viable. In the early days of heart valve banking, the perceived wisdom was that donor cell viability was essential to the success of the graft as donor cells survived transplantation and contributed to the healing process. This lead to a preference for 'homovital' grafts, which had been stored refrigerated for a short period of time in nutrient medium. Current opinion is that donor cell viability is not essential (and may be disadvantageous due to provocation of cell-mediated immune responses). Earlier data that suggested donor cells survived in the recipient for long periods have not been replicated, and evidence suggests that any viable donor cells present in the graft die very soon after transplantation. Therefore, the vast majority of heart valve banks today use cryopreservation to bank heart valves. The long-term storage afforded by cryopreservation permits thorough screening of the donor and the tissue prior to transplantation.

Hearts for valve donation may be obtained from deceased tissue donors during a traditional tissue retrieval, or in an operating theatre if organs are being donated. If a heart taken for transplantation proves unsuitable the valves can be used, or the heart is taken specifically for valve donation. Removal in an operating theatre is preferable as it permits organs to be taken in an aseptic environment immediately post-mortem. This is important as, perhaps more so than any other tissue, hearts are exposed to contamination from intestinal contents through the circulatory system or directly from the abdominal cavity. Where this is not possible, as in the case of tissue donors referred post-mortem, the heart is generally retrieved in a mortuary environment. Following retrieval, either in theatre or mortuary, the heart is transported to the tissue bank in a buffered, physiological transport solution on wet ice.

As the valve dissection is a delicate procedure that takes some time, the entire heart is retrieved rather than attempting valve dissection at retrieval. Adherent fatty tissue is removed from the heart and great vessels and the pulmonary and aortic valves dissected from the body of the heart. The mitral valve may also be banked; however, this is rarely required today. Every effort is made to retain as much vessel as possible, the ascending aorta and aortic arch in the case of the aortic valve, and the pulmonary trunk and pulmonary arteries in the case of the pulmonary valve. Following dissection, a thorough examination of the valve pathology is made. The internal walls of the valve vessels and coronary arteries are examined visually and with palpation for the presence of atheroma and calcification. Atheromatous plaques, which can cause calcification of vessel walls, are a common pathology associated with ageing, and lifestyle factors such as smoking and poor diet. Generally, any indication of calcification will render a valve unsuitable for transplantation, as will heavy atheroma; however, light atheroma would not preclude transplantation. A thorough examination is also made of the valve leaflets (cusps). These are checked for fibrosis (thickening of the leaflets which can reduce flexibility) and fenestrations (holes) which can cause the valves to leak. Any gross pathological abnormalities, for example bicuspid or quadricuspid valves, will also be noted and will generally contraindicate transplantation. The competency of the valves will be assessed by filling the lumen with physiological saline and checking for any leakage. Any observed pathology will be recorded, and valves may be rejected at this stage based on this. See Figure 11.3.

The valves are then decontaminated with an antibiotic solution, with similar microbiological testing as described for skin grafts above. Following decontamination, the valves are measured. The annular diameters of the valve roots and any branching arteries are measured with obturators, and the length of the vessels associated with the valve recorded too. This is done post-decontamination as valves can contract post-mortem. They are then packaged utilizing packaging resistant to low temperatures and a cryoprotectant solution added. For heart valves, this is generally dimethylsulphoxide in a concentration of 10–20% (w/w), dissolved in a buffered physiological solution. This may contain nutrients and/or animal serum, depending on the individual protocol. A zwitterionic buffer such as HEPES is generally used as these remain effective at low temperatures. A secondary overwrap package is then added, and the valves cryopreserved as above. They may then be stored in quarantine pending completion of both donor and tissue related checks.

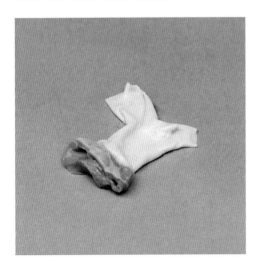

FIGURE 11.3
Pulmonary heart valve graft.

Key points

Cell viability of heart valves is not thought to be critical. The vast majority of heart valves used today are cryopreserved and this long-term storage allows thorough screening of the donor and the tissue prior to transplantation.

SELF-CHECK 11.4

What are the three main reasons for processing tissues? Briefly outline the two methods commonly used to preserve tissues.

Bone

For many types of tissue allograft, in particular musculoskeletal allografts, the presence of viable cells is not required and may in fact result in worse clinical performance. Typically, bone and tendon/ligament grafts are used as structural allografts, giving immediate mechanical support whilst providing a framework which is gradually reabsorbed and replaced by the recipient's cells. In this case, viable donor cells, or to a lesser extent cell remnants, are immunogenic and may provoke an immune response that weakens the graft material. In the interests of balance, it should be noted that it has also been suggested that this immunogenic response may enhance graft incorporation by provoking more rapid revascularization, but this is not based on sound clinical data. Most banking protocols for deceased donor bone therefore focus on removing the cellular elements whilst retaining the structural extracellular matrix.

Bone allografts can be deep frozen immediately following retrieval, as viability is not required. This enables all relevant information relating to the donor to be collated and checked before the tissue is processed, avoiding wasting resources processing tissue which may be unsuitable for clinical application. When the donation has been accepted, the tissue is processed. Following thawing, adherent soft tissue is dissected away from the bone. Depending on the type of graft required, the bone may then be cut using powered saws into a variety of shapes and sizes. These vary from large structural allografts, such as hemi pelvis, or distal or proximal femur, to fine powders composed of morsellized cortico-cancellous bone. Morsellized bone is prepared from larger chunks of bone that are mechanically ground. See Table 11.2.

The grafts are then cleaned, generally using a combination of chemical and physical processes. The overall objective of the cleaning process is to remove donor blood and marrow from the graft. A variety of different chemicals may be included in 'bone washing' protocols, including

TABLE 11.2 Bone products.

Role	Type of graft	Typical application
Structural	Hemi pelvis, cortical strut, femoral head	Replacement of large bone masses following trauma or tumour resection. Reinforcement and replacement of bone weakened by artificial prostheses.
Space filling	Morsellized granules and powders of different sizes	Filling of large gaps in bone. Often impacted to form a solid support for prosthetic placement.
Osteoinductive	Demineralized bone matrix	Oral and maxillofacial repairs, spinal fusion.

solvents and detergents to remove protein and lipid components, and active oxygen compounds that reduce bioburden and improve the cosmetic appearance of the graft. Physical processes, such as increased heat, negative and positive pressure, and centrifugation are often incorporated to improve the efficacy of the washing process. Many of the chemicals and physical treatments are also antimicrobial, and some bone washing protocols have been claimed to achieve sterilization of the graft in addition to marrow and blood depletion.

A more specialized type of processing is used to prepare a type of bone graft called demineralized bone matrix (DBM). This type of graft takes advantage of the fact that cortical bone contains small quantities of powerful **morphogens** called bone morphogenetic proteins (BMPs). These can actively induce the formation of new bone through initiating the 'osteogenic cascade', a sequence of events that involves the attraction of stem cells to the graft, induced differentiation of the stem cells into bone forming cells (osteoblasts), which then proceed to form new bone. This process is strikingly demonstrated in a mouse model, where subcutaneous implantation of DBM causes the formation of an ossicle of bone, replete with its own marrow cavity, independent of the skeletal system. Demineralized bone matrix is prepared by removing the mineral and lipid phases of bone with dilute acids and solvents, which leaves a collagenous matrix containing small amounts (in the order of picograms per gram) of BMPs. The process must be strictly controlled so as not to overexpose the BMPs to acid, which can damage them. Demineralized bone matrix is a unique type of bone graft in that its principal property is biological (active induction of bone formation) rather than biomechanical (passive support and provision of a framework for new bone generation).

Morphogen
Molecule that influences undifferentiated cells to differentiate into specialized cells capable of making specific tissues.

Following completion of the processing protocols, the grafts must be preserved for long-term banking, and may also be sterilized. Preservation may be accomplished using either lyophilization or freezing, there being no requirement for the more sophisticated preservation protocols needed for viable grafts. Lyophilization involves placing the grafts in a vacuum in the frozen state. Vapour is drawn off under the vacuum, and the graft dries at freezing temperatures, avoiding the possibility of damage occasioned by drying at higher temperatures. Lyophilized grafts may be stored and transported at room temperature, which permits for cheaper and less resource intensive storage infrastructure, and renders them more amenable for transport to, and local storage in, hospitals. See Figure 11.4.

It is also common practice for bone allografts to be sterilized prior to issue. This is because (unlike with viable grafts) there is no need to retain cell viability and use of harsh sterilization processes is feasible. This adds to the overall safety of the graft. The most commonly used sterilization process is gamma irradiation, a relatively inexpensive, reliable, and controllable process which permits sterilization of the graft in its final packaging. It does, however, cause a dose-dependent weakening of the bone structure, and should be employed with caution when applied to grafts which are intended to have a weight-bearing role. Where irradiation is utilized, it is good practice to minimize the required dosage by assessing the bioburden of the graft prior to sterilization. The harmful effects of irradiation may be ameliorated by the addition of radioprotectant chemicals to the graft prior to irradiation. Other protocols that may be used to sterilize bone grafts include chemical sterilization, with liquid chemicals, gases, or gas plasmas. Where chemical sterilization is employed, it is important that residual amounts of the sterilizing chemicals are eluted from the graft before it is implanted. Gas and gas plasma sterilization are only practical for lyophilized grafts. As has been previously mentioned, the chemical treatments applied during marrow and blood depletion may also be sufficient to sterilize the graft.

Tendons and ligaments

Tendons and ligaments may also be donated by deceased donors. Technically, a tendon joins muscle to muscle, or bone to muscle, whilst ligaments join bone to bone. Thus, certain types

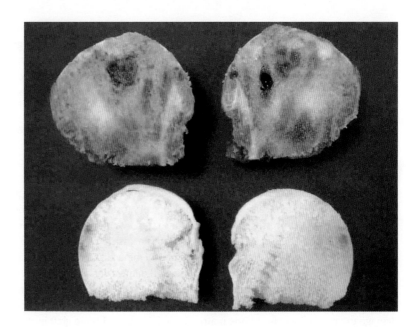

FIGURE 11.4
Cross sections of femoral head grafts before (above) and after (below) marrow depletion.

of tendon/ligament graft will have a bone block at one or either end. As with bone, tendon/ligament grafts may be stored frozen following retrieval pending completion of donor assessments. Processing of tendons is aimed at removing non-essential donor material whilst retaining the essential soft tissue matrix and any bone blocks. As the bone blocks contain the soft tissue insertion points, they need to be processed and banked as composite bone-tendon/ligament grafts. Processing generally commences with a dissection of the graft. In some cases, for example the patellar ligament, the graft may be retrieved as part of the larger knee joint, so the first step is to cut out the bone blocks with a powered saw. The bone blocks may also be dissected to defined sizes, with suture holes pre-drilled, to facilitate placement during transplantation. It is also necessary to remove any adherent muscle and fat. There are then a variety of protocols that may be used to clean the graft, and deplete donor cellular components. However, the soft tendon/ligament matrix is more vulnerable to damage than the hard, mineralized bone matrix, and care must be taken to ensure that the processing protocol does not damage this. Solvents and detergents are generally used in cleaning protocols. However, elevated temperatures (above 37°C) should be avoided as these can damage the soft tissue matrix. A further challenge with tendon/ligament grafts is sterilization. It may be possible to demonstrate that the washing protocol utilized achieves sterilization, but if not, the only widely used option for sterilization is gamma irradiation. This is problematic as the balance of evidence suggests that irradiation damages the structure of the soft tissue matrix, although this may be ameliorated by adjusting the dose applied, irradiating at low temperatures or using radioprotectant chemicals.

Key points

Bone and tendon/ligament grafts are generally used as structural allografts, giving immediate mechanical support whilst providing a framework which is gradually reabsorbed and replaced by the recipient's cells. As viability is not required, bone allografts can be deep frozen immediately following retrieval and processed only when all relevant information relating to the donor is collated and checked. Bone is made available as morsellized, structural bone, and demineralized bone matrix.

How is bone processed and stored?

11.6 **Storage and distribution**

Current clinical practice

The design and growth of human tissues outside the body for later implantation to repair or replace diseased tissues has seen well-established methods and interventions develop over the last 15 years.

Implantation of cell-containing or cell-free devices that induce the regeneration of functional human tissues has further led to the purification and large-scale production of appropriate 'signal' molecules, e.g. growth factors and other proteins, to assist in biomaterial-guided tissue regeneration. Novel polymers are being created and assembled into 3D configurations, to which cells attach and grow to help reconstitute affected tissues. The development of external or internal devices containing human cells and tissues has been designed to replace the function of diseased or failing organs, e.g. left-ventricular assist devices (LVAD) for patients with heart failure who are awaiting transplantation. This approach involves isolating cells from the body, using such techniques as stem cell therapy, placing them on or within structural matrices, and implanting the new system inside the body or using the system outside the body, e.g. the cardiovascular system or for the musculoskeletal system.

Synthetic, biomimetic materials and bioprosthetic devices have also been created by biomedical engineers and scientists to try to replicate, augment, and extend functions performed by natural biological systems (see Section 11.7).

It has become quite apparent, therefore, that the choice of scaffold is crucial to enable the cells in question to function in an appropriate manner to produce the required extracellular matrix, and thus tissue, of a desired geometry and size and normal functional capability. There are, however, legislative and ethical hurdles which need to be cleared, e.g. consideration and implementation of the Human Tissue Act (2004), in order to ensure the continued acceleration of this exciting field of research. Clearly, the potential health benefits to individuals and health services are vast. Stern challenges lie ahead when one considers that, for all the research groups in many different countries and the numbers of materials being investigated, very few examples of biomaterials are in clinical use at present. Some of the issues that need to be addressed comprise the native tissues and organs and the variety of tissue structures. Do scientists need to consider two-dimensional culture techniques as possibly being obsolete as more and more groups switch to three-dimensional bioreactor culture? Furthermore, the question of critical-sized defects comes into play, i.e. do we consider microscale vs. nanoscale; various cell types; culture systems including perfusion of scaffolds; vascularity; waste and nutrient consumption biomonitoring? These are important features of any future improvement of metrology within tissue engineering systems and the development of the next generation of scaffolds.

Researchers within the field are striving to improve the understanding of cell/material interactions; the ability to control the host response, enable the standardization of functional assays/protocols by limiting types of cells in use and by standardizing isolation methods. This can be assessed by using the same markers of biological function and developing a national (and ultimately international) group of reference materials. The adoption of standards is vital as it will lead to innovation, reduced development, processing and manufacturing costs, and more products to market and highlight previous intellectual property problems in indus-try by encompassing validation and accurate measurement modalities. In due course, these considerations need to involve numerous stakeholders, namely the major research councils and government departments (i.e. DTI, DoH) as well as the main standard's authorities and regulatory bodies (ASTM, ISO, BSI, NIBSC, MHRA). The long-term impact will help direct and form development of local ideas to be accepted nationally/internationally. These measures will provide 'best practice' methods in order to create safe, high-quality performance-related products. Educating regulatory authorities and end-users about the technical standards can only lead to long-term benefits to the health sector and, ultimately, the end-users, i.e. the patients.

Purpose of tissue biobanks

A variety of relevant tissue resources such as human tissues, cells, blood and blood products, and serum have played a critical role in academic research helping investigators discover a host of diagnostic tests and assays as well as therapeutic options for a variety of human diseases and conditions. Until relatively recently, biomedical research activity was based on biomaterial resources created by single investigators or research groups. Furthermore, large clinical trials and epidemiological studies have contributed to a better understanding of certain diseases, but the marked pace at which biotechnology, genomics, and other platforms of medical research have revealed further detailed insight to various diseases particularly centred around cancer, neurological disorders, and cardiovascular issues has been evident in the last decade.

We may regard biobanks as a relatively new concept in medical research but the original idea for them can be traced back through modern medical history. Take Burke and Hare, for exam-ple, the Edinburgh-based murderers who 'provided' bodies to anatomists in the early 19th century for dissection. One could argue that they were providing whole cadavers to a 'biobank' of sorts for education purposes, albeit illegally! In fact, their misdemeanors led to the Anatomy Act of 1832 which gave legal license to medical doctors, anatomists, and medical students to dissect donated bodies for their teaching and studies.

The need to understand the clinical and epidemiological prominence of different diseases and the consequences these aspects would present in the further development of more efficient ways to cure and even prevent serious illness made the need for modern-day biobanks ever greater. Biobanks could be considered then to be a refined system that consists of a specific automated storage of a variety of biological materials (relevant human tissues and cells) and their corresponding data, be it clinical, genomic or epidemiological.

Biobanks have been created and developed for use in a variety of significant areas such as basic medical research, clinical and translational medicine, and in national healthcare pro-grammes, e.g. UK Biobank and Future Healthcare Biobank. Over the last 20–25 years several large biobanks have been set up worldwide, to support and innovate modern research direc-tions with particular emphasis on personalized medicine and the numerous –omics disciplines that have emerged. During the latter period of this rapid development and expansion, the personalized medicine theme took on a more individual approach with respect to the use of embryonic cells and adult stem cell populations for a variety of therapeutic interventions, as well as future potential therapies intended for illnesses and conditions patients may develop in the future.

Quality assurance and control are vital considerations when dealing with biobanks. Moreover, a complete and version-controlled series of protocols and policies are required such that the relevant tissues are processed in a manner that allows standardization with other biobanks that preserve samples in the same manner.

One could consider the central principle behind the development of a successful biobank is the requirement to centralize and facilitate the flow of information required by a more complex approach in modern research because of a large bioinformatics need. By definition then, a biobank is a long-term storage and custodial facility for biological specimens, to support future research development. Biobanks essentially consist of two operatively distinct sections: (1) the relevant human cells and tissues that are collected, processed, and archived; and (2) the subsequent holding database that includes all relevant information of the clinical, demographic, and source data per specimen. While there are several types of biobank available across the world, their function is essentially consistent, i.e. the collection, processing, storage, recording, and distribution of biologically relevant material for human therapeutic use and/or research or cell therapies.

Legislation and the Human Tissue Act

The whole process of tissue banking is now covered by a variety of legislation. The EU Directive on Tissues and Cells (2004/23/EC) and its associated Commission Directives (2006/17/EC and 2006/86/EC) have been transposed into UK law as the Human Tissue Regulations 2007. These regulations lay down standards of quality and safety for all aspects of banking of human cells and tissues intended for human applications. In addition, the Human Tissue Act 2004 applies throughout the UK (except Scotland which is legislated by the Human Tissue (Scotland) Act 2006). All tissue establishments need to be licensed by a regulated authority, i.e. the Human Tissue Authority (HTA) here in the UK. Under this parliamentary act, the HTA issues its expected standards in the form of 'Directions' and 'Codes of Practice' to establishments such as universities and medical research institutes. The HTA standards require periodical updating.

The Human Tissue Authority (HTA) was set up to regulate the removal, storage, use, and disposal of human bodies, organs, and tissues for a number of scheduled purposes—such as research, transplantation, education, and training as described in the Human Tissue Act 2004. The Act covers England, Wales, and Northern Ireland and came into force on 1 September 2006.

Key points

- The purpose of modern tissue and biobanks is to centralize storage under controlled conditions and to ensure that samples are free of microbiological contaminants.
- In the UK the Human Tissue Act and Authority regulate the storage and processing of human organs.

Consent for using human tissues

This is essential as the main purpose of the Human Tissue Act 2004 makes consent the fundamental principle underpinning the lawful storage and use of human bodies, body parts, organs, and tissue and the removal of material from the bodies of deceased persons. From an historical perspective, the Human Tissue Act of 1961 applied only to the deceased and there were no penalties or mention of consent when it came to utilizing human tissues for research and education or storage. Indeed, the legislation surrounding this was conspicuous by its absence in training of individuals. Furthermore, the Coroner's rules of 1984 meant that there was no obligation to inform relatives or express their wishes when referring to human tissues from cadavers.

This meant that consent to retain 'tissue' was often interpreted as sufficient authority to retain 'organs' and that any retained tissues for bona fide teaching and research reasons were beyond the coroner's authority. The most fundamental issue here was that families of the deceased were not informed about what had been retained and any disposal of such tissues was deemed as 'clinical waste'. There were several episodes reported by the media (Bristol Royal Infirmary, 1998; Alder Hey (Liverpool) Children's Hospital, 1988–1996; Birmingham Children's Hospital, 2000) where numerous organs were retained without consent for many years and were used for non-descriptive research or organs were sold to the pharmaceutical industry.

When considering consent, particular consideration should be given to the needs of individuals and families whose first language is not English. Consider other formats, such as video or audiotape and, wherever possible, professional translators. If identifiable tissue is to be used for research, patients should be informed about any implications this may have. For example, they may be asked for access to their medical and clinical records. Patients should be told whether the consent is generic (i.e. for use in any future research project which has ethical approval) or specific. If it is the latter, detailed information about the research project should be provided, in line with good practice. Patients should also be told if their samples will or could be used for research involving the commercial sector.

Biobanks

A biobank typically acts as a physical depository for various collections of biological samples as well as clinical data for research purposes obtained from patients that have given informed consent. They often incorporate prospective collections of stored samples as well as historical collections. It provides a unique opportunity to advance biomedical and dental research by making access to tissue surplus to requirements easier, more efficient, and with a high level of governance compliant with HTA standards.

Biobanks typically support projects principally involved in the study of human disease and the normal physiology of the human body. Biobanks will store normal and pathological specimens from relevant tissues in a variety of formats; this could be fresh frozen tissues, histological slides, or wax blocks, for example. The establishment of a core programme of research is advisable and will enable an integrated approach to the management and assimilation of all research groups working within a variety of institutions, providing appropriate structure and support.

Any biobank should ideally aim to encourage several objectives; to facilitate collaborative research; to enhance availability useful tissue holdings to researchers. This would enable and support primary research within an institution and encourage various partners and stakeholders associated with that particular institution, as well as researchers both nationally and internationally. In addition the biobank can serve to assist with regulatory compliance (principally via the HTA) and finally improve research governance.

Management of the biobank

Every tissue establishment must designate a responsible person (termed the Designated Individual (DI)) who shall be responsible for ensuring that all activities relating to human tissues and cells are in accordance with UK enforcement laws. It is therefore the responsibility of the DI, along with various deputies, Designated Persons (DPs), to ensure that all the requirements of the HTA are met in a timely and comprehensive manner and that all personnel working within the scheme and with human cells and tissues are fully trained and comply with the necessary governance, policies, and legislation.

Governance of the biobank

The biobank must comprise its own regulatory policies and guidelines to guarantee compliance with HTA legislation and to ensure quality standards will be maintained. Any biobank will be governed by a local Ethical Review Committee (ERC) which will represent a range of stakeholders, including lay members, who will work together to maximize the potential of the samples stored and registered with the biobank. The committee will ensure that there is appropriate governance, suitable links to relevant communities, and that progress, output, and the development of the biobank is regularly monitored. It will consider the concerns of sample donors as well as tissue depositors and make recommendations to ensure direct benefit of the biobank to ongoing biomedical research. The ERC also must review requests for new sample collections and applications for use of samples/data for research, including those which do not have ethical approval and ensure they satisfy conditions laid down by the Integrated Research Application System (IRAS), which is a single system for applying for the permissions and approvals for health research in the UK before giving approval for the release and use of tissue. It is essential that any such ERC has well-defined terms of reference to ensure the committee fulfils its role.

- The ERC represents a range of stakeholders who will work together to maximize the potential of the samples stored or registered with the biobank.

- The ERC should ensure that there is good governance, appropriate links to the relevant communities, and that progress, output, and the development of the biobank is regularly monitored.

- The ERC will consider the concerns of sample donors and the tissue depositors and make recommendations to ensure direct benefit of the biobank to ongoing biomedical research.

- The ERC will review requests for new sample collections and also requests for use of samples/data for research, including those which do not already have ethical approval and ensure they satisfy conditions laid down by National Research Ethics Service (NRES; part of the Health Research Authority) for the release of tissues by the biobank.

Meetings of the biobank ERC will be chaired by an elected member of the review committee and should, as a minimum, consist of the Designated Individual (DI) for HTA/biobank licence of the institution in question; the biobank facilitator; the institute's Director of Research, if appropriate, or a delegate thereof; a representative of the local NHS Trust, if appropriate; a person representing the biobank users; at least one lay member and an external member representing another stakeholder e.g. a charity or other biobank. As in other similar organizations requiring diligence and governance individuals will be invited to be members of the Ethical Review Committee for a minimum of three years and may be extended as required by agreement. This ensures some longevity and development of experience for the board. It is the responsibility of the ERC to ensure that at all times the biobank follows regulatory (Human Tissue Act 2004) and ethical guidelines and fulfils the standards of best practice. Examples of this include the maintenance of the appropriate Human Tissue Authority licences; controlled and monitored storage of all samples within the biobank under appropriate conditions; the quality and safety of all technical and administrative procedures as well as policies on data protection and the withdrawal, disposal, and transfer of relevant tissues.

It is also an essential requirement that biobanks put in place appropriate service level agreements (SLAs) as well as material transfer agreements (MTAs) ensuring that any biobank has working contracts with those stakeholders depositing collections and requesting samples. This will ensure that appropriate consent is documented for the banking of all samples/data along with written policies and protocols to support these activities. Furthermore, it is essential that samples being transferred to or taken out of the biobank follow regulations governing the transport of biological samples. Moreover, the appropriate disposal of any samples released to users by the biobank must follow strict guidelines and protocols. This includes any material passed on to a third party for ethically approved research studies, which should be covered via a MTA with the third party stating either disposal or return options. This ensures good governance and audit of any tissues outside of the biobank.

It is essential that intellectual property (IP) and any commercial rights are appropriately addressed in contracts, particularly in relation to tissue requests from commercial companies. Thus, compliance with the biobank's policies on storage, health and safety, security, quality management, data protection, access, training, consent, and an audit of compliance must be maintained.

The status of the biobank as a potential research tissue bank requires that the ERC reviews and approves requests from researchers for use of samples and data in research, for which they do not have project-specific ethical approval. This will be carried out under conditions laid down by IRAS in its ethical review of the research tissue bank. Projects will only be reviewed if the sample/data collector agrees in principle to supply the relevant samples and data. Researchers can then make a formal application to the biobank ERC via the biobank administrator indicating the type and amount of material required; the data required to accompany the material; project title and the justification that the research presents no material ethical issues.

11.7 The future–regenerative medicine

As with any clinical science, tissue banking continues to develop and evolve. In its most basic form, tissue banking involves taking a tissue from a living or deceased donor, storing it for a period, then transplanting it into a recipient. We have discussed in this chapter many ways in which the tissue can be processed to make it safer and more clinically effective during the period between donation and transplantation, and one of the areas in which tissue banking has a key role is the emerging field of regenerative medicine, or tissue engineering, as it is also known.

The aim of the procedures discussed above is to replace a damaged tissue or organ with a graft that does not grow, but tissue engineering aims to regenerate and repair the damaged tissue.

This is achieved by either adding a matrix into which cells can grow or by stimulating some of the remaining tissue to divide and regrow, or a combination of the two.

The *Vacanti* mouse

One of the first (and famous) landmark studies that demonstrated the emergence of the possibility of tissue engineering was the production of the *Vacanti* mouse. This was where a scaffold was produced using polyglycolic acid and polylactic acid using a plaster template from a human ear. The scaffold was seeded with chondrocytes and cultured for seven days, and then implanted subcutaneously onto the back of a mouse recipient. The graft became extensively collagenized, and when blood flow was supported with stenting, the new tissue became stable in the animal.

Regenerative medicine has begun to impact on tissue transplantation. This currently includes the areas of orthopaedics and wound healing, but the overall aim is to reduce the dependence on solid organ transplantation, even replacement of it.

The current approaches can be resolved into three broad categories discussed below: tissue/organ regeneration, graft vascularization and innervation, and localized induction of host cell responses.

Tissue/organ regeneration

Damaged tissues have their cellular and protein components removed by a process called decellularization, using detergents and mechanical agitation leaving the structure and properties of the tissue relatively preserved, and in addition to extracellular matrix (ECM) components which are essential for the recellularization process. ECM components are critical to bind integrins, widely expressed adhesion molecules on lymphocytes and other cell types. In animal models, lung, heart, pancreas, kidney, and liver have been used in this process, and coupled with bioreactors to recellularize. The process has also been used in human tissues, for example vascular tissue has been decellularized, and used as a scaffold in patients that are dependent on kidney dialysis allowing the patient's own cells to recolonize the scaffold. Artificial scaffolds have also been used, and have included ECM components, alginate or collagen/fibrin hydrogels, and artificial polymers such as polyethylene glycol and poly lactide-coglycolide. The hydrogens in particular have been used in heart repair, injected into the site of cardiac damage.

It is critical that the decellularization process is optimized, and failures of such engineered tissues are due to suboptimal decellularization and recolonization of the resultant scaffold. The scaffolds themselves can be generated by imaging techniques, often from the patient themselves using such techniques as computerized tomography.

Graft vascularization and innervation

To achieve effective engraftment of engineered tissue, full integration must include the supply of adequate blood vessels and nerves (especially in skeletal muscle grafts) to appropriate structures within the tissue. Vascularization is achieved by a process called angiogenesis and is driven by a number of growth factors, notably VEGF (vascular endothelial growth factor); PDGF (platelet-derived growth factor); angiopoetin; bFGF (basic fibroblast growth factor). Localized delivery of these growth factors greatly enhance vascularization and subsequent success of the graft. However, this is not without problems, maintaining the local delivery is challenging but not impossible. Innervation also involves VEGF, and axonal guidance has been achieved in humans using engineered skeletal muscle grafts on a biomaterial scaffold.

Localized induction of host cell responses

The use of transplanted cells can have a fundamental impact on the tissue repair of an individual, especially following stroke and cardiac arrest. Umbilical cord-derived blood progenitor cells have been used in stroke victims and have shown to enhance angiogenesis, which in turn may have enhanced repair by attracting neuroblasts to the site of injury. Mesenchymal stem cells (MSCs) have been used in patients to induce cardiac repair, brain injury, and nerve repair in multiple sclerosis. A number of preclinical and clinical studies have been reported in the literature regarding this developing area (see the Mao and Moody 2015 review in Further Reading). Another approach currently under investigation is to prevascularize a site where the tissue/organ is to be transplanted. This can be achieved by integrating a scaffold and endothelial and tissue specific cells in a manner to promote angiogenesis in the target area.

3D printing and tissue engineering

The relatively recent mass scale application of 3D printing has offered opportunities in tissue engineering. This may be achieved by the 3D printing of scaffolds to adhere stem cells and regenerate tissues and/or bone structures that can be completely personalized, and based on the scanning of an individual and the defective structure. Whilst this is undoubtedly a future technology, successful bioprinting of human mesenchymal stem cells has been achieved, and neuronal-like cells have been generated after bioprinting the cells onto preformed scaffolds (see Chia & Wu, 2015). It is hoped that with improvements in printing (especially within the 3-4 micrometre range) then such structures as bone, cartilage, blood vessels, nerves, indeed perhaps whole organs, if the complex microvasculature can be suitably scanned and printed at sub-micrometre resolution. Such approaches are being adopted clinically (see Mao & Mooney, 2015).

 Chapter summary

- Diseases and injuries occasioning, or caused by, damaged tissues are a significant clinical and financial burden on the healthcare system.

- Allografts have a key role in treating these conditions, having attributes that cannot be replicated by prosthetic or other biological graft materials.

■ Allografts can be donated by deceased or living donors. Appropriate and informed consent is a key legal requirement for donation to occur.

■ Many different kinds of tissue may be banked, for example skin, heart valves, bone, tendons, and ligaments. The key difference between organ and tissue donation is that tissue grafts can be preserved for long periods.

■ Allografts may be processed prior to being banked to make them safer and/or more clinically effective. Sometimes a compromise must be drawn between processes that improve safety, but may detract from clinical performance.

■ They are different methods available for tissue preservation. The methodology chosen is informed by the need to preserve those qualities of the tissue important for clinical efficacy. Ultra-low temperature storage systems are required for storage of viable grafts.

■ Tissue allografts can serve as excellent scaffolds for the generation of tissue engineered grafts that aim to regenerate and repair damaged tissue not just replace it.

■ Various approaches are being adopted in clinical trials for using engineered tissue as a replacement for the use of directly transplanted organs/tissues.

 Further reading

● **Chia HN & Wu BM. Recent advances in 3D printing of biomaterials.** *J Biol Eng* 9 (2015), 4.

Recent review describing the impact of bioprinting on the tissue engineering field

● **Galea G (ed.)** *Essentials of Tissue Banking*. **Springer, London (2010).**

A publication covering technical, medical, and scientific aspects of tissue banking.

● **Karimi-Busheri, F (ed.)** *Biobanking in the 21st Century*. **Springer, London (2015).**

● **Mao AS & Mooney DJ. Regenerative medicine: current therapies and future directions.** *Proc Natl Acad Sci USA* 112 (2015), 14452–14459.

Excellent review on the current applications of regenerative medicine/tissue engineering.

● **Phillips GO (Series Editor).** *Advances in Tissue Banking*. **Volumes 1–7. World Scientific, Singapore (1997–2004).**

A series of books comprising invited review articles covering all aspects of tissue banking.

● **Salih V (ed.).** *Standardisation in Cell & Tissue Engineering: Methods & Protocols*. **Elsevier, Amsterdam (2013).**

● **The Journal of Cell and Tissue Banking.**

A quarterly journal, published since 2001, containing articles on all aspects of tissue banking.

● **UK Blood Transfusion Services.** *Guidelines for the Blood Transfusion Services in the UK*, **8th edition. The Stationery Office, London (2013).**

UK Blood Service guidelines covering the selection of tissue donors, and the retrieval and processing of tissue grafts, known as the 'red book'.

The Human Tissue Authority **https://www.hta.gov.uk/**

The Journal of Biopreservation and Biobanking **(http://www.liebertpub.com/overview/ biopreservation-and-biobanking/110/)**

British Association for Tissue Biobanking **http://www.batb.org.uk/**

UK Biobank **http://www.ukbiobank.ac.uk**

Answers to the questions in this chapter are provided on the book's accompanying website:

 Go to www.oup.com/uk/avent2eMarfan's syndrome

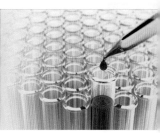

12

Quality Issues

Joan Jones

Learning objectives

After studying this chapter you should be able to:

■ Understand how the contributions of experts have shaped quality issues.

■ Understand how the concepts of quality control, quality assurance, quality assessment, and good manufacturing practice (GMP) are related.

■ Outline the basic ideals of GMP.

■ Outline the GMP Standards required by the Medicines and Healthcare products Regulatory Agency (MHRA) to conform with the Blood Safety and Quality Regulations (BSQR).

■ Understand the requirements of the BSQR, Human Tissue Act, Clinical Pathology Accreditation (CPA), United Kingdom Accreditation Service (UKAS), European Federation for Immunogenetics (EFI), Joint Accreditation Committee-ISCT and EBMT (JACIE), and their relationship to legislation.

■ Describe what a quality management system (QMS) is and how it maintains and improves quality within blood transfusion and transplantation departments.

■ Outline current haemovigilance systems in the UK.

Introduction

This chapter considers how blood transfusion and transplantation departments can satisfy the various standards and regulations that govern these disciplines, and guarantee the quality of the services they provide. It will also describe how a department can prove it is maintaining these standards to the regulatory bodies and demonstrate that it isimproving the quality of the service. It will discuss quality assurance, quality assessment, quality management systems, and how the principles of GMP are an integral part of maintaining the system. The chapter also discusses **haemovigilance** and the current systems in place within the UK.

> **Haemovigilance**
> Is defined as a set of surveillance procedures covering the whole transfusion chain (from the collection of blood and its components to the follow up of recipients) intended to collect and assess information on unexpected or undesirable effects resulting from the therapeutic use of labile blood components and to prevent their recurrence.

12.1 **Evolution of quality**

The move of *quality* to the top of organizational agendas has risen dramatically over the past 20 years. Much of the background stems from a number of industrial experts moulding managers' attitudes to quality within the workplace. Experts such as W Edwards Deming, Joseph Juran, and Philip Crosby have introduced concepts which although initially designed for consumer products, have spread into public services, such as the National Health Service. Many of the theories, such as Deming's 14 points and 'plan do check act' (PDCA) cycles, still hold true today, and although initially ignored by many industrialists they have become commonplace and the basis of quality management systems across the world. The concepts are designed to stop mistakes, introduce consistency, train staff, and improve processes, all virtues that blood transfusion and transplant professionals aspire to.

Traditionally all diagnostic laboratory tests have included *controls*, to ensure that the test has worked satisfactorily. With blood grouping, samples of known group are used as positive and negative controls, for example A and B cells for ABO grouping, K+ and K− cells for K typing.

In a test or assay where a numerical value is obtained, such as a haemoglobin estimation, there is an accepted level of experimental error and controls are used to ensure the accuracy and precision of that assay. In the late 1960s there were a number of pilot exercises to assess what variation there was between the same assay but performed by different laboratories. The value of such exercises was soon recognized and led to greater standardization of techniques and the introduction of more, and better, control materials. Initially schemes for haematology and transfusion these were run under the auspices of the British Society for Haematology (BSH) but later they came under the umbrella of the UK National External Quality Assessment Scheme (NEQAS) as they remain today.

Over the years various guidelines have been developed, mainly by committees of BSH, to help those working in the field of transfusion to develop them into *processes* and *procedures* that reflect the current state of technology and therapy. In clinical pathology laboratories, there was a marked improvement in the quality of the assays performed during the 1980s, but there was growing concern about the management and staffing, both scientific and medical, of laboratories. The two major professional bodies involved in clinical laboratories, the Institute of Biomedical Science (IBMS) and the Royal College of Pathologists, cooperated in looking at ways in which these concerns might be addressed. In both Canada and Australia there were already standards written for clinical laboratories and inspection schemes in place. These were used as a basis for a UK scheme and after a number of pilots, Clinical Pathology Accreditation (UK) Ltd (CPA) was launched in January 1992. Although it was not mandatory that laboratories should be accredited under this professionally led scheme, most soon saw its value, especially in the 'market place' atmosphere that was driving the NHS at that time. The diagnostic aspects of the blood centres' work, such as the reference laboratories, were accredited by CPA, but not the donor testing and component preparation as these had already been taken within the scope of the Medicines Inspectorate.

The original quality standards, such as BS 5750, were mainly concerned with the *product*; did it conform to the agreed specifications? But the later standards, the ISO 9000 series, also took account of the *process*, the steps taken to produce the product or result. Until 1988 all government run organizations, such as the NHS, had general immunity from prosecution for anything they did wrong or harm they did to patients. When it was proposed that this Crown privilege was to come to an end and blood was deemed to be a product within the scope of the Consumer Protection Act of 1987, the Blood Transfusion Services in the UK got together to produce some specifications for the blood components that they produced and agreed criteria for who could or could not give a blood donation. These were published in 1989 as the first edition of what came to be known as the Red Book—the *Guidelines for the Blood Transfusion Services in the UK*.

This first edition also contained a brief chapter on 'guidelines for a quality system for the collection and processing blood and blood products' that were in turn based on a British Standard 5750 for Quality Systems. This was the beginning of what some now describe as a quality culture, or the cynical as a quality industry, in the field of transfusion and transplantation.

The 1989 Red Book outlined for the first time details of what a bag of red cells, for example, should contain, and how many and how often such units should be tested to see if they complied with the standard. The main criterion for a unit of red cells was that the haematocrit or packed cell volume should be between 0.55 and 0.75, and that 1% of all units should be tested.

Many more and stricter standards then followed. To ensure products met these standards, quality monitoring laboratories were set up in blood (transfusion) centres to test the required number of units and to evaluate and validate any new processes introduced. The general quality standard BS 5750 became more rigorous as the ISO 9000 series was introduced, and to meet its requirements all aspects of the blood centres' activities came under the ever watchful eye of a new breed of employee, the quality manager and their new quality systems. These standards were for blood centres only and were not related to hospital blood banks. However, this soon changed with the introduction of the legally binding Blood Safety and Quality Regulations, 2005. The Human Tissues Act of 2004, brought transplant laboratories into the regulatory fold, with inspection and accreditation by the Human Tissues Authority. These are considered in more detail below.

The Department of Health has also produced a number of circulars aimed at improving transfusion practice across the country. The first circular known as *Better Blood Transfusion* (HSC 1998/224) was introduced following the recommendations of a symposium held by the UK Chief Medical Officer on evidence-based blood transfusion in 1998. These recommendations were designed to promote best practice by introducing local sets of rules based on national guidelines looking at the appropriate use of blood. The circular introduced the compulsory requirement for a hospital transfusion committee and the concept of transfusion practitioners in all trusts so that a multi-professional team could introduce and monitor these local guidelines. Other aspects looked at the training of staff, encouraging laboratories to become CPA accredited, the use of audit, and giving patients more information about transfusion. The circular has since been replaced by a number of new circulars, one in 2002, *HSC 2002/009 Better Blood Transfusion—Appropriate Use of Blood*, and one in 2007, *HSC 2007/001: Better Blood Transfusion—Safe and Appropriate Use of Blood*. All these recommendations are sent to the chief executive of NHS hospital trusts to be implemented by the transfusion laboratory within five years. The aims of the last circular were to:

- Build on the success of previous *Better Blood Transfusion* initiatives to further improve the safety and effectiveness of transfusion.
- Ensure that *Better Blood Transfusion* is an integral part of NHS care.
- As part of clinical governance responsibilities, make blood transfusion safer.
- Avoid the unnecessary use of blood and blood components (fresh frozen plasma and platelets) in medical and surgical practice.
- Avoid unnecessary blood transfusion in obstetric practice and minimize the risk of haemolytic disease of the fetus and newborn (HDNF).
- Increase patient and public involvement in blood transfusion.

Key points

Quality systems have been evolving over several decades and are now essential tools in the management of a laboratory to ensure that the product or service provided is fit for purpose.

12.2 **Quality management systems**

Quality has always been a requirement within the blood transfusion department due to the serious consequences that an error may cause to a patient. Therefore, there is a need to prove that quality is an integral part of the daily work and departments are continually striving to improve the quality of the service they provide. This growth has been driven by legislation, such as the Blood Safety and Quality Regulations (BSQR) and has also been influenced by regulatory bodies such as the Medicines and Healthcare products Regulatory Agency (MHRA), and Clinical Pathology Accreditation (CPA), all requiring certifiable compliance and demonstrable improvements in quality. In 2009 CPA became a wholly owned subsidiary of UKAS as part of a strategy to modernize pathology services in the UK. UKAS is currently managing the transition of all CPA-accredited laboratories to UKAS accreditation to the internationally recognized standard ISO 15189:2012, *Medical Laboratories—particular requirements for quality, competence,* and the transition of CPA-accredited External Quality Assurance Providers (EQA) to ISO/IEC 17043:2010, *Conformity Assessment—General requirements for proficiency testing.* Other bodies such as the NHS Commissioning Board Special Health Authority and the **Serious Hazards Of Transfusion** (SHOT) scheme are there to help us learn from our mistakes and prevent them from re-occurring. These are each dealt with in further details later in this chapter.

Blood transfusion is a key part of modern healthcare and it is the responsibility of the National Blood Services and hospital laboratories to provide an adequate supply of blood and components for all patients requiring transfusion. It is also vital that these products are safe, clinically effective, and of appropriate and consistent quality, so that patients are not put at risk. It is the responsibility of the management and staff at all levels to achieve these goals and make sure that the blood supply is 'fit for its intended use' and that it conforms to the required standard.

To achieve its quality objectives, laboratories must have well-designed, structured, and organized quality in place that assures the user that the product or service provided is safe and efficient—a **quality management system**.

To accomplish this, the department must implement a **quality assurance** scheme that incorporates all the planned and systematic actions necessary to provide confidence that the product or service will satisfy the required standards. And to ensure that the laboratory is consistently producing a quality product or service the system needs standards that must be regulated by using good manufacturing practice (GMP) as part of this quality assurance programme. Good manufacturing practice provides a model on which to base a documented quality system and it describes the practical activities and controls which need to be in place so that the product or service achieves the appropriate standard.

Quality assurance

As stated above, quality management is a system to ensure both the accuracy and reproducibility of working practices are maintained and also to allow for improvement to be made. For

Quality management system (QMS)

Is a system of processes that ensures consistency and improvement of working practices, which in turn provides products and services that meet customer's requirements (e.g. a safe unit of blood).

Quality assurance

Is the prevention of quality problems through planned and systematic activities designed to detect, correct, and ensure that consistent quality is achieved. Good manufacturing process (GMP) is that part of the quality assurance system that assures that results and products are consistently produced, achieving the required standard and are 'fit for purpose'.

consistency to be achieved, departments require protocols, called 'standard operating procedures' (SOP) that all staff can follow. An example of this could be how to perform a blood group test using manual techniques. Staff will be trained and their competency to follow these protocols assessed, before being allowed to perform the test unsupervised.

The department will use a number of methods to assure themselves that the results they are reporting are accurate, and therefore safe. **Quality control** is essentially a way of assuring that the techniques used, and described by the SOPs, achieve and maintain the expected outcome.

A commonly used control is to test a number of samples with known blood groups in each batch of tests to make sure that the analyser is giving the expected result. These controls should also show up underlying trends in the assay by, for example, plotting optical density data from an analyser, so that remedial action can be taken before a problem arises. This type of control is an example of **internal quality control (IQC)** that can be defined as a set of procedures for continually assessing each assay, and the results they produce, to decide if they are good enough to be released. This means that IQC has an immediate effect on the laboratory's activities and actually controls the output of the department. If the IQC fails then the results of a test, reagent, or process should not be released and an investigation should be initiated to find the cause of the problem and rectify it. Internal quality control is, therefore, controlling the day-to-day consistency of the laboratory's results and processes.

Another way of checking the quality of a department is to compare the results of the assays performed with other laboratories, thus monitoring the performance and effectiveness of their IQC measures. This inter-laboratory comparability is known as **external quality assessment (EQA)**. The various United Kingdom external quality assessment schemes help ensure that the results of investigations are reliable and comparable wherever they are produced. To achieve this, samples of known but undisclosed results are sent to laboratories who are members of the scheme. The department then tests the samples, using their normal procedures and processes, and returns the results to the scheme organizer. The results are then compared to the actual result and those from other laboratories so they can receive independent, objective, and impartial reports on their performance, enabling them to identify weakness and take appropriate action.

The UK Blood Services produce some three million units of blood and components every year, each one must be of a certain standard as laid down by the *Guidelines for the Blood Transfusion Service in the UK* (the Red Book). An example of this would be a standard level of Factor VIII in units of FFP so that users can expect that level of quality in each component. To maintain this quality, each service will perform quality monitoring tests and participate in the EQA scheme for each assay. However, it is not possible to test every product and therefore **statistical process control (SPC)** techniques are employed using data from usually 1% of components that are tested. This statistical method is used to observe the performance of the production process in order to predict significant deviations that may later result in a rejected product. An example of this is leucodepletion of whole blood, where 1% of all whole blood donations are tested to make sure that the volume of the donation is 470ml (±50 ml) in a minimum of 75% of tests, and that 99% of leucocyte-depleted components have less than 5×10^6 leucocytes per unit. If this is not achieved then it identifies a problem somewhere in the process that must be investigated and corrected.

Statistical process control was pioneered by Walter Shewhart in the early 1920s. W Edwards Deming later applied SPC methods, in the USA during the Second World War, and successfully improved quality in the manufacture of munitions and other strategically important products. The power of SPC lies in its ability to look at a process, and variation within that process, to give a numerical value that can be used to assess the quality of the procedure and to allow the early detection of problems and thereby their prevention.

Quality control

Is any technique employed to achieve and maintain the quality of product, process, or result.

Internal quality control (IQC)

Is a set of procedures for continually assessing laboratory work and the results they produce to decide if they are good enough to be released.

External quality assessment (EQA)

Is a system of objectively checking the results of one laboratory with those from other, similar laboratories by the testing of undisclosed samples, thus ensuring that results are comparable wherever they are produced.

Statistical process control (SPC)

Is a method of quality control for a product or a process that relies on a system of analysis of an adequate sample size without the need to measure every product of the process.

These three quality control mechanisms strengthen the quality assurance process, with IQC and SPC looking at the continuous process, and EQA assessing and comparing quality across laboratories. Once a department can establish that its procedures and processes are capable of meeting the expected quality another question now needs to be asked, 'Can we continue to do the job correctly?'

To answer this question, we have to monitor the processes and the controls on them. This does not only mean the detection of quality problems, but also how we can prevent them from occurring; in other words, can we *assure* quality?

Good manufacturing practice (GMP)

To obtain this quality objective a department needs to design and implement a QA system incorporating good manufacturing practice. Good manufacturing practice is that part of the quality assurance system that assures that results and products are consistently produced achieving the required standard and are 'fit for purpose'.

GMP is the basis of the UK *Rules and Guidance for Pharmaceutical Manufacturers and Distributors*, known as the 'Orange Book'. The basic requirements of GMP are (Table 12.1):

- All processes are approved, documented, reviewed, and tested to produce the expected results to the appropriate quality.
- All critical steps and critical changes are validated.
- All necessary facilities for GMP are provided, including:
  - Appropriately qualified and trained staff to carry out procedures correctly
  - Adequate space and premises

TABLE 12.1 **Basic principles of good manufacturing practice.**

1.	All processes are clearly defined and controlled. All critical processes are validated to ensure consistency and compliance with specifications.
2.	All processes are controlled, and any changes to the process are evaluated. Changes that have an impact on the quality of the blood/component are validated as necessary.
3.	Instructions and procedures are written in clear and unambiguous language.
4.	Operators are trained to carry out and document procedures.
5.	Records are made that demonstrate all the steps required by the defined procedures and instructions were in fact taken and that the quantity and quality of the blood/component was as expected. Deviations are investigated and documented.
6.	Records of testing and distribution that enable the complete history of an issued unit of blood to be traced are retained in a comprehensible and accessible form.
7.	The storage and distribution of blood minimizes any risk to their quality.
8.	A system is available for recalling any blood product.
9.	Complaints about products are examined, the causes of quality defects are investigated, and appropriate measures are taken with respect to the defective product and to prevent recurrence.

- Suitable equipment and services
- Correct materials, containers, and labels
- Approved procedures and processes
- There are suitable storage and transport facilities.

- Records for instrument and storage devices used in processes are recorded and any problems/deviations are recorded.
- A complete audit of the processes is required.
- A recall system of a product/result is required.
- Complaints and quality problems are corrected and changes introduced to stop them reoccurring.

A more comprehensive detailed breakdown of the chapters can be found in Table 12.2.

TABLE 12.2 **Details of GMP requirements.**

Quality management	Requires: (a) Commitment and support of management (b) Quality policy defining the department's intentions in respect of quality (c) Quality manual which is a description of the quality system (d) Fully documented policies and procedures
Personnel	Requires: (a) Appropriate numbers of qualified and competent staff (b) Well-defined responsibilities (c) Personal development plan for every member of staff (d) Understanding of the requirements of health and safety
Premises and equipment	Requires: (a) Premises suitable for their intended use (b) Efficient workflow (c) Clean and temperature controlled (d) Equipment designed and maintained for its intended purpose (e) All changes must be controlled (f) Ensuring validated equipment, systems, and processes
Documentation	Requires: (a) Well-structured, easy to follow procedures (b) Controlled and reviewed on a regular basis (c) Fully audited amendments (d) Stored in a secure area
Service provision	Requires: (a) Work areas are secure (b) No unauthorized access (c) Documented procedures for all tasks (d) Traceability of all products from receipt to final fate (e) Inventory records
Quality control	Requires: (a) Internal quality control of all tests (b) Participation in external QC (c) Wrong results must be reviewed and actioned

(Continued)

TABLE 12.2   Continued

Contract manufacture and analysis	Requires: (a) Scheduled equipment maintenance (b) Formal service level agreements with all contractors and users
Complaints and product recall	Requires: (a) Procedure for managing complaints (b) Procedure for recalling products not 'fit for purpose' (c) Investigation of complaints and recalls
Self-inspection	Requires: (a) Internal audits with all non-conformances addressed (b) Formal documentation of audit (c) Closure on all actions

Within the Orange Book there are also various annexes that give additional information on procedural activities and validation processes for computerized systems and the use of ionizing radiation of blood components. The qualification and validation annex describes the principles of qualification and validation that are applicable to blood transfusion/transplantation laboratories to prove control of the critical aspects of particular operations. If there are any significant changes to the facilities, equipment, or the processes that may affect the quality of the product, then they must be validated prior to their introduction or reinstatement. A risk assessment approach should be used to determine the change in process to maintain the system in a validated state. In other words if you change any part of a process you must assess whether the system will give the same quality of result, this is known as *change control*.

Key points

Quality assurance in broad terms is the prevention of problems through planned and systematic activities (including documentation) so that the department can achieve control of its processes and achieve the consistent quality required by the patient.

SELF-CHECK 12.1

Can you name three differences between IQC and EQA?

12.3 Blood safety and quality regulations

Several years ago, the European Commission (EC) agreed that for several reasons it would be worthwhile to 'set standards of quality and safety for the collection and testing of human blood and blood components. This would cover their processing, storage and distribution when intended for transfusion'. In effect the standard was to cover the whole process from donor to patient—from 'vein to vein'.

The main directive was 2002/98/EC—*Setting Standards of Quality and Safety for the Collection, Testing, Processing, Storage, and Distribution of Human Blood And Blood Components* (and amending

Directive 2001/83/EC). It was supplemented by Technical Directive 2004/33/EC—*Implementing Directive 2002/98/EC as regards certain technical requirements for blood and blood components.*

These two directives were transposed into UK law on 8 February 2005 as the Blood Safety and Quality Regulations (BSQR). Two further technical directives, on Haemovigilance and Quality Systems, were published and these were transposed into law in 2006.

The two directives, which became law in 2005, had an impact on all the UK blood services, but the impact was greater on the hospital blood banks as, for the first time, their activities came within legally binding regulations. It is the responsibility of the competent authority, currently the MHRA, to oversee compliance with BSQR by both the blood services and individual hospital blood transfusion laboratories. The latter are required to complete a compliance report every year for the MHRA, based on the principles of GMP, including being accredited by CPA, now undertaken by UKAS with accreditation to ISO 15189 standards.

The MHRA can inspect a laboratory if they feel, on review of their annual compliance report, that there might be a problem, or if a **serious adverse reaction** or **serious adverse event** has been reported that they deem might indicate some underlying problem. If an inspection is warranted the inspector will visit the department and perform an audit based on the GMP standards. All non-conformances identified at audit must be corrected within a specified timeframe before the department is deemed compliant. It is therefore essential that all personnel involved in blood transfusion understand the principles of GMP so that quality is built into the organization and the processes within it (see Figure 12.1). The MHRA also has the power to instigate a 'cease and desist' order or prosecute the 'responsible person' (nominally the chief executive) under criminal law if the standards are not met or information has been falsely submitted.

Serious adverse reaction (SAR)

Is defined within the regulations as: 'An unintended response in a donor or in a patient that is associated with the collection or transfusion of blood or blood components that is fatal, life threatening, disabling, or incapacitating, or which results in, or prolongs, hospitalization or morbidity'.

Serious adverse event (SAE)

Is defined as: 'Any untoward occurrence associated with the collection, testing, processing, storage and distribution of blood or blood components that might lead to death or life-threatening, disabling, or incapacitating conditions for patients, or which results in, or prolongs hospitalization or morbidity'.

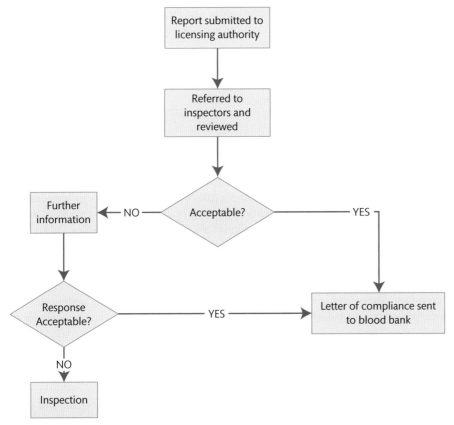

FIGURE 12.1
Annual compliance form review by MHRA.

12.4 The *In Vitro* Diagnostic Medical Devices Directive

One of the major elements of any laboratory assay is the reagent, or reagents, used. Over the years a number of countries developed their own criteria or standards for the commonly used reagents, such a blood grouping sera. With the advent of monoclonal antibodies there was a move away from grouping reagent produced in small batches from human sera, to producing large batches of monoclonal reagents by fewer manufacturers. Although these monoclonal reagents were more consistent batch to batch, and generally better than those from human sources, the differing standards made it difficult for one reagent to be sold in all countries. Within Europe some standards were agreed for the major reagents used in clinical tests, such as testing for HIV, hepatitis B and C, and for ABO and RhD blood grouping, and these became incorporated into the European *In Vitro* Diagnostic Medical Devices Directive (98/79/EC). The Directive was initially implemented into UK law by the In Vitro Diagnostic Medical Devices Regulations 2000, which have now been consolidated into the Medical Devices Regulations 2002.

The aim of the Directive was to deliver common regulatory requirements dealing specifically with the safety, quality, and performance of *in vitro* diagnostic medical devices (IVDs), and to ensure that IVDs do not compromise the health and safety of patients, users, and third parties, and attain the performance levels attributed to them by their manufacturer.

The Directive defines an IVD as:

> ...any medical device which is a reagent, reagent product, calibrator, control material, kit, instrument, apparatus, equipment, or system, whether used alone or in combination, intended by the manufacturer to be used *in vitro* for the examination of specimens, including blood and tissue donations, derived from the human body, solely or principally for the purpose of providing information ...

The legislation mainly affects the manufacturers of reagents and other diagnostic devices, but users within Europe should ensure that any diagnostic device they use has the appropriate CE marking to show that it complies with these regulations.

12.5 Clinical laboratory accreditation

Within the UK there were two laboratory accreditation bodies, operating in complementary fields, the United Kingdom Accreditation Service (UKAS) and Clinical Pathology Accreditation (UK) Ltd (CPA). Clinical Pathology Accreditation is now part of UKAS and this has enhanced the development of accreditation policy, facilitation of the exchange of best practice and accreditation, and also has avoided the proliferation of accreditation standards for laboratories.

UKAS focuses on the requirements for quality systems and competence as detailed in the *International Standards for Medical Laboratories*, ISO 15189-2012. Accreditation involves an independent assessment of the laboratory to determine if the tests being performed have demonstrated quality and reliability to the required ISO standard. These standards are for all clinical laboratories, not just blood transfusion laboratories, but help to ensure good quality systems are not just in place but are actually working.

ISO 15189 aims at creating a standard measure of quality in medical laboratories and covers the organization and quality management system, the resources, and the evaluation and quality assurance activities required to ensure that pre-examination, examination, and post-examination activities of the laboratory are conducted in such a manner that they meet the needs and requirements of the users. To ensure that these objectives are being met laboratories are assessed against 15 management and 10 technical standards on an annual basis by surveillance visits, with a full re-assessment every fourth year.

The following are the basic requirements for ISO 15189 certification and the assessors evaluate all factors in the laboratory that affect the quality of the test result including:

- Well-documented laboratory procedures
- Identifying and correcting non-conformities or breaches in standards
- Auditing the departmental processes
- Performance monitoring the laboratory
- Training and competency assessment of staff
- Equipment maintenance, calibration, and traceability of measurements to relevant standards
- Validation and verification of procedures
- Ensuring the quality of the results meet the required standard
- Ensuring that the Laboratory Information Management System (LIMS) meets the needs and requirements of the users
- ISO 15189 requires an effective detailed analysis of medical laboratory procedures in a bid to make sure that all weaknesses have been identified.
- Detailed evaluation reports of the existing quality management system as well as other monitoring and evaluation reports.
- A detailed audit of management reviews.

If on an assessment visit non-compliances are found, which is often the case, then the laboratory has to agree a timeframe in which to rectify the shortcomings. If these are not done, or the assessors feel that the laboratory has major failings then the laboratory is not accredited, or its previous accreditation is revoked.

12.6 The Blood Stocks Management Scheme

Another important aspect of quality is to ensure resources are used properly, and blood components, being a valuable resource, are no exception. The Blood Stocks Management Scheme (BSMS), was established to understand and improve blood inventory management across the blood supply chain and fits in with the *Better Blood Transfusion* objectives of avoiding unnecessary blood transfusion.

The BSMS is a partnership between hospitals and blood services, with an aim to maximize the use of donated blood by increasing the understanding of blood supply management. It was established in 2001 in England and now includes the blood services and hospitals in Wales, Northern Ireland, Scotland, and the Republic of Ireland. Central to the work of the BSMS is VANESA, a data management system where hospital and blood service data are collected, that now has a large bank of data on the blood supply chain and this has provided detailed knowledge of its various elements. Hospital participants can view real time data and charts and have the opportunity to benchmark performance against other users, for example those with similar blood usage. This has led to improvements in stock management. The BSMS provides inventory practice surveys and reports, publications, meetings, and training events, as part of its drive to improve stock management. More information about the work of the BSMS can be found at www.bloodstocks.co.uk.

Key points

Blood services and hospital transfusion laboratories now have to conform to certain legal regulations and these are enforced by a series of inspections. UKAS accreditation assessments help laboratories maintain their quality systems in good order.

SELF-CHECK 12.2

(a) What standards are used for medical laboratory accreditation? (b) What standards are used by the MHRA to assess compliance to the BSQR?

12.7 Other legislation and regulatory bodies

The Human Tissue Act 2004

Following some highly publicized irregularities with the collection and use of hearts from children, the Human Tissue Act was passed to regulate the removal, storage, use, and disposal of human bodies, organs, and tissues specifically for research, transplantation, education, and training. Laboratories involved in collecting and processing stem cells, bone marrow transplantation, or the retrieval of any human tissue are required to be licensed under this Act and are subject to inspection by the regulatory authority, the Human Tissue Authority.

Joint Accreditation Committee-ISCT and EBMT (JACIE)

This is a non-profit body established in 1998 to assess and accredit haemopoietic stem cell (HSC) transplantation. It aims to promote high-quality patient care and laboratory performance and is an internationally recognized system of accreditation. It has established standards, conducts inspections, and accredits programmes to encourage organizations to meet these standards. This is a voluntary not legislative system to accreditation. Centres can demonstrate they have a QMS and will be issued with a certificate of accreditation.

European Federation for Immunogenetics (EFI)

EFI was formally founded in March 1985 with these aims:

- To advance the development of immunogenetics in Europe as a discipline of medicine and support research and training.
- To provide a forum for exchange of scientific information and to reinforce the skills and knowledge of young scientists and others working in the field.
- To create a formal organization of workers in the field of immunogenetics, histocompatibility testing, and transplantation.
- To elaborate recommendations for standardization of techniques, quality control, and criteria for accreditation and to support their implementation.

- To promote the organization and use of immunogenetic databases.
- To develop relations with similar organizations.

The EFI publish standards for histocompatibility testing, which provide a basis for the EFI accreditation process.

12.8 Guidelines

As stated at the beginning of this chapter, the British Society for Haematology (BSH) develop and review many guidelines covering both laboratory and clinical aspects of transfusion medicine. These guidelines are accessed by following the link: www.b-s-h.org.uk/guidelines.

It is recommended that all laboratories comply with these guidelines and although it is not mandatory, regulating bodies are using these guidelines as standards that they expect a department to achieve.

12.9 Haemovigilance

In Chapter 7 we considered the two haemovigilance schemes that operate in the UK, SHOT and SABRE. The main aims of the SHOT scheme when it was launched in November 1996, were to improve the quality and safety of blood transfusions, and this was reinforced with the Blood Safety and Quality Regulations (BSQR); together they are a powerful tool in transfusion quality management systems.

From the cases referred to SHOT, which are analysed and reported annually, the four initial objectives of the scheme, listed below, have been realized and have had a positive impact on transfusion quality and safety in the UK.

The initial objectives of SHOT were:

- Improving safety of the transfusion process
- Informing policy within transfusion services
- Improving standards of hospital transfusion practice
- Aiding production of clinical guidelines for the use of blood components

More than a decade later these objectives are still relevant and the lessons learnt are also applicable to blood services outside the UK. The International Haemovigilance Network (IHN), with members from 28 countries, has the aim to develop and maintain a worldwide common structure with regards to safety of blood/blood products and haemovigilance of blood transfusion. The International Haemovigilance Network has established an international database so that in future comparisons can be made between the adverse events reported in various countries.

As said in Chapter 7, over the first decade of reporting, the trends observed by SHOT have demonstrated how an effective vigilance system can increase patient safety through a learning and improvement culture, rather than a punitive approach to errors, with the focus on safety and quality, monitoring, and audit. The number of events reported overall has risen, whilst the frequency of the most serious events, and the mortality directly related to transfusion, has fallen.

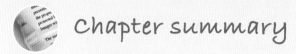

Chapter summary

- Over the past few decades methods have been introduced to improve the quality of blood transfusion/transplant departments by controlling and assuring that the blood, product, or result is of a high standard, fit for purpose, and is maintained at that level.

- As part of a planned quality assurance programme which is designed to detect, correct, and ensure that consistent quality is achieved, techniques such as internal quality control and statistical process control look at the continuous process, while EQA assesses and compares quality across laboratories.

- Statutory bodies like the MHRA inspect laboratories to determine conformance to legislation such as the BSQR. GMP is an important part of conforming to BSQR.

- All these processes combine to produce a QMS which helps provide products and services that meet the customers' requirements, for example a safe unit of blood to be transfused.

- The requirements of various expert committees, accrediting bodies, and legislation all help to improve the quality of the services provided by transfusion and transplant departments.

- Haemovigilance schemes such as SHOT use surveillance procedures to collect and assess information on unexpected or undesirable effects of blood and products to prevent their recurrence.

Further reading

BSH Guidelines covering many aspects of blood banking and transfusion: **http://www.b-s-h.org.uk/guidelines.**

- **Beckman N, Nightingale MJ & Pamphilon D. Practical guidelines for applying statistical process control to blood component production.** *Transfusion Med*, 19 (2009), 329–39.

Blood Stocks Management Scheme reports: **www.bloodstocks.co.uk.**

- **De Vries RRP, Faber J-C & Strengers PFW. Haemovigilance: an effective tool for improving transfusion practice.** *Vox Sang*, 100 (2011), 60–7.

Guidelines for the Blood Transfusion Services in the United Kingdom, other guidelines, useful information, and links: **www.transfusionguidelines.org.uk.**

International Haemovigilance Network (IHN) website: **www.ihn-org.com.**

MHRA guidance for reporting incidents (SABRE): **www.mhra.gov.uk/Safetyinformation/Reportingsafetyproblems/Blood/index.htm.**

Serious Hazards Of Transfusion (SHOT) annual reports: **www.shotuk.org.**

Answers to the questions in this chapter are provided on the book's accompanying website:

 Go to www.oup.com/uk/avent2e

Glossary

Acanothocytes From Greek *Acantha* meaning thorn—abnormal red cell shape associated with some conditions (see McLeod syndrome). Red cells have thorny like projections on their surface.

Adaptive immune response The arm of the immune response that reacts specifically to antigens. Divided into the humoral (e.g. immunoglobulins) and cellular (e.g. T cells) immune responses.

Adult stem cells Undifferentiated cells that are found throughout the body and replace damaged or dying organs/tissues by cell proliferation.

Allele One of two or more alternative forms of a gene that arise by mutation and are found at the same place on a chromosome.

Alloantibodies Antibodies that react with an inherited antigenic characteristic that is lacking in the recipient.

Alternative pathway An arm of the complement cascade where complement components (C3) are bound by bacterial membranes leading to activation.

Amnion The innermost of the two membranes surrounding the placenta.

Amniocentesis The invasive procedure of sampling amniotic fluid (containing fetal cells and hence DNA) from the amnion.

Anastomosis The connection of two structures, for example, a blood vessel graft to a native blood vessel.

Annealing (relating to the PCR). The process of cooling the reaction to such a temperature so that PCR primers can bind to the denatured DNA.

Anterior cruciate ligament A ligament located within the knee joint that plays a crucial role in stabilizing the joint and is commonly damaged in sporting injuries.

Anticoagulant A substance which when it is added to the blood inhibits clotting.

Anti-D prophylaxis programme The routine screening procedure of all D-negative mothers in most countries. D-negative mothers are screened for anti-D, and if identified receive further attention. Prophylactic anti-D (a blood product) is given to mothers carrying D-positive infants antenatally and at birth. In many countries the fetus is genotyped to permit only mothers with D-positive babies receiving such treatment.

Antigen Any foreign structure capable of eliciting an immune response to both T and B cells.

Antigenic vestibule (RhD) The open domain of the RhD protein responsible for expression of all D epitopes.

Antiglobulin test Also known as the Coomb's test, where anti-human immunoglobulin is used to bridge bound IgG to red cells so that they agglutinate.

Antisera Blood serum containing polyclonal antibodies.

Antithetical One of two or more alternative antigens.

Apheresis Collection of different blood cells using a machine.

Apoptosis Programmed cell death—the process in which cells control their own demise.

Articular cartilage Hard, smooth cartilage that lines bone in joint surfaces.

Autoantibodies Antibodies directed against antigens on one's own cells, which can lead to an increased rate of cell destruction as in autoimmune haemolytic anaemia.

Autoimmune neutropenia An autoimmune disease in which the antibodies form target granulocytes. These antibodies can recognize HNAs, especially in children.

Batch pre-acceptance testing Tests performed to show batch of test kits/reagents received meets pre-defined criteria such as sensitivity and specificity and has not deteriorated during transportation.

Biallelic The two alternative alleles of a gene.

Bioprosthetic graft A composite graft, comprising both prosthetic and biological materials.

Biotin A water-soluble B complex vitamin, necessary for the growth of cell, production of fatty acids, and metabolism of protein and fat. It is used in the laboratory because it interacts strongly with streptavidin. Thus, molecules labelled with biotin can be detected with streptavidin conjugated to a reporter molecule.

Buffy coat The layer of leucocytes sitting on top of the red cell layer after centrifugation.

Cancellous bone Open 'spongy' bone, mostly present in the ends of long bones.

Cellular immunity That part of the immune system that is initiated by the recognition of a foreign protein or cell and leads to its removal or destruction by the interaction of complement, or cytokines produced by cytotoxic or killer T cells.

Chorionic villous sampling (CVS) The invasive obstetric procedure of sampling chorionic villus used early in pregnancy for prenatal diagnosis.

Classical pathway The primary arm of the complement cascade that leads to red cell destruction when complement components bind to immunoglobulin bound to red cells and other cell types (e.g. bacteria).

Clinically significant antibody An antibody capable of causing red cell destruction *in vivo*.

Codominant Allelic genes whose products are all expressed equally.

Codons Three base pairs that code for a particular amino acid.

Cold ischaemia time During transplantation this time begins when the organ is cooled with a cold perfusion solution after organs are harvested and ends after the tissue reaches physiological temperature during the implantation procedure.

Compatibility testing Compatibility testing within the laboratory covers the processes by which donor red blood cells (RBCs), plasma and/or cellular components are either tested or checked to ensure that incompatible RBCs or blood components are not issued or released from the laboratory for transfusion to patients.

Congenic Organisms produced as the result of specific inbreeding in an experimental setting so that they only differ in one gene locus.

Continuous epitope An epitope confined to a single domain of an antigen.

Cortical bone Hard, compact bone forming the external part of all bones and providing strength and stiffness to the skeleton.

Costal cartilage Hyaline cartilage, located between the ribs. Utilized as a graft material in reconstructive surgery.

Cytosol The aqueous component of the cytoplasm in an intact cell.

Cytotoxic The ability to kill cells either by loss of membrane integrity, necrosis, or programmed cell death, apoptosis.

Deformability The elastic ability of the erythrocyte imparted by its membrane. Erythrocytes can negotiate microcapillaries half their diameter due to their deformability.

Denaturing (relating to the PCR) In the PCR reaction heating to 94/95°C so as to melt the template DNA into two strands, breaking the hydrogen bonding between complementary base pairs.

Discontinuous epitope An epitope that is structurally dependent on at least two spatially discrete regions of the antigen. But, importantly, must be close to one another to permit binding by the paratope of an antibody.

Doppler ultrasonography A method of ultrasound that measures the blood flow in vessels non-invasively (see middle cerebral artery)

Drug-dependent antibodies Antibodies that react with a drug directly or with an antigenic structure created when the drug binds to a naturally occurring structure (referred to as haptenization).

Endoloop A cytoplasmic localized loop structure of a polytopic membrane protein.

Endosome A membrane-bound intracellular compartment providing an environment for material to be sorted before degradation by the lysosome.

Engraftment when infused donor cells embed in the bone marrow and start producing new haematopoietic cells.

Epitope The specific region on an antigen which the immunoglobulin binds via its paratope. Also known as an **antigenic determinant.**

Eryptosis The process by which senescent red cells are removed by splenic macrophages.

Exoloop An externally localized loop domain of a membrane protein.

Extension (relating to the PCR) The process where the PCR reaction is heated to the optimum temperature for the thermostable DNA polymerase to allow the synthesis of new PCR products.

Extravascular haemolysis Immune-mediated cell removal that takes place outside the circulation in the liver or spleen.

External quality assessment (EQA) A system of objectively checking the results of one laboratory with those from other, similar laboratories by the testing of undisclosed samples, thus ensuring that results are comparable wherever they are produced.

FcRN The fetal/neonatal IgG transporter expressed in the placenta and gut lining to absorb maternal antibodies to protect the fetus. In the case of HDFN and NAITP this process is pathogenic.

Fetal genotyping The prenatal determination of blood groups using DNA based techniques (e.g. PCR). Now uses predominantly free fetal DNA found in maternal plasma.

First field resolution This is how a low resolution HLA type is described because the numerals describing the HLA molecule are in the first field before the colon, for example HLA-DRB1*12.

Fluorescent bead based assay Assays which use fluorescently dyed beads which have been coupled with either recombinant or isolated human glycoproteins from platelet or granulocyte membranes.

Free fetal DNA (ffDNA) Placentally derived DNA found in maternal blood that is >150 bp and used now extensively in the non-invasive prenatal diagnosis of blood groups.

Granulocyte agglutination test A simple test that brings together small volumes of isolated granulocytes and human test or control where the agglutination endpoint is measured by eye using a microscope.

Glycosyltransferase Golgi membrane bound enzyme that catalyses the transfer of a monosaccharide from its nucleoside derivative to a growing carbohydrate chain.

Glycophosphotidylinositol (GPI) anchor A chemical linkage between glycoproteins and the cell membrane which can be readily cleaved under certain conditions thereby releasing the glycoprotein from the cell surface.

Graft versus host disease (GVHD) The most common cause of graft failure that is caused by donor immune cells, especially T lymphocytes, reacting against recipient tissue. The characteristic symptoms are the presence of a rash, diarrhoea, and abnormal liver function tests.

Granulocyte chemiluminescence test (GCLT) A biological assay that utilizes human monocytes to detect granulocyte antibodies bound to the membrane surface.

Granulocyte immunofluorescence test (GIFT) A whole-cell immunofluorescence assay capable of detecting granulocyte reactive antibodies.

Haemolytic disease of the newborn and fetus (HDNF) A disease associated with the fetomaternal transfer of red cell antibodies that cause haemolysis and red cell destruction in the fetus or infant. Originally HDN, but 'F' added as most management now occurs *in utero*.

Haemopoietic Blood cells produced in the bone marrow.

Haemovigilance Is defined as a set of surveillance procedures covering the whole transfusion chain (from the collection of blood and its components to the follow up of recipients) intended to collect and assess information on unexpected or undesirable effects resulting from the therapeutic use of labile blood components and to prevent their recurrence.

Haplotypes Linked genes, the alleles contributed from one or the other parent, in a blood group system that are passed on together.

Hapten A substance that is unable to elicit an immune response by itself (usually because it is too small) but which can do so when combined with a larger molecule.

Human leucocyte antigen (HLA) The highly polymorphic class 1 and class 2 HLA molecules give rise to the prime cause of organ rejection.

Human neutrophil antigen (HNA) The term given to allelic forms of granulocyte glycoproteins that give rise to an allo-immune response.

Human platelet antigen (HPA) The term given to allelic forms of platelet glycoproteins that give rise to an alloimmune response.

Humoral immunity That part of the immune system that is initiated by the recognition of a foreign protein or cell and lead to its removal or destruction through the interaction of a specific antibody.

Hyperhaemolysis Characterized by marked reticulocytopenia (a significant decrease from the patient's usual absolute reticulocyte level), hyperbilirubinemia, and haemoglobinuria.

Iliac crest Part of the pelvic bone, often used as a source of bone autograft.

Immediate spin technique A serological method whereby red cells and antisera are spun without incubation to detect agglutination.

Immune response The body's ability to recognize and defend itself against substances that appear foreign and harmful such as bacteria and viruses.

Immunocompetent The ability to produce an immune response following a challenge with an antigen.

Immunogenic The likelihood that an antigen will stimulate an immunological response.

Immunoprecipitation The isolation of immune complexes (usually with monoclonal antibodies) to identify membrane or intracellular components.

In utero Literally within the uterus.

Innate immune response The arm of the immune response that does not respond to specific antigens, for example Toll like receptors on macrophages and neutrophils, and the soluble components of complement.

Intercostal arteries Small arteries, branching off the thoracic aorta and supplying blood to the intercostal space.

Internal quality control (IQC) Is a set of procedures for continually assessing laboratory work and the results they produce to decide if they are good enough to be released.

Intracellular Within the cellular milieu.

Intravascular haemolysis Cells being lysed within the circulation by antibodies that activate the complement pathway, especially anti-A and anti-B.

Irradiation A process for inactivating donor lymphocytes using gamma (or X-ray) irradiation to prevent transfusion-associated graft versus host disease (TA-GVHD), a rare but potentially fatal consequence of blood transfusion.

Isoantibodies Antibodies that react with an antigen that is normally found in all individuals but which is lacking in the recipient.

Kernicterus Pathogenic deposit of bilirubin in the fetal brain, a sign of severe haemolytic disease of the newborn.

Law of mass action Chemical term for when two substrates come together and react to reach an equilibrium, and is dependent on the concentrate of both substrates.

Lectin A sugar-binding protein or glycoprotein of non-immune origin, which can agglutinate cells and/or precipitate glycoconjugates.

Lectin pathway An arm of the complement pathway where mannose binding lectin and proteins binds to bacterial or viral mannose containing oligosaccharides and initiates the binding of further complement components and activation of the cascade.

Leucodepletion A process for removal of white blood cells from blood components to less that 5×10^6 per unit through an in-line filter.

Linkage disequilibrium The tendency of certain alleles at different loci to occur on the same chromosome more often than expected by chance, for example HLA-A*01-B*08-DRB1*03:01 are in positive linkage disequilibrium as the observed frequency of this haplotype is greater than the expected frequency.

Macrophage A major immune phagocytic cell that is associated with red cell turnover or destruction. Found in huge numbers in the spleen.

Marfan's syndrome A genetic disorder, causing weakness of the connective tissue. A contraindication for donation of soft tissue allografts.

McLeod syndrome Caused by a gene defect in the *XK* gene (and others) leading to acanthocytic red cells and depression of Kell system antigens. Individuals have neural defects leading to peripheral neuropathy, cardiomyopathy, and anaemia.

Membrane plasticizer The presence of cholesterol in membranes inducing the physical characteristic that they maintain their fluidity in the microcirculation by prevention of gelling in the extremities.

Membrane skeleton The mesh-like network of proteins that give erythrocytes their extreme flexibility. Comprising predominantly of α-and β-spectrins, protein 4.1R, ankyrin, actin, and p55.

Memory cells Types of B or T lymphocytes that remember exposure to antigen and are thus primed to response on re-exposure to it producing a secondary immune response.

Meniscal cartilage Crescent-shaped fibrocartilage structures within the knee joint, which distribute weight and reduce friction during movement.

Microarray techniques An assay system using labelled probes to simultaneously identify a range of different characteristics.

Mimotopes Short synthetic peptides that mimic natural epitopes of the individual blood group antigens that are being developed to be used in microarray antibody detection systems without the need for intact red cells.

Monoclonal antibody immobilization of granulocyte antigens (MAIGA) assay An ELISA assay which uses monoclonal antibodies against granulocyte antigens as the basis of detection and identification of granulocyte-specific antibodies.

Monoclonal antibody immobilization of platelet antigens (MAIPA) assay An ELISA assay which uses monoclonal antibodies against platelet antigens as the basis of detection and identification of platelet specific antibodies.

Monoclonal antibody (MAb) Produced from a single clone of B cells.

Monoclonal Produced from one clone of (normally B) cells.

Morphogen Molecule that influences undifferentiated cells to differentiate into specialized cells capable of making specific tissues.

Morsellized bone graft Bone graft milled to granules or powders of different diameters.

Multipotent Multipotent progenitor or stem cells can give rise to many but limited types of cell.

Myeloablation Chemotherapy treatment given prior to a stem cell transplant that completely removes all haematopoietic and cancer cells.

Natural killer cells (NKCs) An immune cell of the innate immune response. They detect depression of class I HLA antigens on infected or tumerous cells and kill them by inducing apoptosis.

Naturally acquired antibodies Normally referring to anti-A, -B, or anti-galactosyl epitope, those antibodies present in an individual with blood group specificity that have been made by previous exposure to similar bacterial structures in the gut.

Necrotizing fasciitis A serious infection of the skin and subcutaneous tissue, requiring aggressive debridement of infected tissue.

Neonatal alloimmune neutropenia (NAIN) Neutropenia in a neonate (or fetus) caused by the maternal fetal transfer of granulocyte specific antibodies recognizing either HNAs or granulocyte glycoproteins inherited by the fetus from the father but absent in the mother.

Neonatal alloimmune thrombocytopenia (NAIT) Thrombocytopenia in a neonate (or fetus) caused by the maternal fetal transfer of platelet-specific antibodies recognizing either HPAs or platelet glycoproteins inherited by the fetus from the father but absent in the mother.

Next generation sequencing (NGS) First emerging in 2006, a replacement sequencing chemistry coupled with sequencing millions of DNA molecules in parallel. Several sequencing instruments on the market utilize NGS–e.g. Illumina, Ion & Proton torrent, Oxford nanopore, Pacific Biosystems.

Neutropenia Low numbers of neutrophil leucocytes.

Neutrophils Together with eosinophils and basophils these circulating white cells are collectively known as granulocytes or polymorphonuclear cells. In normal healthy adults, neutrophils account for >90% of all granulocytes. Most laboratories do not attempt to separate these three cell types prior to antibody testing so any antibodies detected are more correctly called granulocyte-specific. Nonetheless, some HNA, i.e. HNA-1 and -2, have been shown to be truly neutrophil-specific in that they are expressed on neutrophils but not eosinophils or basophils.

Non-haemolytic febrile transfusion reactions (NHFTRs) An increase in temperature ≥1°C following a blood transfusion but which is not associated with red cell haemolysis.

Non-myeloablative Chemotherapy treatment given prior to a stem cell transplant that does not completely remove haematopoietic and cancer cells but instead depends on donor cells to kill the cancer.

Null allele A mutant gene that does not function like the normal gene. Many null HLA alleles lack cell surface expression and cannot present peptides to the immune system.

Osteochondral graft A composite graft, comprising bone plus an intact articular cartilage surface.

Ovalocytes Abnormal ovoid red cells associated with membrane skeletal defects, e.g. complete glycophorin C deficiency (Leach phenotype) or South Asian Ovalocytosis (band 3 defect).

Palmitoylation A post-translational protein modification that adds palmitic acid to cysteine side chains.

Pancytopenia Low numbers of all blood cell lines (RBC, WBC, and platelets)

Paratope The epitope binding region of the immunoglobulin molecule.

Pathogen inactivation A process for removal of infectious agents in blood components/products through chemical or heat treatment and filtration.

Pathogen reduction Process for reducing or eliminating most infectious agents in blood components/products.

Philadelphia positive status Leukaemic cells that show the presence of a translocation between chromosomes 9 and 22 to create the BCR-Abl (tyrosine kinase) fusion protein. The derivative chromosome 22 is much smaller than usual and is termed the 'Philadelphia' chromosome.

Phycoerythrin (PE) A red protein found in red algae and cyanobacteria. It is used as a fluorescent label for antibodies used in the laboratory for the detection of specific markers on cell surfaces, in the cytoplasm, or on DNA, by utilizing its ability to absorb blue green light and emit orange-yellow light ($475 \pm 10nm$).

Plasticity The ability of cells to become cell types which they are not normally recognized to become.

Platelet immunofluorescence test (PIFT) A whole-cell immunofluorescence assay capable of detecting platelet reactive antibodies.

Platelet transfusion refractoriness A suboptimal increase in circulating platelet count following platelet transfusion.

Pluripotent Is the ability of the human stem cell to differentiate or become almost any cell in the body.

Polyclonal antibodies These are produced by more than one clone of cells.

Polymerase chain reaction (PCR) An enzyme reaction utilizing Taq polymerase to amplify the copy number and hence enable detection of a genetic characteristic.

Polymerase chain reaction with sequence-specific primers (PCR-SSP) or allele-specific PCR The polymerase chain reaction using primers that recognize a DNA sequence encoding a unique heritable genetic characteristic—typically an SNP.

Polymerase chain reaction and restriction fragment length polymorphism (PCR-RFLP) The PCR amplifies a polymorphic sequence which is then recognized by a restriction endonuclease that cleaves on allele and the other intact. Normally detected by gel electrophoresis.

Polymorphism The occurrence of more than one form of the antigen.

Polyspecific AHG (anti-human globulin) reagents A blend of antibodies that recognize immunoglobulins and anti-C3d of complement used in the Coomb's (antiglobulin) test.

Polytopic A membrane protein that spans the membrane bilayer multiple times.

Post-transfusion purpura (PTP) An unexpected thrombocytopenia occurring 5–12 days after a blood transfusion that is associated with the presence of platelet-specific antibodies.

Prophylactic anti-D A preparation of human anti-D that is administered either during or after giving birth to a RhD positive infant to prevent alloimmunization.

Proteasome An intracellular proteolytic complex that degrades cytosolic and nuclear proteins.

Public epitopes A region of an antigen shared by many different antigens that is recognized by antibodies, B cells, or T cells.

Quality assurance Is the prevention of quality problems through planned and systematic activities designed to detect, correct, and ensure that consistent quality is achieved. Good manufacturing process (GMP) is that part of the quality assurance system that assures that results and products are consistently produced, achieving the required standard, and are 'fit for purpose'.

Quality control Is any technique employed to achieve and maintain the quality of product, process, or result.

Quality management system (QMS) Is a system of processes that ensures consistency and improvement of working practices, which in turn provides products and services that meet customer's requirements (e.g. a safe unit of blood).

Rh$_{null}$ (regulator type) The null phenotype of the RH system, with red cells expressing no Rh or LW antigens, and have a defect in the Rh-associated glycoprotein gene *RHAG*.

Rhesus box Repeated 9 Kb DNA sequences that flank the *RHD* gene in D-positive individuals. The *RHD* deletion type D-negative genotype results in a hybrid Rhesus box where crossover that generated the deletion produces a hybrid *Rhesus box*.

Second field resolution This is how a high resolution or allele level HLA type is described because the second field after the first colon is populated, for example HLA-DRB1* 12:01.

Sensitivity This is the proportion of people who have a disease/infection (or products such as antibodies to it) which is correctly identified by a screening test.

Serious adverse event (SAE) Is defined as: 'Any untoward occurrence associated with the collection, testing, processing, storage and distribution of blood or blood components that might lead to death or life-threatening, disabling, or incapacitating conditions for patients, or which results in, or prolongs hospitalization or morbidity'.

Serious adverse reaction (SAR) Is defined within the regulations as: 'An unintended response in a donor or in a patient that is associated with the collection or transfusion of blood or blood components that is fatal, life threatening, disabling, or incapacitating, or which results in, or prolongs, hospitalization or morbidity'.

Serious Hazards Of Transfusion (SHOT) The UK haemovigilance scheme.

Serological crossreactivity This is where antibodies react with a public epitope shared by different HLA molecules. These HLA molecules that share a public epitope are often described as Cross Reactive Groups (CREG), for example anti-HLA-B7 antibodies can crossreact with a shared epitope on HLA-B42, B55, and B56.

Single nucleotide polymorphism (SNP) A single nucleotide substitution in the DNA reading frame that encodes a particular inherited characteristic.

Specificity This is the proportion of people who are correctly identified by a screening test as negative for the disease/infection.

Spherocytes Abnormal-shaped red cells associated with membrane skeletal defects (e.g. Spectrin) in hereditary anaemias. Erythrocytes gradually lose their biconcave disc morphology and become more spherical.

Statistical process control (SPC) Is a method of quality control for a product or a process that relies on a system of analysis of an adequate sample size without the need to measure every product of the process.

Streptavidin A bacterial protein purified from *Streptomyces avidinii* that has a high affinity for biotin.

Telomeres Repeated DNA sequences at the ends of chromosomes that stabilize the DNA and chromosome structure. They are considered 'biological clocks' and control the number of times chromosomes can replicate.

Ternary complex The key protein–protein interactions that govern the assembly of the erythrocyte membrane, comprising the major players, Spectrin, actin, protein 4.1R, p55, and ankyrin.

Thromobocytes Alternative term for platelets (especially in Europe).

Thrombocytopenia Low numbers of platelets in the circulation.

Thrombogenic Material which causes blood to clot on contact.

Toll-like receptors Present on macrophages and neutrophils and recognize bacterial components—part of the innate immune system.

Toxic epidermal necrolysis A serious life-threatening condition, usually caused by reaction to medication, resulting in the detachment of the epidermis from the dermis.

Transdifferentiation The ability of cells to change into a completely different cell type of another tissue.

Transfusion reactions This is a systemic response produced by the body to the infusion of blood or blood components/products. The adverse reaction may be to proteins in the blood or incompatible cellular components such as leucocytes, platelets, or erythrocytes.

Transfusion-related acute lung injury (TRALI) Difficulty in breathing associated with de novo chest X-ray changes observed within six hours of transfusion that is not associated with transfusion overload or cardiac insufficiency.

Transfusion-related alloimmune neutropenia (TRAIN) A transient neutropenia following infusion of a blood product due to the action of neutrophil-specific antibodies but which does not develop the symptoms of TRALI.

Validated Having documentary evidence to show that a system/equipment or process meets pre-defined requirements for its intended use.

Warm ischaemia time The time elapsing between death and a body being placed into a refrigerated environment.

Window period This is the period between the onset of the infection and the appearance of the detectable infectious agent or antibodies to it. For a virus, the window period is shorter for the detection of the viral RNA/DNA than antibodies which are produced later in the infection.

Abbreviations

2,3,DPG	2,3 diphosphoglycerate
A&E	Accident and Emergency
Ab	antibody
ACD	acid citrate dextrose
ADCC	antibody-dependent cell-mediated cytotoxicity
ADP	adenosine diphosphate
ADU	avoidable, delayed and under transfusion events
Ag	antigen
AHG	anti-human globulin
AHTR	acute haemolytic transfusion reaction
AIHA	autoimmune haemolytic anaemia
AIDS	acquired immune deficiency syndrome
ALG	anti-lymphocyte globulin
ALL	acute lymphoblastic leukaemia
ALLO	alloimmunization
AML	acute myeloid leukaemia
Anti-HBc	antibody to hepatitis B core antigen
Anti-HBe	antibody to hepatitis B e antigen
Anti-HBs	antibody to hepatitis B surface antigen
APC	antigen presenting cells
APTT	activated partial thromboplastin time
ARDS	acute respiratory distress syndrome
ATG	anti-thymocyte globulin
ATL	adult T cell leukaemia/lymphoma
ATP	adenosine triphosphate
ATR	acute transfusion reactions
BAT	bottom and top
BBMR	British Bone Marrow Register
BBTS	British Blood Transfusion Society
BGS	blood group system
BHK	baby hamster kidney
BM	bone marrow
BMP	bone morphogenetic protein
BPAT	batch pre-acceptance testing
BSBMT	British Society for Bone Marrow Transplant
BSE	bovine spongiform encephalitis
BSH	British Society for Haematology
BSQR	Blood Safety and Quality Regulations
BTS	blood transfusion service
BWS	British Working Standard
CAD	compound adsorption device
CAM	cell adhesion molecules
CAPA	corrective and preventative actions
CAT	column agglutination technology
CCP	complement control proteins
C-CAMP	cyclophosphamide, vincristine, adriamycin, and methylprenidolone
CD	cluster distribution
CFS	colony stimulating factor
CFU	colony forming units
CH	chromosome
CHO	Chinese hamster ovary
CHIKV	chikungunya virus
CLIA	chemiluminescence immunoassay
CML	chronic myeloid leukaemia
CMV	cytomegalovirus
CNS	central nervous system
CPA	Clinical Pathology Accreditation
CPD	citrate phosphate dextrose
CQC	Care Quality Commission
CR1	complement receptor 1
CRYO	cryoprecipitate
CS	cell salvage
CSP	cryosupernatant plasma
CPDA-1	citrate phosphate dextrose containing adenine
DAT	direct antiglobulin test
DBM	demineralized bone matrix
DHTR	delayed haemolytic transfusion reaction
DI	designated individual
DIC	disseminated intravascular coagulation
DL	Donath-Landsteiner
DLI	donor lymphocyte infusion
DMSO	dimethyl sulphoxide
DNA	deoxyribonucleic acid
dNTP	deoxynucleotide triphosphate
DoB	date of birth
DTT	dithiothreitol
E	erythroid
eBDS	enhanced bacterial detection system
ECM	extracellular matrix

EFI	European Federation for Immunogenetics
EI	electronic issue
EIA	enzyme immunoassay
ELISA	enzyme-linked immunosorbent assay
EPO	erythropoietin
EQA	external quality assessment
EU	European Union
ffDNA	free fetal DNA
FBS	fetal blood sampling
FFP	fresh frozen plasma
FMH	feto-maternal haemorrhage
FNHTR	febrile non-haemolytic transfusion reactions
FRALE	frangible anchor linker effector
FTA	fluorescent treponemal antibody
FTA-abs	fluorescent treponemal antibody-absorbed
GCLT	granulocyte chemiluminescence test
GCSF	granulocyte colony stimulating factor
GIFT	granulocyte immunofluorescence test
GM	granulocyte-monocyte
GMP	good manufacturing practice
GP (1)	glycoprotein
GP (2)	general practitioner
GVHD	graft versus host disease
GVL	graft versus leukaemia
GVT	graft versus tumour
HAM	HTLV-I associated myelopathy
HAS	human albumin solutions
Hb	haemoglobin
HBc	hepatitis B core
HBcAg	hepatitis B core antigen
HBeAg	hepatitis B e antigen
HBsAg	hepatitis B surface antigen
HBV	hepatitis B virus
HCT	haemopoietic cell transplant
HCV	hepatitis C virus
HDFN	haemolytic disease of the fetus and newborn
HDN	haemolytic disease of the newborn
HEPES	4-(2-hydroxyethyl)-1-piperazineethanesulfonic acid
HIV	human immunodeficiency virus
HLA	human leucocyte antigens
HMWK	high molecular weight kininogen
HNA	human neutrophil antigens
Hp	haptoglobin

HPA(1)	Health Protection Agency
HPA(2)	human platelet antigens
HPC	haemopoietic progenitor cells
HSC	haemopoietic stem cells
HSE	handling and storage errors
HT	high titre
HTA	Human Tissue Authority/act
HTLV	human T cell lymphotropic virus
HTLV-1	human T cell lymphotropic virus-1
HTR	haemolytic transfusion reaction
IAT	indirect antiglobulin test
IBCT	incorrect blood component transfused
IBGRL	International Blood Group Reference Laboratory
ICH	intra-cranial haemorrhage
ID	individual donation
IFA	indirect fluorescent antibody
IL	interleukin
INR	international normalized ratio
IQC	internal quality control
ISBT	International Society of Blood Transfusion
ISCT	International Society for Cellular Therapy
ISXM	immediate spin crossmatch
ITP	idiopathic thrombocytopenia
IUT	intrauterine transfusion
IVDD	In Vitro Diagnostics Device
IVIg	Intravenous immunoglobulin
JACIE	Joint Accreditation Committee-ISCT and EBMT
Kg	kilograms
LDH	lactate dehydrogenase
LIMS	laboratory information management system
LISS	low ionic strength solution
MAC	membrane attack complex
MAIGA	monoclonal antibody immobilization of granulocyte antigens
MAIPA	monoclonal antibody immobilization of platelet antigens
MB	methylene blue
MBFFP	methylene blue-treated FFP
MCP	monocyte chemoattractant protein
MDS	myelodysplastic syndromes
MegK	megakaryocytic
MHC	major histocompatibility complex
MHRA	Medicines and Healthcare products Regulatory Agency
MOP	metoxypsoralen

MTU	multi-tube unit		PT	prothrombin time
NAIN	neonatal alloimmune neutropenia		PTP	post-transfusion purpura
NAIT(P)	neonatal alloimmune thrombocytopenia		QA	quality assurance
NAT	nucleic acid testing		QMS	quality management system
NBTC	National Blood Transfusion Committee		RBCs	red blood cells
NEQAS	National External Quality Assessment Scheme		rBGPs	recombinant blood group proteins
NetCord-FACT	International Standards for Cord Blood Collection, Processing, Testing, Banking, Selection and Release		RCOG	Royal College of Obstetricians and Gynaecologists
			RES	reticulo-endothelium system
NFAT	nuclear factor of activated T cells		RIBA	recombinant immunoblot assays
NIBTS	Northern Ireland Blood Transfusion Service		RNA	ribonucleic acid
			RPR	rapid plasma reagin
NGS	Next Generation sequencing		RT	reverse transcriptase
NHFTR	non-haemolytic febrile transfusion reactions		SABRE	serious adverse blood reactions and events
NHSBT-TS	National Health Service Blood and Transplant Tissue Services		SaBTO	Advisory Committee on the Safety of Blood, Tissues and Organs
NHSLA	National Health Service Litigation Authority		SAE	serious adverse event
NIBSC	National Institute of Biological Standards and Control		SAG	saline, adenine, and glucose
			SAG-M	saline, adenine, glucose, and mannitol
NK	natural killer cells		SAR	serious adverse reaction
NMDP	National Marrow Donor Program		SCD	sickle cell disease
NP	nurse practitioner		S/CO	sample optical density to cut-off ratio
NPSA	National Patient Safety Agency		SDS-PAGE	sodium dodecyl sulphate polyacrylamide gel electrophoreis
NRC	National Referral Centre			
NTMRL	National Transfusion Microbiology Reference Laboratory		SEAC	Spongiform Encephalopathy Advisory Committee
PBSC	peripheral blood stem cells		SHOT	Serious Hazards Of Transfusion
PCR	polymerase chain reaction		SNBTS	Scottish National Blood Transfusion Service
PCR-SSP	polymerase chain reaction with site specific primers		SNP	single nucleotide polymorphism
PCR-RFLP	Polymerase chain reaction with restriction fragment length polymorphism		SOP	standard operating procedure
			SPC	statistical process control
			SPU	sample preparation unit
PCT	photochemical technology		TACO	transfusion-associated circulatory overload
PDCA	plan, do, check, act			
PI	pathogen inactivation		TA-GvHD	transfusion-associated graft versus host disease
PIFT	platelet immunofluorescence test			
PK	prekallikrein		TBI	total body irradiation
PLTS	platelets		TMA	transcription mediated amplification
PNH	paroxysmal nocturnal haemoglobinuria		TNBP	tri-(n-butyl)-phosphate
PR	pathogen reduction		TNFα	tumour necrosis factor α
PrPc	cellular form of prion protein		TPHA	*Treponema pallidum* haemagglutination assay
PrPsc	abnormal prion protein			
PSM	platelet suspension medium		TPO	Thrombobopoetin

TPPA	*Treponema pallidum* particle assay	URD	unrelated donor
TRAIN	transfusion-related alloimmune neutropenia	vCJD	variant Creutzfeldt–Jakob disease
TRALI	transfusion-related acute lung injury	VDRL	Venereal Diseases Research Laboratory
TRT	turnaround time	vWF	von Willebrand factor
TSP	tropical spastic parapheresis	WBC	white blood cells
TTI	transfusion-transmitted infection	WBS	Welsh Blood Service
UCT	unclassified complications of transfusions	WHO	World Health Organization
UGT	UDP-glucoronosyltransferase	WNV	West Nile virus
UKAS	United Kingdom Accreditation Service	WP	window period

Index